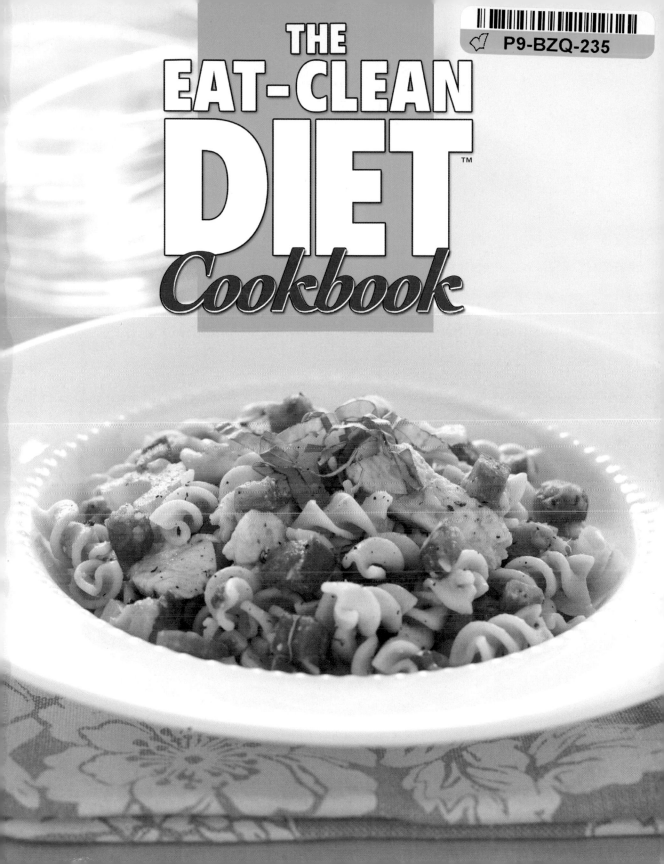

THE EAT-CLEAN DIET™ Cookbook

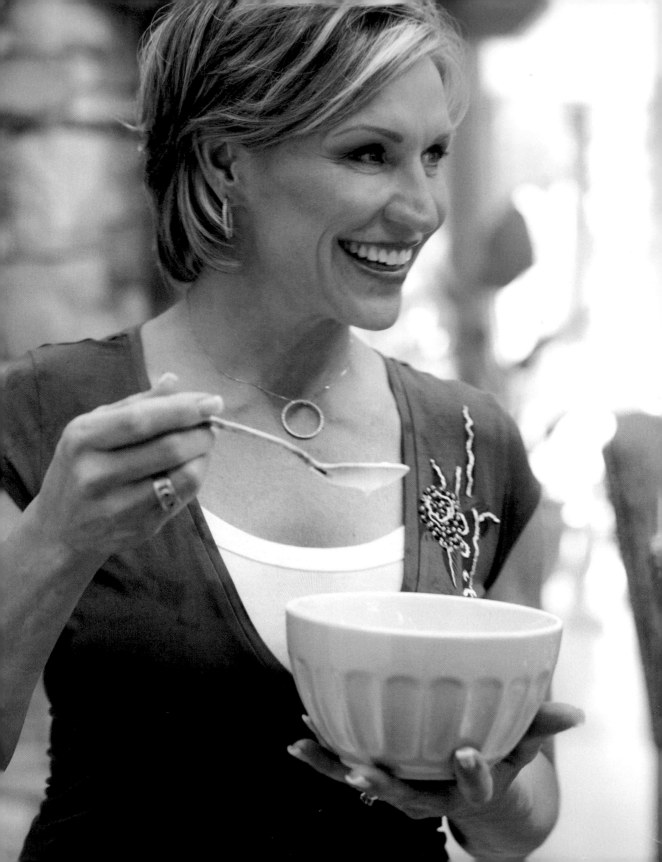

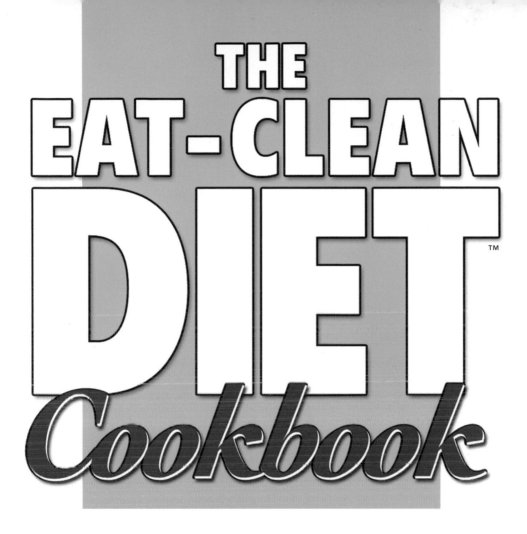

THE EAT-CLEAN DIET™ Cookbook

Great-Tasting Recipes that Keep You Lean!

TOSCA RENO

FOREWORD BY Dr. Lisa Hark, PhD, RD

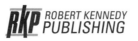

ROBERT KENNEDY PUBLISHING

Published by Robert Kennedy Publishing
5775 McLaughlin Road
Mississauga, ON
L5R 3P7 Canada
Visit us at **www.eatcleandiet.com**
and **www.toscareno.com**

Design by Gabriella Caruso Marques
Edited by Wendy Morley and Rachel Corradetti

National Library of Canada Cataloguing in Publication

Reno, Tosca, 1959-
        The Eat-Clean Diet Cookbook : Great-Tasting Recipes that Keep You Lean! / Tosca Reno;
foreword by Lisa Hark.

ISBN-13: 978-1-55210-044-8
ISBN-10: 1-55210-044-8

        1. Reducing diets- Recipes. 2. Cookery (Natural Foods) I. Title.

RM222.2.R464 2007   641.5′635   C2007-904401-8

10 9 8 7 6 5 4 3

Distributed in Canada by
NBN (National Book Network)
67 Mowat Avenue, Suite 241
Toronto, ON
M6K 3E3

Distributed in USA by
NBN (National Book Network)
15200 NBN Way
Blue Ridge Summit, PA
17214

Printed in the United States of America.

IMPORTANT

The information in this book reflects the author's experiences and opinions and is not intended to replace medical advice.

Before beginning this or any nutritional or exercise regimen, consult your physician to be sure it is appropriate for you. Ask for a physical stress test.

Writing a successful book is never the work of just one person. I want to thank my better half Robert Kennedy for his guidance, love, passion and patience – without him there would be no cookbook. To our extended family Braden and Chelsea, and my children Kelsey-Lynn, Rachel, and Kiersten, a big hug for all your input, especially Rachel whose long hours of proofing and indexing keep my efforts looking professional.

This book is made by its images; photographers Robert Reiff, Cathy Chatterton and Donna Griffith have surpassed themselves.

I owe a debt of thanks to the tireless efforts of Wendy Morley for her constant stream of ideas and promotional planning.

To N.B.N.'s Les Petriw, and Bev Greene and Trevor Ratz of Robert Kennedy Publishing, I appreciate your high interest, suggestions and hands-on involvement.

And to the beautiful Gabby Caruso, whose dedication to perfection of design is evident throughout this book, I offer my heartfelt appreciation.

ACKNOWLEDGMENT

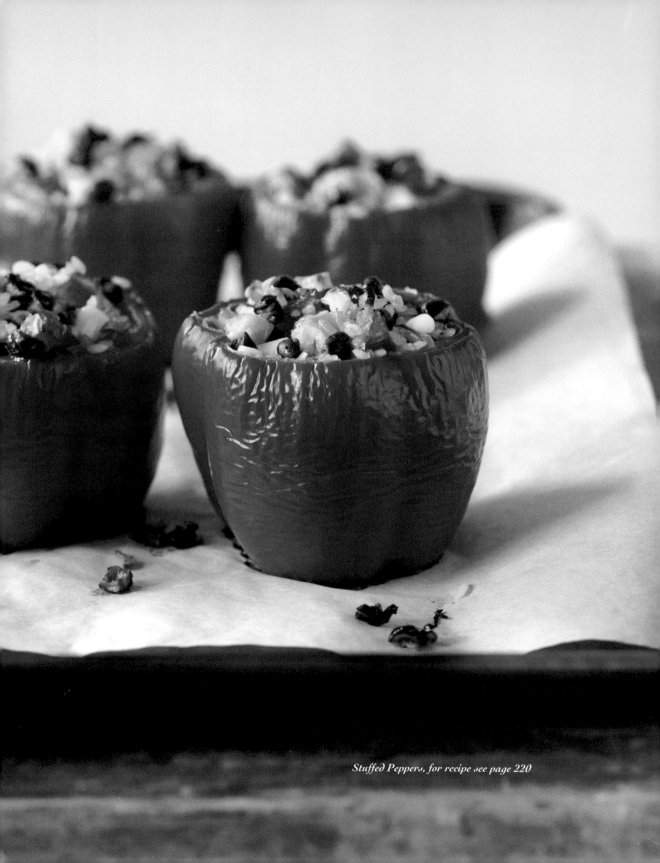

Stuffed Peppers, for recipe see page 220

CONTENTS

Tosca Reno's story is one of inspiration, motivation, and hope for anyone trying to improve his or her lifestyle. Like so many others, Tosca's story began while she was a busy mother who spent all of her time caring for everyone but herself. Weighing more than 200 pounds before turning 30, Tosca realized after many years that she needed to reclaim her life by making major changes in her diet and lifestyle. But rather than attempting to follow a restrictive diet that would leave her feeling hungry and deprived, Tosca chose to reshape her life by eliminating all foods that were processed and nutritionally devoid. She replaced junk food with fruits and vegetables, and white bread with whole grains. Today, Tosca has crafted an entire lifestyle that is centered upon the foundation of Eating Clean. Her transformation from an obese twenty-something to a forty-something swimsuit model is proof that *The Eat-Clean Diet* can transform your health, looks, and self-esteem.

Eating Clean is a lifestyle based on dietary logic. It is a nutritional plan that maximizes one's intake of protein, fiber, vitamins, minerals, and antioxidants by incorporating "whole foods" from every food group. Because foods that are processed lose a significant portion of their nutritional content, Eating Clean focuses on foods that have been minimally processed and are as close to nature as possible. I believe that by eating foods that are fresh and from their natural source, you can feel better, look better, and surely have more energy. You may even live longer because you are reducing your risk of developing chronic diseases such as high blood pressure, high cholesterol, and diabetes.

> *By eating foods that are fresh and from their natural source, you can feel better, look better, and surely have more energy.*

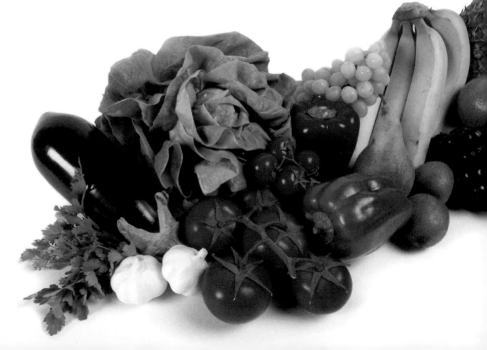

Her ingredient list brimming with whole grains, lean protein sources, and fresh fruits and vegetables, it is no wonder Tosca was able to come up with recipes that are as delicious as they are nutritious. Instead of relying on saturated fats like butter and cream to make her dishes savory, Tosca uses a spectrum of innovative ingredients like herbs, fruits, and spices. As a result, her recipes are loaded with new flavors and unexpected combinations you and your family will love.

Tosca knows that finding the time and energy to cook for a family can be a challenge, especially for busy moms who don't have time to fuss over complicated recipes and obscure ingredient lists. That's why Tosca made certain to create fast, easy recipes for *The Eat-Clean Diet Cookbook*. Some of my favorites are the Applesauce Pumpkin Muffins, Sesame Roasted Broccoli, and Quinoa with Sundried Tomatoes. She makes it simple for anyone to follow the program. In fact, many of her recipes can be made in advance or tossed together in less time than it takes to have a pizza delivered!

In this era, when obesity prevalence has reached an all-time high and cardiovascular disease is the number-one killer of women, it's certainly time for all of us to get our priorities straight. Rather than looking toward another fad diet, Tosca Reno has hit the mark by developing a lifestyle based on good nutrition and exercise. Eating Clean is not a plan that will abandon you once you lose a few pounds, but one to live by, and to raise your family by. This collection of recipes makes the task of overhauling your diet and transforming the way you think about food infinitely easier. The recipes are quick, simple, and will allow you to achieve your goals of health, wellness, and weight loss in a way that is both casual and delicious. Enjoy!

Lisa Hark, PhD, RD

Family nutrition expert, TV host, bestselling author, and mother of two.
www.lisahark.com

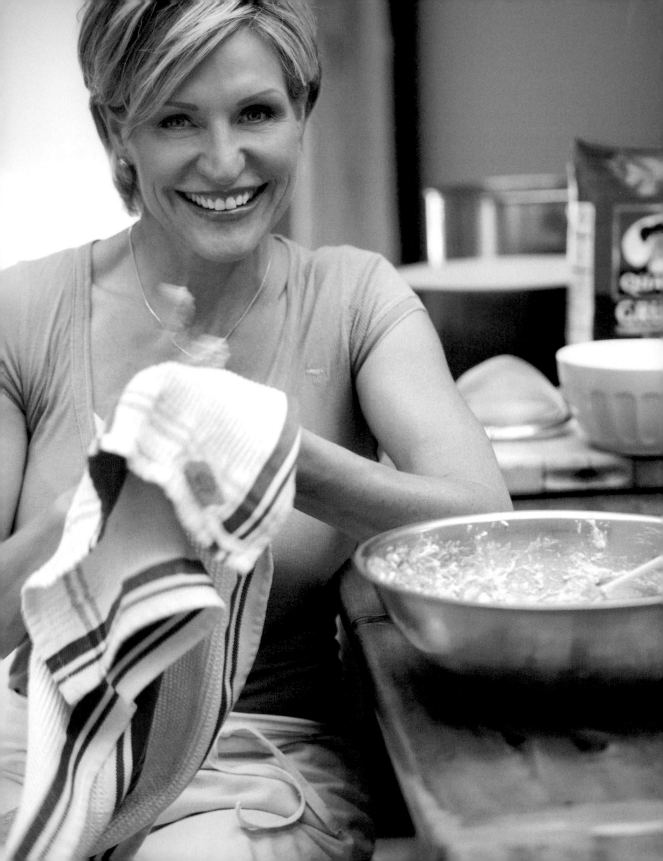

Introduction

· ·

WHY EAT CLEAN?

Millions of you are overweight and dieting right now. Numbers released by the *Journal of the American Medical Association* suggest that 65 percent of North Americans are overweight. Will this number ever stop growing? We are firmly in the grip of a "globesity" crisis and can expect hundreds of thousands of obesity-related deaths in North America in the coming years. But it isn't just the weight we need to worry about; the real concern is what's happening to our bodies at the microscopic level. With an increase in weight comes an array of diseases, including diabetes, hormonal imbalances, osteoporosis, heart disease, stroke, unstable blood sugar, metabolic syndrome X, high blood pressure, arthritis and more.

Yet if you've ever attempted to diet you know there are stages you go through, including starting, starving and stopping. Chances are once you stopped dieting your weight bounced right back to where it was before you started… and picked up a few extra pounds along the way. We call that yoyo dieting. It doesn't work! It happens every time we fall off the diet wagon and most of us do just that because most diets are not sustainable. There's just too much punishment involved.

Enter Eating Clean. When I turned 40 and had over 70 pounds to lose, I succeeded by Eating Clean. Clean Eating is a lifestyle that works, and I'm living proof. I went from weighing over 200 pounds and being an ordinary, depressed housewife to losing over 70 pounds and becoming a cover model for *Oxygen* magazine. I could hardly believe how amazing I felt – loaded with energy, vitality and blazing self-esteem. I did not feel like a middle-aged frump any more. Friends who hadn't seen me in a while said I looked 20 years younger.

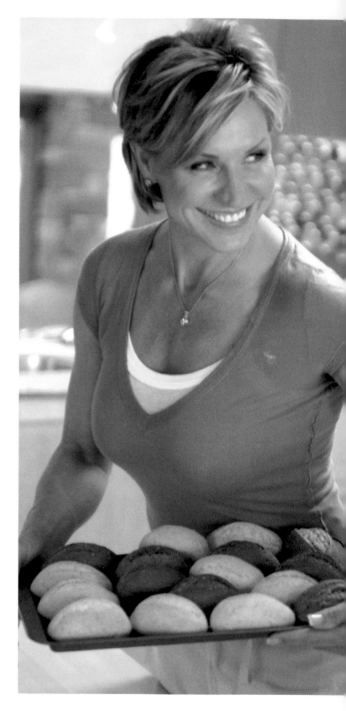

"I want to live a long, healthy life with my three daughters and my new stepfamily, so I work hard at Clean Eating. I don't want to miss a single day God has planned for me."

I admit, in the beginning I wondered how following a plan that had you eat six times per day could help you lose weight. It was nothing like any other diet I had tried. It didn't even feel like a diet because I wasn't hungry. In my mind dieting involved avoiding all foods but celery and carrot sticks. It also meant feeling hungry a lot! Along with that hunger came the inevitable binge when I just couldn't take depriving myself anymore.

Now I've kept my weight off for several years. I've never been so hungry or felt so deprived that I binged in revenge. I feel in control of my eating and know exactly what to eat every day. It's a wonderful feeling to know that you have the upper hand over food. I know what I am supposed to eat and have guidelines set for me. Clean Eating does just that and so does *The Eat-Clean Diet Cookbook.* The foods, quantities and timing are laid out in an easy-to-follow pattern. I love it!

Not only will Clean Eating prevent you from becoming (or remaining) one of the several hundred million North Americans struggling with overweight or obesity, it will vastly improve your health, energy level and appearance. As part of my health crusade I schedule yearly checkups with my doctor. When I started Eating Clean she began to notice changes in my blood work. Not only had I lost significant weight, but my blood levels showed marked decreases – in a good way. Here was actual proof that Clean Eating was benefiting my health. My triglycerides, cho-

lesterol, LDL cholesterol, blood pressure and blood sugar levels dropped. My doctor was amazed. My tests are now so good, there is no place to record the results on the standard charts! For me, having good blood work results is like getting an "A" on my report card. I'll take it! And I had special reason to want to change my health for the better. My dad had had a heart attack at 64. Far too young for a father to die. I obviously know how dangerous and deadly a poor diet can be. I want to live a long, healthy life with my three daughters and my new stepfamily, so I work hard at Clean Eating. I don't want to miss a single day God has planned for me.

My decision to write *The Eat-Clean Diet Cookbook* evolved naturally after writing *The Eat-Clean Diet.* So many of those who read my book asked for Clean-Eating recipes to have on hand. Since I had the recipes as well as a passionate desire to share what I know with appreciative readers, the cookbook grew.

From a practical point of view, millions of us panic at the thought of preparing any kind of meal. That fear combined with a lack of time paralyzes the cook and leaves him or her, young or old, reaching for the quickest thing available, usually pasta or chicken nuggets and more often than not, ordering out. After viewing the vanguard movie, **Super Size Me**, I can no longer summon the courage to eat or serve a chicken nugget ever again and I don't want you to eat it either.

With *The Eat-Clean Diet Cookbook* sitting on your kitchen counter, meal planning and preparation becomes a breeze. I think you'll agree with me, meal planning is the worst! Skim through the pages of my book. Earmark a few recipes or ask your kids to do it. Get interested and get started today. Make your next meal a Clean-Eating meal. I'll be doing the same, every day and every night, right along with you.

I would like you to enjoy mealtimes again. I want you to re-embrace your family and friends, taste food and learn to love to eat properly once more. Are you one of the many who believes healthy food tastes like cardboard? You'll never think that way again after reading *The Eat-Clean Diet Cookbook*. Best of all, you will learn to eat nutritionally while rediscovering the body you once had – the one that disappeared after years of horrific eating habits.

Having a cookbook filled with Clean-Eating recipes is like having life insurance – it's a plan for you to follow which gives you the rules, the results and the outcomes for a healthier life. I believe you'll enjoy the Clean-Eating recipes and cooking as much as I do. The recipes are easier than you think and the flavors are stunning because the foods are natural, wholesome and Clean. It's enjoyable and rewarding to prepare Clean-Eating meals because I know for sure I am serving foods brimming with health and nourishment. My children, aged 13 to 21, are in the kitchen right along with me, cooking Clean-Eating foods and having a grand time. They don't want to eat pizza pockets, whatever they are. They ask for my Roasted Red Pepper Soup (page 45) instead. We strap on aprons on a Sunday morning, fire up the stove and prepare a delicious breakfast of Caledon Baked Oatmeal (page 20) and Kiwi Citrus Smoothies (page 37) or Egg White and Turkey Scramble (page 13). We are a Clean-Eating family. Welcome!

Tosca Reno

P. S. I'm a visual person so I have included easy-to-identify symbols that help you plan and prepare meals in a snap!

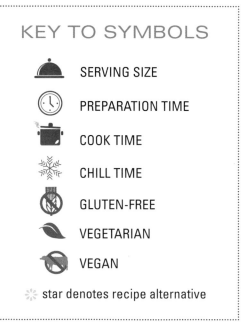

KEY TO SYMBOLS

SERVING SIZE

PREPARATION TIME

COOK TIME

CHILL TIME

GLUTEN-FREE

VEGETARIAN

VEGAN

star denotes recipe alternative

CLEAN-EATING PRINCIPLES

Remember, to lose or gain weight you must eat more! However, your food choices need to be clean and healthy. These are the Clean-Eating principles that will guide you through your physique and health transformation. Photocopy this page and stick it on your fridge or in a cupboard where you will be reminded to follow the habits until they become your lifestyle.

- Eat 5 – 6 small meals every day.

- Eat every 2 – 3 hours.

- Combine lean protein and complex carbs at every meal.

- Drink at least 2 liters, or 8 cups, of water each day.

- Never miss a meal, especially breakfast.

- Carry a cooler loaded with Clean-Eating foods to get through the day.

- Avoid all over-processed, refined foods, especially white flour and sugar.

- Avoid all saturated and trans fats.

- Avoid sugar-loaded colas and juices.

- Consume adequate healthy fats (EFAs) each day.

- Avoid alcohol – another form of sugar.

- Avoid all calorie-dense foods containing no nutritional value.

- Depend on fresh fruits and vegetables for fiber, vitamins and enzymes.

- Stick to proper portion sizes – give up the super sizing!

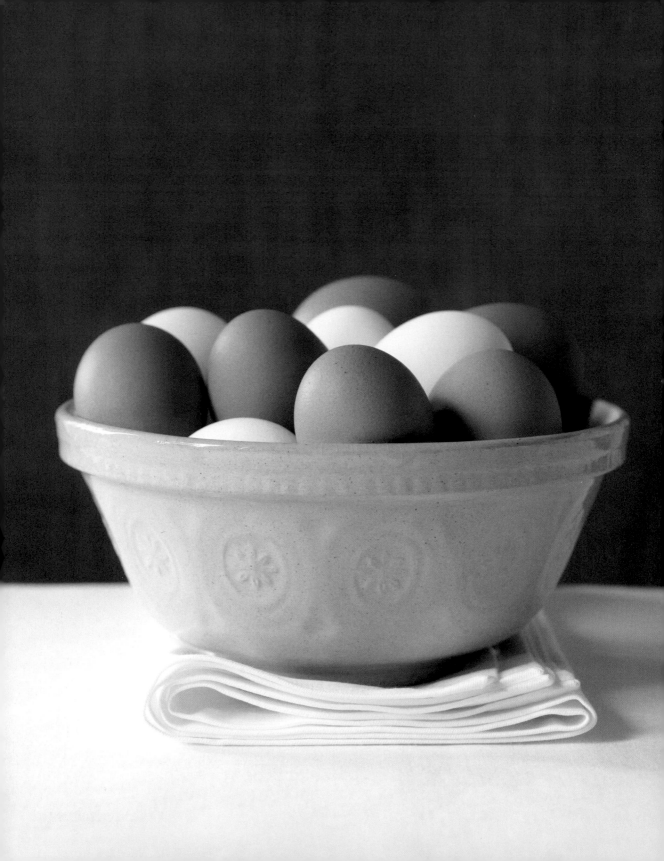

Breakfast

Breakfast is the meal most of us choose to skip. Yet it is the meal most needed to get your day off to an energized start. Assuming you have gone all night without food or water, you should be feeling your tummy by now. In fact, with regular Clean Eating, you may even be awakened by a tummy demanding food.

The only answer is to fill it with delicious Clean-Eating breakfast options such as Swiss Muesli (page 32), an Oh-My-Gosh Omelet (page 24) or an Egg White and Turkey Scramble (page 13). These breakfast choices are so satisfying, lean and mighty, you won't ever skip breakfast again.

CROCK-POT PORRIDGE

W hole grains are essential for building strong, lean bodies. What better way to start your day than with a crock pot loaded with the best of the body-building whole grains? Set it all up the night before, plug in and wake up to "instant" home-cooked goodness. Jazz up the porridge with fresh berries, flax seed, wheat germ and bee pollen. Guess who's buff now?

INGREDIENTS:

½ cup / 120 ml cracked wheat

1 ½ cup / 360 ml steel-cut oats

½ cup / 120 ml rye flakes

½ cup / 120 ml brown rice

¼ cup / 60 ml wheat germ

6½ cups / 1.5 L water or any combination of liquids
   including rice milk, soy milk, almond milk,
   goat's milk and/or water to equal 6½ cups

½ cup / 120 ml raisins

½ cup / 120 ml chopped dates

1 Tbsp / 15 ml best-quality bourbon vanilla

1 ½ tsp / 7.5 ml vanilla

Pinch nutmeg

PREPARATION:

1 Place all ingredients in a 3-quart-or-greater crock pot. Stir well to combine all ingredients. Cover.

2 Set on lowest cooking temperature and cook over-night. If your crock pot cooking time is set by length of cooking time, set for the longest cooking time and lowest heat.

3 Spoon into cereal bowls in the morning and serve piping hot!

REMEMBER: Try unsweetened applesauce instead of sugar as a sweetener – delicious!

HINT: Add any dried fruit or unsalted nuts you may like to this dish, it is very forgiving.

NUTRITIONAL VALUE PER SERVING:
Calories: 313 | Calories from Fat: 29 | Protein: 10g | Carbs: 63g
Dietary Fiber: 8g | Sugars: 12g | Fat: 3g | Sodium: 3mg

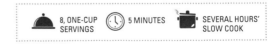

8, ONE-CUP SERVINGS   5 MINUTES   SEVERAL HOURS' SLOW COOK

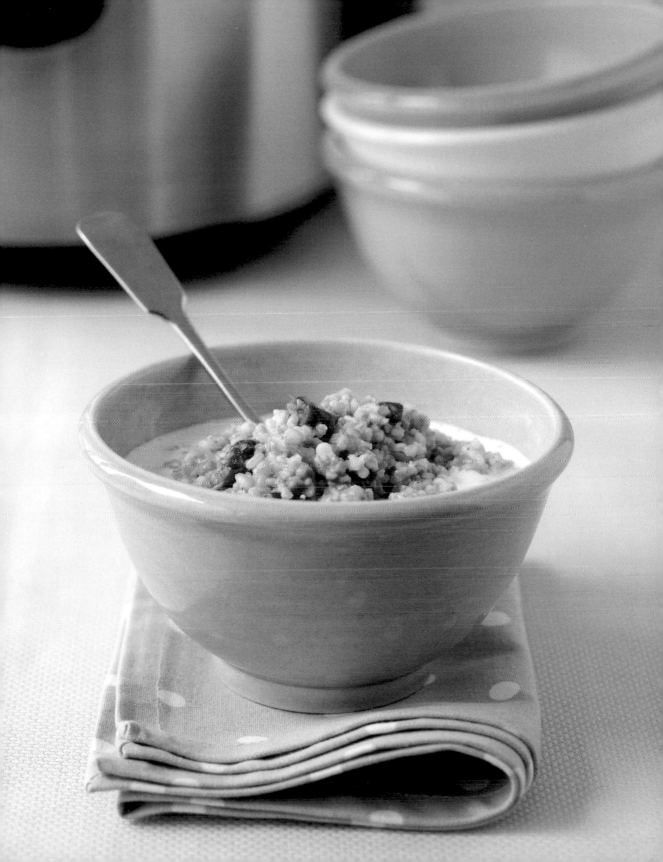

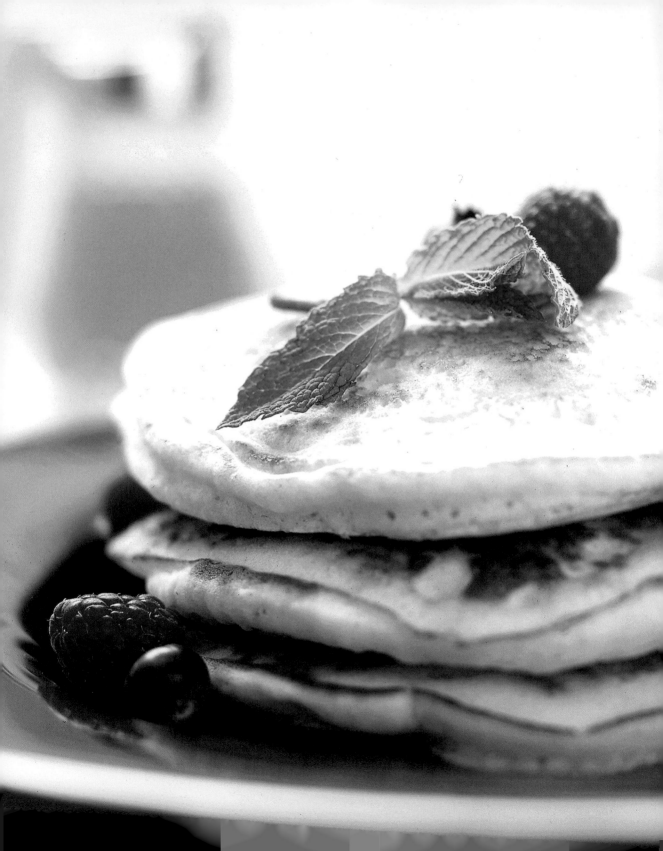

COTTAGE CHEESE PANCAKES

Raise the Bar reader, Laura Wilkins, shared her favorite childhood pancake recipe with me. Her version called for two tablespoons of sugar but I substituted maple sugar flakes as a healthier Clean-Eating sweetening ingredient. It is an excellent Clean-Eating pancake recipe because it calls for nonfat cottage cheese, which is an excellent source of lean protein, as is the fat-free yogurt. Egg whites make the pancakes fluffy and a good source of protein. Yum!

INGREDIENTS:

Dry:

1¼ cups / 300 ml whole-wheat flour

1 tsp / 5 ml baking powder

2 Tbsp / 30 ml maple sugar flakes

½ tsp / 2.5 ml ground cinnamon

¼ tsp / 1.25 ml sea salt

Wet:

8 egg whites

1 cup / 240 ml fat-free cottage cheese

1 cup / 240 ml fat-free plain yogurt

Cooking spray

Thanks Laura! Now we can all enjoy this healthy and delicious version of your pancakes.

PREPARATION:

1 Combine first five ingredients in a medium bowl. Make a well in the center.

2 Combine eggs, cottage cheese and yogurt in small bowl. Pour into well. Stir until just moistened.

3 Heat a nonstick pan or griddle or prepare a skillet with cooking spray. Heat should be medium high. Use ¼ cup of batter for each pancake. Cook until lightly browned on both sides. Keep warm in oven until all the batter has been used up.

4 Serve with fruit.

TIP

Bring egg whites to room temperature first. This helps make them fluffier.

NUTRITIONAL VALUE PER PANCAKE:

Calories: 81 | Calories from Fat: 2 | Protein: 7g | Carbs: 12g
Dietary Fiber: 1g | Sugars: 3g | Fat: 0.3g | Sodium: 112mg

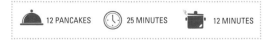

12 PANCAKES   25 MINUTES   12 MINUTES

EGG WHITE AND TURKEY SCRAMBLE

Who says you can't have turkey for breakfast? Ground turkey is a delicious Clean-Eating alternative to greasy, fat-laden bacon. It tastes wonderful when mixed with scrambled eggs and Clean-Eating spinach and tomato. Now this is the way to start your day!

INGREDIENTS:

8 egg whites

1 pound / 454 g lean ground turkey or tofu

2 cups / 480 ml shredded spinach

2 tomatoes, coarsely chopped

1 clove garlic, minced or pressed through
    garlic press

Sea salt and black pepper to taste

PREPARATION:

1 Cook ground turkey or tofu in a medium skillet until cooked through and lightly browned. Drain excess juices from the pan. Place turkey in a bowl and set aside.

2 Wipe the pan clean with a paper towel. Scramble the egg whites until dry. Add scrambled eggs to cooked turkey.

3 In a small skillet coated with cooking spray, lightly sauté tomatoes, spinach and garlic.

4 In a large skillet combine all ingredients and mix until evenly distributed. Season with salt and pepper and serve immediately.

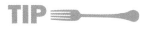

TIP

If you want totally fat-free turkey, rinse the cooked ground meat in boiling water before adding it to the remaining ingredients.

NUTRITIONAL VALUE PER SERVING:
Calories: 114 | Calories from Fat: 8 | Protein: 24g | Carbs: 2g
Dietary Fiber: 0.59g | Sugars: 1g | Fat: 0.8g | Sodium: 120mg

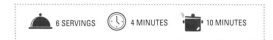

6 SERVINGS   4 MINUTES   10 MINUTES

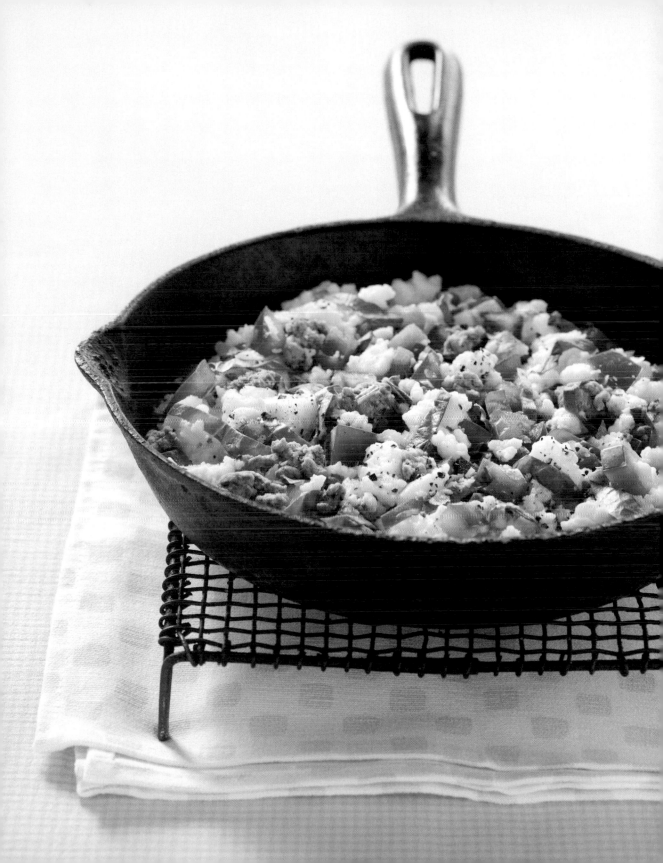

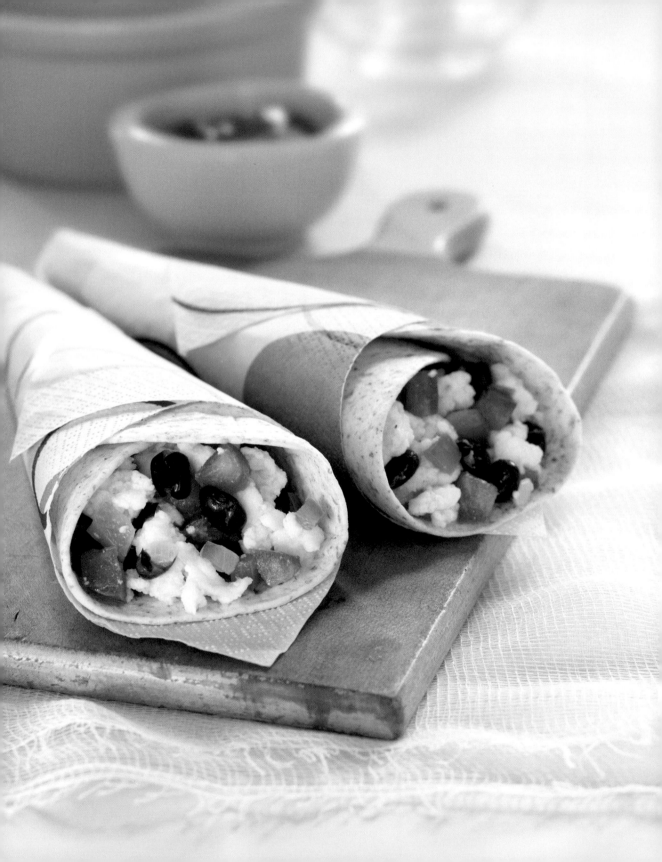

EAT-CLEAN BREAKFAST BURRITOS

The burrito has quickly become a North American favorite, but the traditional version comes with loads of unnecessary calories and fat. Try this low-fat version for breakfast and be amazed at the flavor.

INGREDIENTS:

2 cups / 480 ml egg whites

½ cup / 120 ml nonfat cottage cheese

½ cup / 120 ml chopped tomatoes

½ cup / 120 ml chopped red or green sweet pepper

½ cup / 120 ml chopped sweet onion – Vidalia or purple

½ cup / 120 ml black beans, rinsed and well drained then mashed coarsely with a fork

4 small Ezekiel grain or other whole-grain tortillas or wraps

Sea salt and fresh ground black pepper to taste

Cooking spray

PREPARATION:

1 Preheat oven to 250°F / 121°C. Place tortillas or wraps in oven to warm while preparing remaining ingredients.

2 In a small bowl whisk egg whites, cottage cheese, salt and pepper.

3 In a medium skillet coated with cooking spray, sauté vegetables and beans until soft. Pour the egg/cottage cheese mixture over vegetables and cook until mixture sets. Once firm, divide egg mixture among the warmed tortillas. Roll each into a burrito. Garnish with low-fat, low-sodium salsa.

TIP

Make extras of these portable burritos for lunch! They are just as delicious cold.

NUTRITIONAL VALUE PER SERVING:

Calories: 198 | Calories from Fat: 36 | Protein: 19g | Carbs: 20g
Dietary Fiber: 2.5g | Sugars: 3.5g | Fat: 4g | Sodium: 466mg

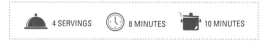 4 SERVINGS   8 MINUTES   10 MINUTES

POWER OATMEAL PANCAKES

Everyone loves pancakes. This light fluffy cake-like breakfast food is traditionally eaten with gobs of butter and syrup. None of this makes for Clean Eating. Try this delicious variation, which is sure to please the palate as well as the waistline.

INGREDIENTS:

6 egg whites, beaten until fluffy

½ cup / 120 ml low-fat cottage cheese

1 scoop whey protein

½ cup / 120 ml oatmeal, uncooked

¼ cup / 60 ml wheat germ

¼ cup / 60 ml flax seed

1 tsp / 5 ml baking powder

1 Tbsp / 15 ml canola oil

½ tsp / 2.5 ml cinnamon

Cooking spray

PREPARATION:

1 Place all ingredients except beaten egg whites in a food processor and pulse or blend until mixture is uniform.

2 Pour blended ingredients into a bowl and add the egg whites. Fold until just blended.

3 Prepare a griddle with cooking spray. Ladle pancake mixture onto griddle and cook until both sides are browned.

How do you eat pancakes Clean-Eating style?

Skip the syrup and place a dollop of unsweetened applesauce on each pancake. Or you can try this little trick: Place ½ cup of blueberries or raspberries in a small saucepan along with 1 tablespoon of water. Mash the berries and bring the mixture to a boil. When the fruit is uniformly hot and beginning to get syrupy, remove from heat and pour into a small jug. Drizzle over pancakes. Delicious!

NUTRITIONAL VALUE PER 2-PANCAKE SERVING:

Calories: 283 | Calories from Fat: 100 | Protein: 21g | Carbs: 24g
Dietary Fiber: 4.5g | Sugars: 0.3g | Fat: 10.5g | Sodium: 198mg

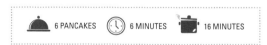 6 PANCAKES   6 MINUTES   16 MINUTES

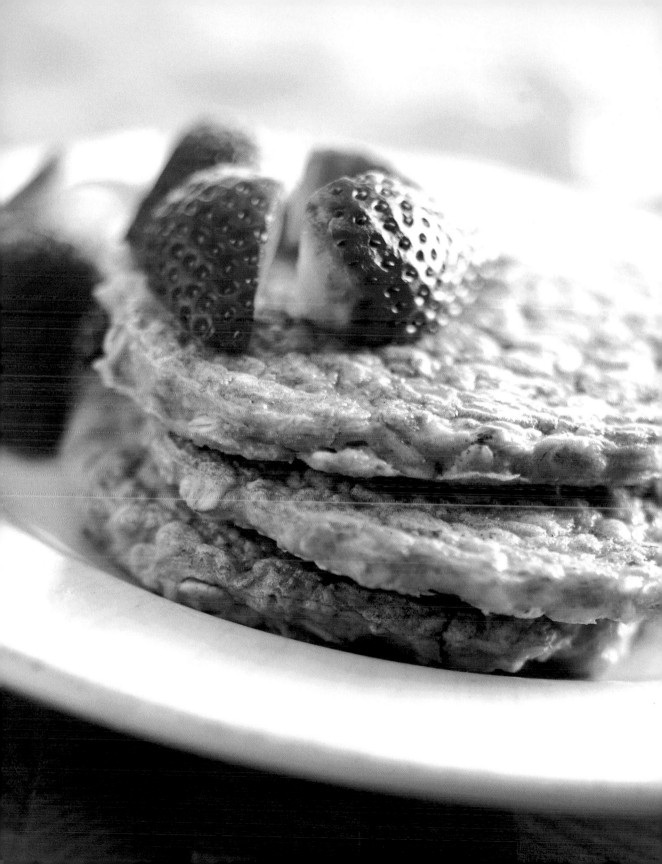

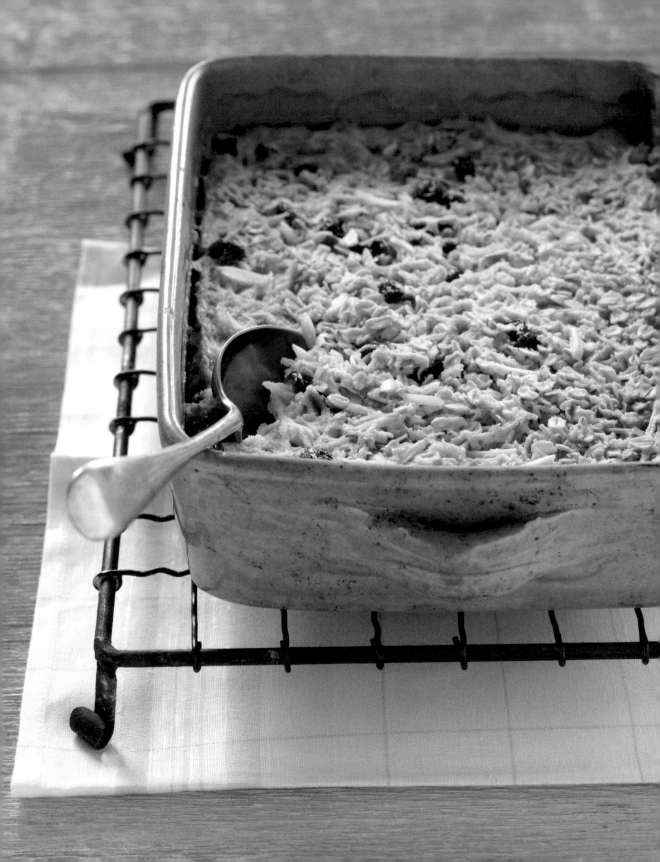

CALEDON BAKED OATMEAL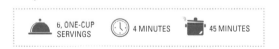

Thihis dish always appears at festive occasions and family get-togethers. I like to vary the ingredients depending on the season. In the winter I'll add dried cranberries and plenty of cinnamon and nutmeg. Cranberries are rich in flavonoids, which have been found to possess anticancer, antibacterial, antiviral and anti-inflammatory properties. In the spring I'll add raisins and vanilla. It's a forgiving dish that can be made to suit your taste. I measure the dry ingredients the night before so all I have to do in the morning is add the liquid ingredients. While it's baking in the oven I have time to prepare other breakfast items.

INGREDIENTS:

2 cups / 480 ml old-fashioned oats

2 cups / 480 ml low-fat or skim milk or soy milk

½ tsp / 2.5 ml best-quality vanilla

½ cup / 120 ml slivered almonds

½ cup / 120 ml dried cranberries or other dried fruit
of your choice

1 large unpeeled MacIntosh apple, grated (apple
should be firm)

4 Tbsp / 60 ml maple syrup

Cooking spray

NUTRITIONAL VALUE PER SERVING:

Calories: 419 | Calories from Fat: 81 | Protein: 15g | Carbs: 71g
Dietary Fiber: 8g | Sugars: 31g | Fat: 9g | Sodium: 85mg

6, ONE-CUP SERVINGS	4 MINUTES	45 MINUTES

PREPARATION:

1 Preheat oven to 400°F / 204°C. Coat a 3 quart (large) casserole dish or baking pan with cooking spray.

2 Combine all ingredients in a large bowl. If you are preparing this the night before don't add the liquid ingredients such as milk and grated apple until morning.

3 Place mixture in a casserole dish. Bake uncovered for 45 minutes.

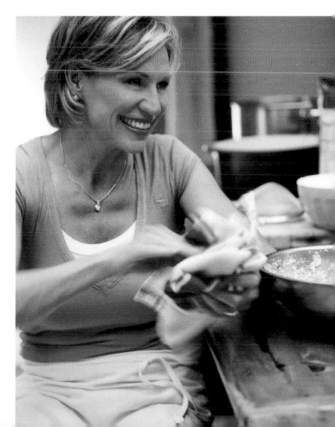

TIP

If you have more people to feed, simply double the recipe.

CAUTION

Those with a severe gluten intolerance or celiac disease are normally able to eat oats, but only if the oats are grown and processed in places guaranteed uncontaminated by grains containing gluten.

CLEAN-EATING MUESLI – *The Super Breakfast*

If more people knew the benefits of muesli and how good it tastes then I am sure more people would eat breakfast. This is a fast and easy breakfast that packs a superior nutritional punch. Make yourself a bowl today! Enjoy it for breakfast with fruit salad or mixed berries. This is one of the meals I like to call an assembly meal because it requires no cooking. Gentlemen, this means you too can be impressive in the kitchen!

INGREDIENTS:

1 cup / 240 ml low-fat quark, kefir, whipped cottage cheese or yogurt

½ cup / 120 ml skim milk soured with 1 tsp lemon juice, or buttermilk

1 Tbsp / 15 ml organic honey

2 Tbsp / 30 ml flax oil

2 Tbsp / 30 ml ground flax seeds

1 unpeeled, grated apple

1 Tbsp / 15 ml coarsely grated walnuts

1 tsp / 5 ml cinnamon

½ cup / 120 ml blueberries, divided

½ cup / 120 ml raspberries, divided

PREPARATION:

1 In a medium bowl blend the quark, kefir, whipped cottage cheese or yogurt with soured milk or buttermilk, honey, flax oil and cinnamon. Set aside.

2 Spoon 1 tablespoon / 15 ml of ground flax seed in each of two smaller cereal bowls. Do the same with the apples, ground walnuts and berries. Divide mixture in first bowl evenly between the two smaller bowls.

TIP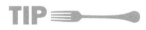

Men, if you want to impress your Clean-Eating women, I suggest you adopt this recipe as your own– hmmm, Valentine's Day, Mother's Day, birthdays. You're going to make her so very happy.

NUTRITIONAL VALUE PER SERVING:

Calories: 409 | Calories from fat: 198 | Protein: 18g | Carbs: 38g
Dietary Fiber: 7g | Sugar: 25g | Fat: 22g | Sodium: 433mg

2 SERVINGS   5 MINUTES   0 MINUTES

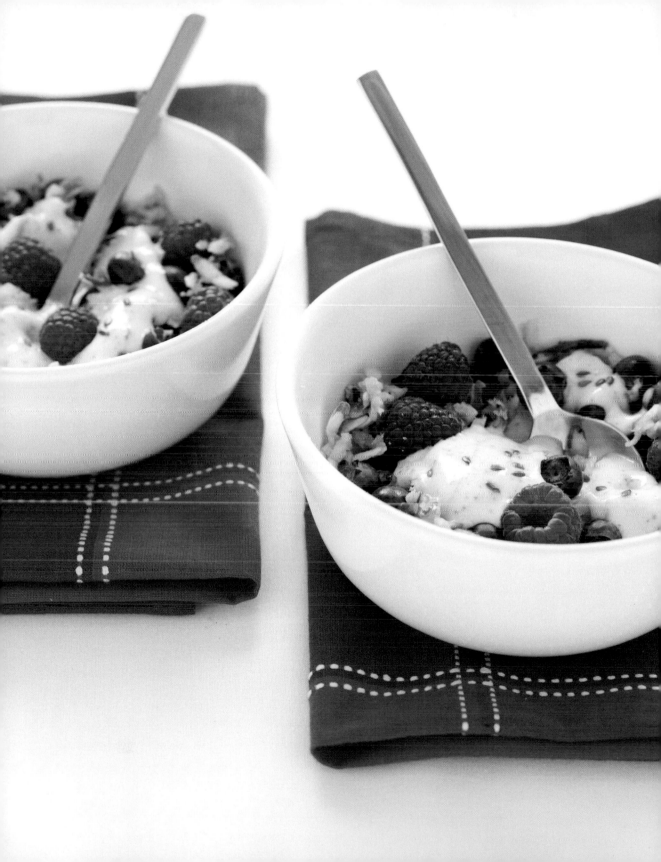

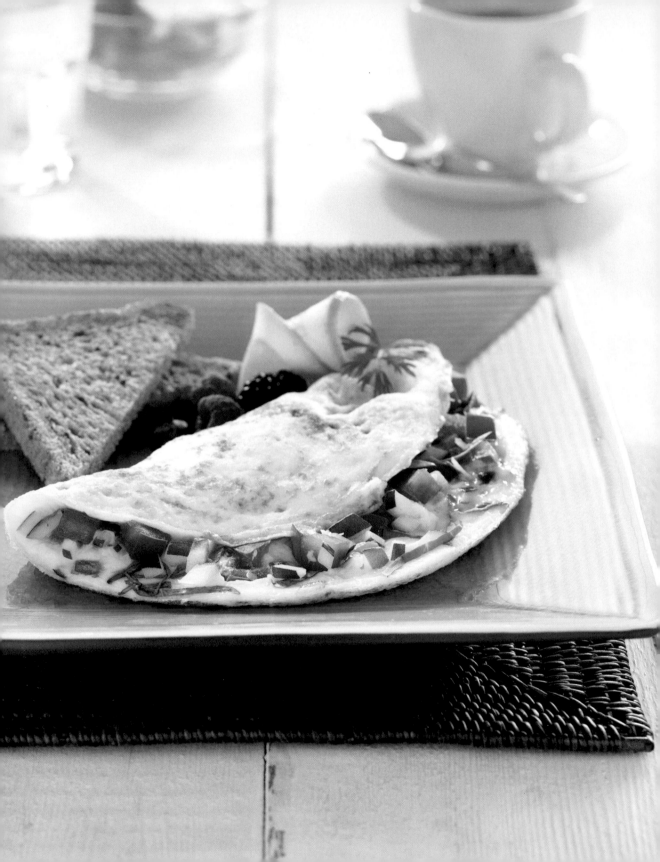

OH-MY-GOSH EGG-WHITE OMELET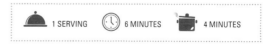

Egg whites provide a nearly perfect protein source. They take on the flavors of your favorite ingredients. Here's a great way to get creative with your morning meal.

INGREDIENTS:

4 - 5 egg whites

1 egg yolk

2 Tbsp / 30 ml skim milk

1 plum tomato, chopped

1 small clove garlic, passed through a press

1 handful shredded spinach

1 Tbsp / 15 ml minced purple onion

Olive oil-based cooking spray

PREPARATION:

1 Beat egg whites with the yolk and skim milk.

2 Quick sauté the vegetables – just till soft.

3 Pour eggs into a small frying pan coated with cooking spray. Cook till firm. Add vegetables on one half of omelet, then fold other half over top. Let sit for 30 seconds or so, then serve.

TIP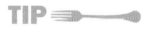

Serve for breakfast, lunch or dinner. This is a simple superb meal not to be missed. Make one in advance to pack in your cooler. Sandwich it in a pita or wrap (gluten free if necessary) and have it for lunch. Reach for it as a late supper idea.

NUTRITIONAL VALUE PER SERVING:

Calories: 203 | Calories from Fat: 47 | Protein: 20g | Carbs: 18g
Dietary Fiber: 2g | Sugars: 8g | Fat: 5g | Sodium: 272mg

1 SERVING   6 MINUTES   4 MINUTES

APPLESAUCE PUMPKIN MUFFINS

Everyone loves a delicious muffin, especially with a steaming cup of coffee, but few of us like the nasty calorie surprise that comes with most commercially made muffins. Did you know some popular coffee chains offer muffins that pack a whopping 600 plus calories? Try these little gems for your morning wake-up call.

INGREDIENTS:

1 cup / 240 ml old-fashioned oatmeal, not instant

½ cup / 125 ml unsweetened applesauce

½ cup / 125 ml canned pumpkin

2 large egg whites + one yolk, lightly beaten

2 Tbsp + 1 tsp / 35 ml canola oil

1 Tbsp / 15 ml double-acting baking powder

½ tsp / 2.5 ml baking soda

1 tsp / 5 ml cinnamon

¼ tsp / 1.25 ml ground nutmeg

1 tsp / 5 ml pumpkin pie spice

½ cup / 120 ml milk or milk alternative or ½ cup apple juice

½ cup / 120 ml amaranth or quinoa flour or flour of your choice

¼ cup / 60 ml whole-wheat flour

¼ cup / 60 ml maple sugar flakes

½ cup / 120 ml dried cranberries or raisins *(optional)*

PREPARATION:

1 Preheat oven to 375°F / 190°C. Line muffin pan with paper or silicon liners or coat with cooking spray.

2 Combine oatmeal, pumpkin, applesauce, juice or milk, eggs and oil. Mix until all ingredients are blended.

3 Measure and mix all dry ingredients. Make a well in the center and pour wet ingredients into dry. Add dried fruit if using. Mix until dry ingredients are just moistened. Fill muffin cups ⅔ full. Bake 15-20 minutes or until lightly browned on top.

ALTERNATIVE: If you don't have pumpkin you can use a sweet potato. Simply microwave the sweet potato and let cool. Remove the skin and mash the flesh. Measure out the required quantity. Voilà!

NOTE: In the photo, light cream cheese is being used as a spread on these muffins. As long as the fat is *at most* 50% that of regular cream cheese, you can enjoy light cream cheese on occasion.

NUTRITIONAL VALUE PER MUFFIN:
Calories: 189 | Calories from Fat: 78 | Protein: 6g | Carbs: 21g
Dietary Fiber: 2g | Sugars: 8g | Fat: 8g | Sodium: 25mg

12 MUFFINS   30 MINUTES   20 MINUTES

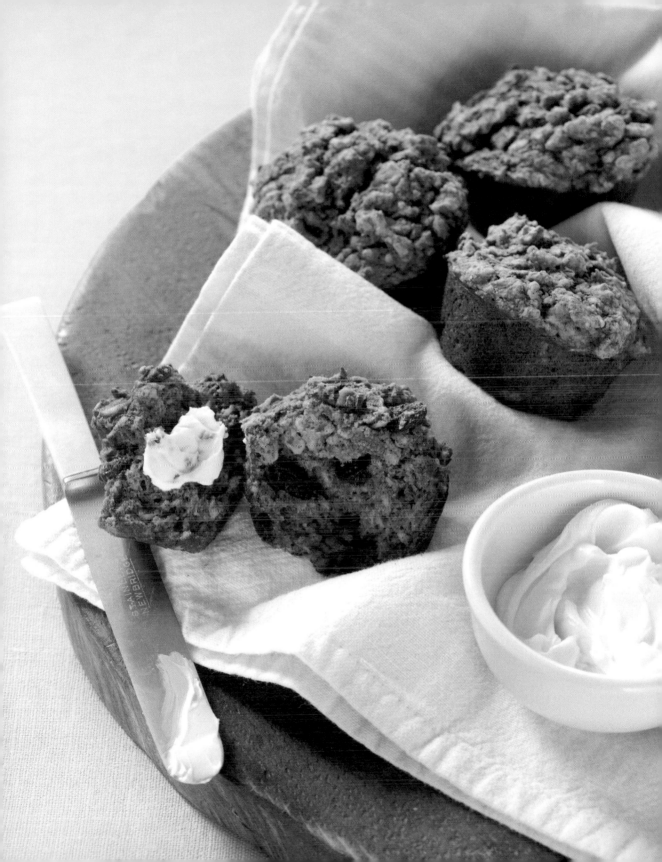

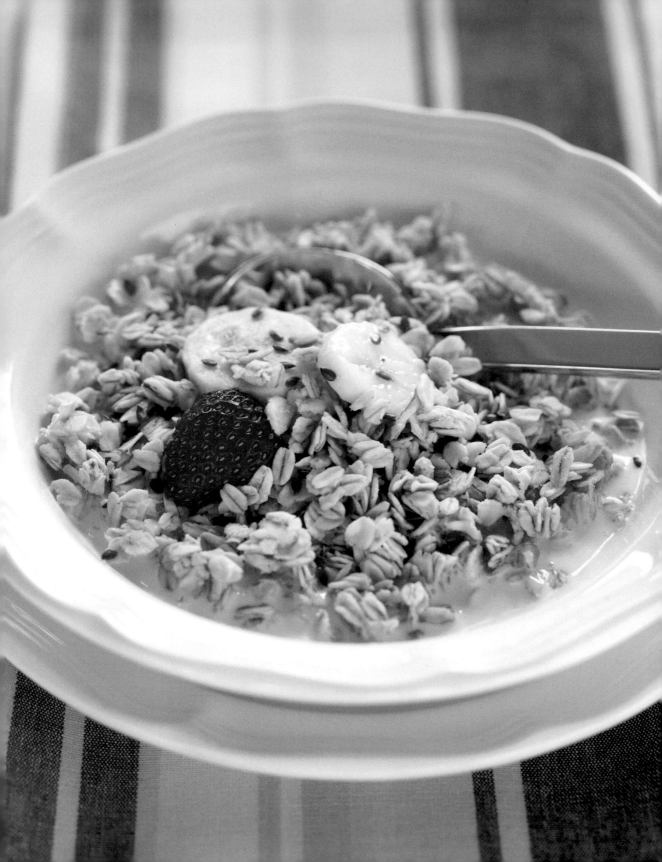

LOADED OATS

There is no better way to start the day than with oatmeal, but who wants oatmeal every day? Make this interesting variation of oatmeal to keep your interest and fuel your body with delicious protein.

INGREDIENTS:

2 cups / 480 ml oatmeal, uncooked

4 Tbsp / 60 ml natural nut butter – almond, peanut, cashew butter or other

2 cups / 480 ml skim milk or milk alternative (soy milk, rice milk or other)

2 cups / 480 ml water

1 tsp / 5 ml cinnamon

2 scoops best-quality protein powder, flavor of your choice

4 Tbsp / 60 ml coarsely ground flax seeds

NUTRITIONAL VALUE PER SERVING:

Calories: 503 | Calories from Fat: 147 | Protein: 28g | Carbs: 64g
Dietary Fiber: 10g | Sugars: 7g | Fat: 16g | Sodium: 140mg

PREPARATION:

1 Bring the four cups of liquid to a boil in a saucepan.

2 Add remaining ingredients except flax seed, and reduce heat. Cook gently for 3 to 5 minutes, until mixture becomes uniform and thick.

3 Ladle into four bowls and sprinkle each with 1 tablespoon ground flax seed. Serve immediately.

4 SERVINGS   5 MINUTES   5 MINUTES

NOTE: This recipe can easily be made for one person by dividing the recipe by four.

CAN YOUR KIDS MAKE OATMEAL?

Introduce your children to the benefits of Clean Eating, too. Start with the most important meal of the day... breakfast! Have you taught your kids how to make oatmeal by themselves? It's easier than you think.

OATMEAL PREPARATION:

1 Fill a kettle with water.

2 Let it come to a full boil. Turn it off.

3 Measure a half cup of dry oatmeal into a cereal bowl – use longer-cooking oats, if possible.
Carefully pour one cup of boiled water into the cereal bowl, making sure every flake is immersed.
BE CAREFUL!! THE KETTLE AND THE WATER ARE HOT.

4 Place a plate over the cereal bowl and let sit for 5 to 10 minutes. Voilà! Your oatmeal is ready!

OATMEAL TOPPINGS:

• Mixed berries
• Chopped apple
• Chopped banana
• Raisins
• Flax seed
• Bee pollen
• Wheat germ
• Unsweetened low-fat yogurt
• Unsweetened applesauce
• Maple flakes

GLUTEN-FREE FLAVOR-FULL PANCAKES

Many of us cannot or choose not to eat gluten. Gluten causes painful digestive issues for those who cannot tolerate it. But everyone loves pancakes. Where can you find a recipe for those who want to eat them but need to avoid gluten? Here's a recipe that works, and tastes so good you won't realize you are not eating the real thing.

INGREDIENTS:

1 cup / 240 ml flour prepared as follows:

- ¼ cup/ 60 ml tapioca

- 1 tsp / 5 ml guar gum

- ¾ cup / 180 ml rice flour

½ cup / 125 ml soy, rice or almond milk

1 tsp / 30 ml organic honey

2 eggs or egg white substitute

1 Tbsp / 30 ml canola or safflower oil

Cooking spray

PREPARATION:

1 Place all dry ingredients in a medium bowl.

2 Using a whisk, mix dry ingredients well. Add milk, honey, eggs and oil. Whisk until all ingredients are well blended. Add more milk if necessary to make batter runny.

3 Pour ¼ to ⅓ (about 70 ml) cup pancake batter on hot griddle or frying pan coated with cooking spray. When bubbles form on top of pancake, flip. Cook until golden on both sides.

TIP

The dry ingredients can be pre-mixed and placed in an airtight container.

NUTRITIONAL VALUE PER 2-PANCAKE SERVING:
Calories: 276 | Calories from Fat: 56 | Protein: 6g | Carbs: 46g
Dietary Fiber: 2g | Sugars: 2g | Fat: 6g | Sodium: 62mg

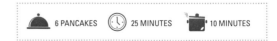
6 PANCAKES   25 MINUTES   10 MINUTES

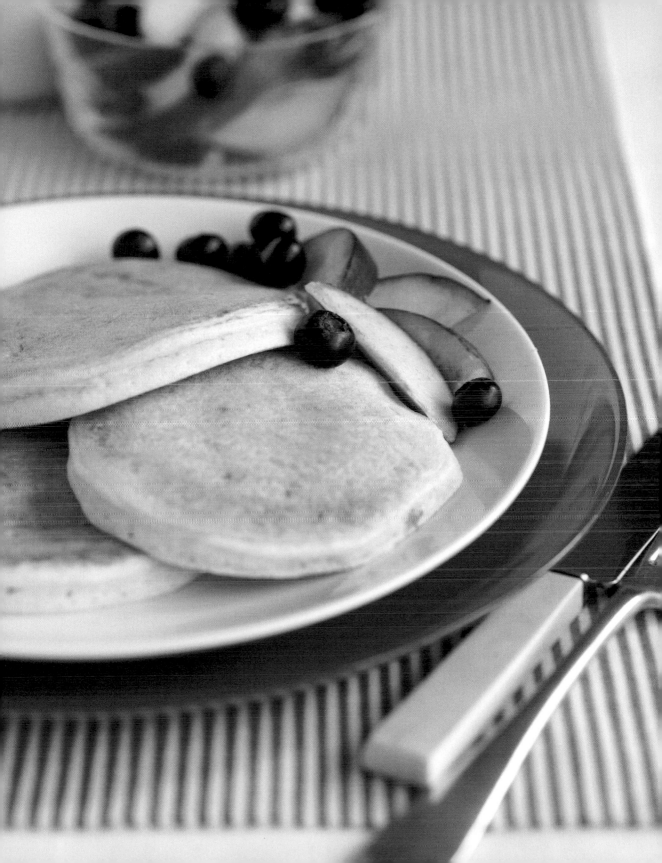

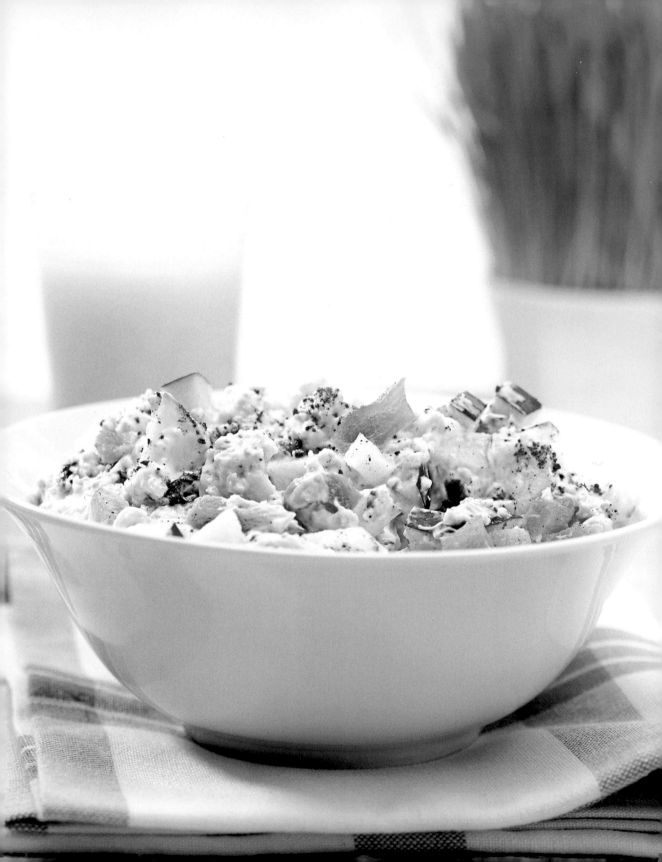

SWISS MUESLI

This is my favorite version of muesli. It tastes and feels as indulgent as the authentic variety, which is loaded with extra calories and fat. This recipe is a slimmer, cleaner version, but oh so delicious! The best part is that you can make it in advance and eat it over the course of two or three days. The flavor actually improves as it sits in the fridge.

INGREDIENTS:

½ cup / 25 ml hot water

½ cup / 120 ml 3 - 5 minute oats

1 cup / 240 ml low-fat or nonfat yogurt or soy yogurt

¼ cup / 60 ml raisins

¼ cup / 60 ml dried cherries or cranberries or both

2 Tbsp / 30 ml natural bran

2 Tbsp / 30 ml wheat germ

2 Tbsp / 30 ml coarsely ground flax seeds

2 Tbsp / 30 ml oat bran

2 Tbsp / 30 ml organic honey

1 apple, unpeeled, cored and diced

3 bananas, peeled and sliced

PREPARATION:

1 In a medium bowl, pour hot water over oats. Let stand for 20 minutes or until water is absorbed.

2 Add remaining ingredients except bananas. Mix well. Cover and refrigerate for up to three days. Serve with sliced bananas.

NOTE: This can serve as breakfast if you eat a one-cup serving. You can mix in your protein powder of choice to make it a complete Clean-Eating breakfast. This recipe also works as a snack before bed if you eat a ½ cup / 120 ml serving.

NUTRITIONAL VALUE PER SERVING:

Calories: 350 | Calories from Fat: 43 | Protein: 10g | Carbs: 72g
Dietary Fiber: 7g | Sugar: 41g | Fat: 4g | Sodium: 50mg

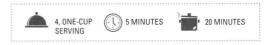

4, ONE-CUP SERVING   5 MINUTES   20 MINUTES

BREAKFAST FRUIT AND NUT COOKIES

Wouldn't it be a treat to have a delicious yet low-fat breakfast cookie with your morning cup of coffee? Try these breakfast cookies for a yummy alternative to muffins.

INGREDIENTS:

½ cup / 120 ml brown sugar

¼ cup / 60 ml melted Olivina or light oil

3 egg whites

¼ cup / 60 ml finely chopped dried figs

¼ cup / 60 ml dried cranberries

1 tsp / 5 ml best-quality vanilla

1 cup / 240 ml all-purpose flour

½ cup / 120 ml whole-wheat flour

½ cup / 120 ml bran flakes

2 Tbsp / 30 ml ground flax seed

½ tsp / 2.5 ml baking soda

¼ tsp / 1.25 ml ground cinnamon

¼ tsp / 1.25 ml ground allspice

¼ cup / 60 ml slivered almonds

PREPARATION:

1 Preheat oven to 350°F / 177°C.

2 Combine sugar, oil and egg whites in a large mixing bowl. Stir in chopped dried fruits and vanilla.

3 Lightly spoon all-purpose flour into measuring cups and level with a knife. Combine whole-wheat flour, bran, baking soda, flax seed and spices. Stir with a whisk or fork.

4 Add flour mixture to egg mixture, stirring until just combined. Fold in almonds.

5 Drop by tablespoon full onto baking sheets lined with parchment paper or Silpat. Bake for 12 minutes or until almost set. Cool on pans and transfer to wire racks to cool completely.

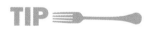

TIP

Make sure to let these cookies cool properly on a rack before placing them in an airtight container.

NUTRITIONAL VALUE PER COOKIE:
Calories: 154 | Calories from Fat: 56 | Protein: 2g | Carbs: 22g
Dietary Fiber: 1g | Sugar: 12g | Fat: 6g | Sodium: 26mg

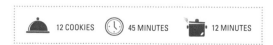

12 COOKIES   45 MINUTES   12 MINUTES

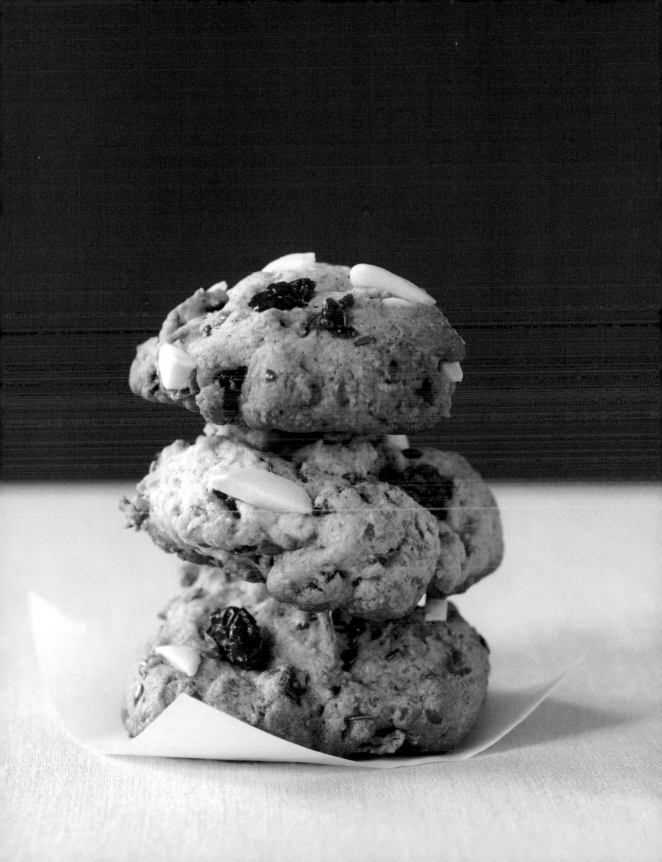

BREAKFAST IN A BLENDER

Each of us has a day when making breakfast is just too much trouble. Yet we know this meal is a must to get our metabolism revved up. How do we manage? One of the best ideas is to put an assortment of ingredients in a blender and push "GO." Breakfast in a blender is your way to a roaring start.

INGREDIENTS:

1 scoop protein powder – your choice

⅓ cup / 80 ml dry oatmeal

⅔ cup / 160 ml water or soy milk, cow's milk, almond or rice milk

1 Tbsp / 5 ml natural almond butter or nut butter of your choice

1 frozen banana (if you don't have a frozen one, use a fresh banana)

2 Tbsp / 30 ml unsweetened applesauce

1 Tbsp / 15 ml flax seed (whole flax seed is fine)

1 Tbsp / 15 ml wheat germ

½ cup / 120 ml ice cubes

PREPARATION:

1 Blend all ingredients. Drink your breakfast!

NUTRITIONAL VALUE PER SERVING:

Calories: 275 | Calories from Fat: 31 | Protein: 8g | Carbs: 55g
Dietary Fiber: 6g | Sugar: 28g | Fat: 3g | Sodium: 37mg

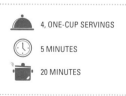

4, ONE-CUP SERVINGS

5 MINUTES

20 MINUTES

EAT-CLEAN WAYS TO
MAKE INTERESTING SMOOTHIES

Smoothies are a superb way to nourish tired muscles after a workout, or a quick way to get loads of nutrients when you don't have time to make a meal.

Here are five quick tips to make a unique smoothie:

1 Don't hesitate to use oatmeal in a smoothie. Adding leftover cooked oatmeal or dry oats boosts the fiber value of a smoothie while adding a host of "get your engine started" nutrients. Throw in frozen or fresh fruits and a scoop of protein powder and whiz it up. Perfect!

2 Love the taste of pumpkin pie? Here's the healthy alternative. Microwave a sweet potato. Let it cool and put the flesh in a blender. Add a dash of vanilla and some cinnamon and nutmeg. Throw in some plain, nonfat yogurt, and purée along with a handful of ice cubes. Delicious!

3 Nut butters add not only healthy fats to your smoothie but also fiber and loads of flavor. Add a tablespoon of your favorite nut butter (mine is almond), frozen banana, ¼ cup / 60 ml dry oatmeal, ½ cup / 125 ml soy or milk of your preference and purée. Toss in a handful of ice cubes for a thinner consistency.

4 Silken tofu makes a beautifully light smoothie. Put ½ cup / 120 ml silken tofu in a blender. Add 1 cup / 240 ml frozen mixed berries and a handful of ice cubes. Blend until smooth. This is better than sorbet!

5 Throat-saver smoothie. Ever had a nagging sore throat and wanted it to feel better? Try this: Place ½ cup / 120 ml alfalfa sprouts (loaded with vitamin C) in a blender. Add 1 scoop hemp protein powder, 1 Tbsp / 15 ml almond butter, ½ cup / 120 ml plain nonfat yogurt and 1 Tbsp / 15 ml pumpkin oil (for zinc). Quickly cook or microwave 2 Tbsp / 30 ml oats in ½ cup / 125 ml water. Once the mixture comes to a boil pour it over the ingredients in the blender. Purée and drink away your sore throat.

SIMPLE SUNSHINE SMOOTHIE

INGREDIENTS:

½ cup / 120 ml nonfat cottage cheese
½ cup / 120 ml milk – skim, soy, almond, rice, goat or milk of your choice
½ tsp / 2.5 ml vanilla
1 tsp / 5 ml lemon-flavored avocado oil
1 scoop whey protein, vanilla or unflavored
1 navel orange, peeled
1 Tbsp / 15 ml wheat germ
Handful ice cubes

METHOD:

Purée all ingredients.

BLUEBERRY BUZZ SMOOTHIE

INGREDIENTS:

½ cup / 120 ml milk – skim, soy, almond, rice or other
½ cup / 120 ml water
½ cup / 120 ml frozen blueberries
1 Tbsp / 15 ml flax seed
½ cup / 120 ml unsweetened applesauce
½ cup / 120 ml plain nonfat yogurt
2 scoops whey protein powder – vanilla or unflavored
Handful ice cubes

METHOD:

Purée all ingredients.

OATMEAL PROTEIN SMOOTHIE

INGREDIENTS:

¼ cup / 60 ml dry, uncooked oatmeal
1 Tbsp / 15 ml natural nut butter – peanut, soy, cashew, almond or nut butter of your choice
1 scoop protein powder, vanilla is best
1 Tbsp / 15 ml organic honey or agave nectar
1 Tbsp / 15 ml flax seed

1 cup / 240 ml milk – skim, almond, goat, soy, rice or milk of your choice
½ tsp / 2.5 ml cinnamon
Ice

METHOD:

Purée all ingredients, adding ice to adjust consistency of smoothie.

VARIATION:

4 Tbsp / 60 ml raw, unsalted sunflower seeds added

KIWI CITRUS SMOOTHIE

INGREDIENTS:

1 kiwi, peeled
1 navel orange, peeled
1 scoop whey protein powder, vanilla or unflavored
½ cup / 120 ml nonfat, plain yogurt
1 tsp / 5 ml lemon flavored avocado oil
Pinch nutmeg
Pinch cinnamon
1 tsp / 5 ml fresh lime juice
½ cup / 120 ml ice cubes

METHOD:

Purée all ingredients. If the smoothie is too thick add more ice and blend again.

VITAMIN BOOSTER SMOOTHIE

INGREDIENTS:

½ cup / 120 ml alfalfa sprouts
¼ cup / 60 ml frozen strawberries
¼ cup / 60 ml frozen mixed berries
¼ cup / 60 ml frozen mango
1 tsp / 5 ml flax oil
1 scoop whey protein powder, vanilla or unflavored
1 Tbsp / 15 ml agave nectar or organic honey
1 cup / 240 ml cold water

METHOD:

Purée all ingredients.

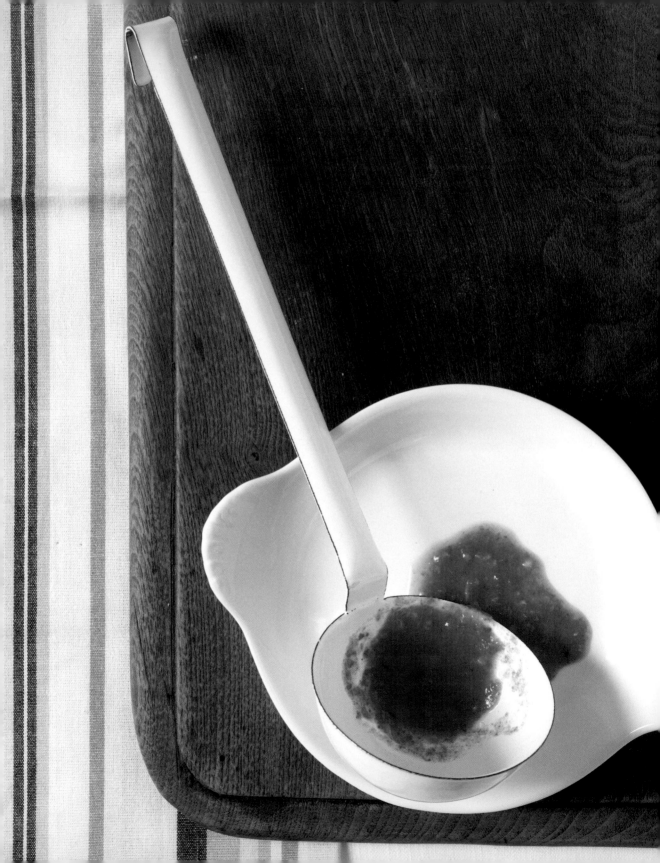

2

Soups

· ·

There is magic in a pot of soup, I always say. I lose myself in the soup-making process – mixing root vegetables, grains, and other nourishing ingredients to create a soul satisfying brew. I love making soup so much I even create a batch when the temps reach into the 80s or higher; not just on a frigid winter day.

Make your own magic or try these soups I have divined just for you. Add a hearty whole-grain bread and one of the spreads (see Sauces, Spreads and Salsas) for a complete meal. An elegant soup can be served all on its own with a delicious wine. When entertaining try Roasted Butternut Squash Soup on page 52.

WILD RICE AND TOFU SOUP

Wehani wild rice is developed by Lundberg Family Farms in California. It is a colorful grain and adds that extra little something to this already mouth-watering soup. Toss in tofu and an assortment of veggies and legumes and you can't go wrong. Enjoy this complete Clean-Eating meal in a bowl!

INGREDIENTS:

1 cup / 240 ml Wehani rice or other wild rice variety

4 Tbsp / 60 ml best quality olive oil

1 cup / 240 ml carrots, peeled and diced

1 cup / 240 ml parsnips, peeled and diced

1 cup / 240 ml sweet Vidalia onion, diced

6 cups / 1.4 L low-sodium chicken or vegetable stock (Make sure it's gluten free if this is an issue)

3 cups / 720 ml low-fat, plain soymilk

1 garlic clove, minced

1 cup / 240 ml white kidney beans, rinsed and drained

1 cup / 240 ml kidney beans, rinsed and drained

1 cup / 240 ml black beans, rinsed and drained

1 cup / 240 ml regular tofu, cubed

Sea salt and black pepper

PREPARATION:

1 Cook rice according to package directions.

2 Meanwhile, sauté carrots, parsnips and onion in olive oil.

3 In large pot place sautéed vegetables, poultry stock and soymilk. Add garlic, beans and tofu. Simmer for 10 minutes. Add cooked rice and stir until just blended. Season with salt and pepper.

TIP

Want to speed up cooking time? Add uncooked rice to the stock at the beginning. Or use planned leftovers (extra rice from the day before).

NUTRITIONAL VALUE PER SERVING:

Calories: 494 | Calories from fat: 161 | Protein: 21g | Carbs: 64g
Dietary Fiber: 13g | Sugars: 7g | Fat: 17g | Sodium: 1278mg

4 SERVINGS · 25 MINUTES · 30 MINUTES

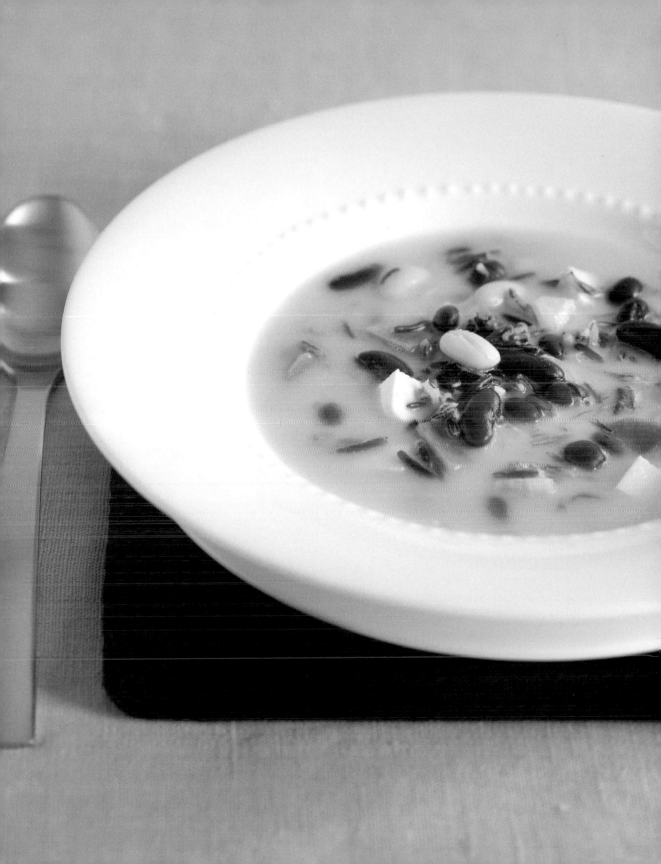

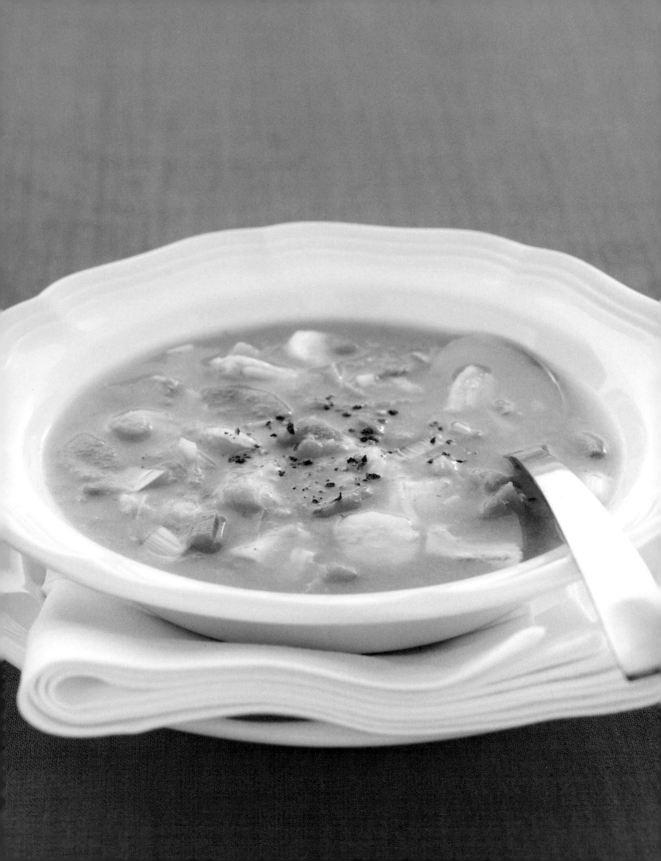

SPLIT PEA SOUP

This is another childhood favorite recipe. My mother used to make this soup for us frequently and I love the heartiness of it. One bowl is a meal in itself— not to mention the oodles of fiber it contains. Traditionally, ham is used in this recipe but I find roasted turkey breast is a delicious Clean-Eating alternative.

INGREDIENTS:

2 cups / 480 ml dried split peas

12 cups / 2.9 L water

4 bay leaves

Sea salt

1 Tbsp / 15 ml olive oil

1 large yellow onion, peeled and chopped

4 ribs celery, trimmed and chopped

3 thick carrots, peeled and chopped

2 cups / 480 ml low-sodium chicken or vegetable broth (gluten free if necessary)

6 cups / 1.4 L water

1 tsp / 5 ml fresh thyme, chopped

1½ cups / 360 ml cubed roasted turkey breast*

* If vegetarian, remove turkey breast.

TIP

The Dutch love their Erwten Soep! Make plenty. There won't be leftovers.

PREPARATION:

1 Put dried peas in large saucepan and cover with 12 cups / 2.9 L of water. Add 2 bay leaves and sea salt and bring to a boil. Let cook on medium heat for 10 minutes. Drain and set aside.

2 In a Dutch oven, place olive oil and heat over medium heat. Add onion, celery and carrots. Sauté for 8 minutes until onion begins to turn translucent.

3 Add chicken broth or preferred cooking liquid and 6 cups / 1.4 L water. Add 2 more bay leaves, peas, and thyme and bring to a boil. Add roasted turkey breast. Reduce heat and cover. Let simmer for an hour. The peas need to be soft. Check the pot now and then, since the peas have a tendency to settle to the bottom and burn. You'll have to break them up by stirring them.

4 Remove the bay leaves and season with sea salt and fresh ground black pepper. Serve hot.

NUTRITIONAL VALUE PER SERVING WITH TURKEY:

Calories: 200 | Calories from Fat: 18 | Protein: 19g | Carbs: 27g
Dietary Fiber: 10g | Sugars: 4g | Fat: 2g | Sodium: 172mg

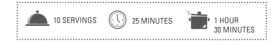

10 SERVINGS   25 MINUTES   1 HOUR 30 MINUTES

ROASTED RED PEPPER SOUP

The flavor of red pepper is enhanced to perfection when it is roasted. In this vibrant soup red peppers burst with nutrition and sweetness. I love to make a pot of soup to last the weekend. Everyone can help themselves, and I know the soup I make is far more nourishing than anything out of a can. Somehow I just can't bring myself to buy the canned varieties knowing how easily I can whip up a much more nutritious soup.

INGREDIENTS:

10 – 12 medium sweet red bell peppers, halved, seeds discarded

3 Tbsp / 45 ml olive oil, rice bran oil or avocado oil

1 medium yellow onion, peeled and finely chopped

1 large sweet carrot, peeled and diced

2 large cloves garlic, peeled and crushed

1 medium Yukon Gold potato or sweet potato, peeled and diced

2 tsp / 10 ml chopped fresh thyme

1 Tbsp / 15 ml chopped fresh basil

4 cups / 960 ml low-sodium, low-fat chicken or vegetable stock (gluten free if necessary)

2 bay leaves

2 tsp / 30 ml red wine vinegar

⅛ tsp / 0.6 ml cayenne pepper

Sea salt and fresh ground black pepper to taste

1 basil leaf (for garnish)

PREPARATION:

1 Preheat broiler. Place red peppers cut side down on baking sheet(s). Lightly coat the outside of each pepper with your oil of choice. Place baking sheet under the broiler and cook until the skins blacken. Remove from broiler and place all peppers in a large bowl immediately. Cover tightly with plastic wrap. This helps the peppers sweat, which loosens the skins. Wait until the peppers are cool enough to handle and gently remove the skin from each. Put skinned peppers in a bowl and set aside.

2 In a Dutch oven or stock pot, heat 1 tablespoon / 15 ml oil of choice over medium heat. Add the onion and carrot and cook until the onion is soft and translucent. Add the garlic and sauté briefly. Add potato or sweet potato, herbs, stock, skinned, roasted peppers, and bay leaves. Simmer until all vegetables are soft. When ready, remove the bay leaves and purée the soup until it is smooth. Add vinegar and cayenne pepper. Season with sea salt and freshly ground black pepper. Garnish with a fresh basil leaf and serve immediately.

TIP

For another Clean-Eating garnish, use a dollop of low-fat plain yogurt.

NUTRITIONAL VALUE PER SERVING:
Calories: 118 | Calories from Fat: 51 | Protein: 2g | Carbs: 15g
Dietary Fiber: 3g | Sugars: 7g | Fat: 5g | Sodium: 190mg

8 SERVINGS   30 MINUTES   40 MINUTES

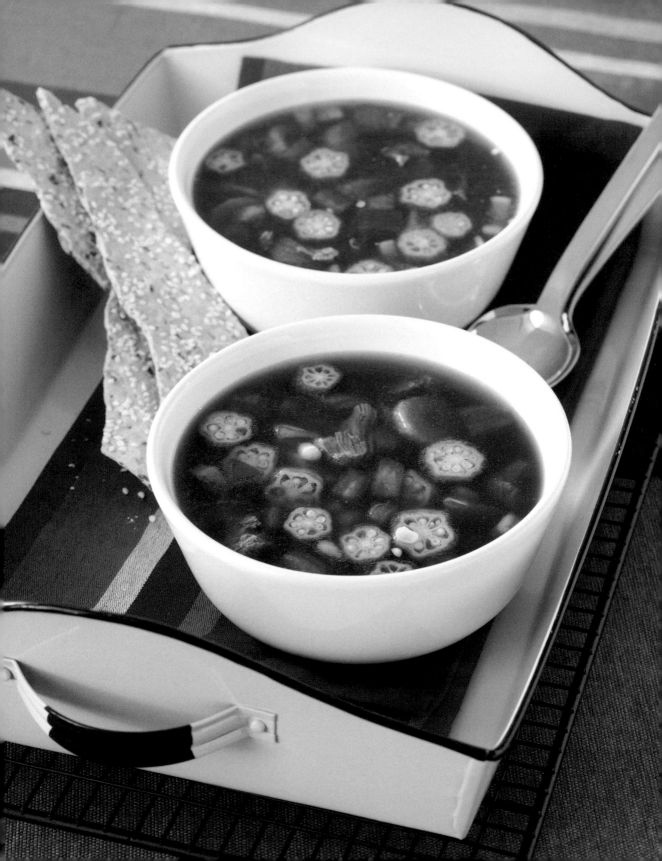

PEPPER POT SOUP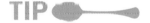

This filling soup has its origins with First Nations peoples, who made the most of available ingredients to feed themselves. The soup is simple to make and provides a colorful alternative to more ordinary fare.

INGREDIENTS:

2 pounds / 908 g venison or bison ribs or shanks

2 large onions, peeled and quartered

2 large carrots, peeled and cut into chunks

4 ribs celery

4 bay leaves

2 quarts / 1.9 L water

3 Roma tomatoes, seeded and coarsely chopped

1 large red bell pepper, seeded and chopped

1 cup / 240 ml okra, sliced

½ cup / 120 ml sliced carrots

¾ cup / 180 ml fresh corn kernels

½ cup / 120 ml chopped celery

Sea salt and black pepper

PREPARATION:

1 Place meaty bones in a Dutch oven or large soup pot. Add onions, celery, carrots, bay leaves and water. Bring to a boil. Reduce heat and let simmer for 3 hours.

2 Remove meat from hot liquid and allow to cool. Once cooled, remove meat in bite-sized pieces. Discard bones. Remove bay leaves and discard. Add remaining ingredients to soup and simmer for 1½ hours, partially covered. Add meat, simmer for another five minutes and serve.

TIP

Don't be afraid to try okra in this soup. The flesh helps create a beautiful thick liquid.

NUTRITIONAL VALUE PER SERVING:

Calories: 307 | Calories from Fat: 101 | Protein: 35g | Carbs: 16g
Dietary Fiber: 3g | Sugars: 5g | Fat: 11g | Sodium: 156mg

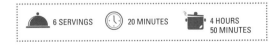

6 SERVINGS   20 MINUTES   4 HOURS 50 MINUTES

NOT-SO-BASIC TOMATO SOUP

I could eat tomato soup any time any day, but it has to be homemade. Nothing beats the intense crimson color of this stunning soup. Serve it as part of an ideal Clean-Eating meal or wow your guests with it as an appetizer when entertaining.

INGREDIENTS:

5 lbs / 2.3 kg fresh tomatoes – use a mixture of
Romas, field and cluster or heirloom tomatoes
1 Tbsp / 15 ml olive oil
½ cup / 120 ml water
¼ cup / 60 ml fresh basil leaves
1 tsp / 5 ml organic honey
Sea salt and fresh ground black pepper
Juice of one fresh lemon

PREPARATION:

1 Wash tomatoes under cold running water. Remove green crowns.

2 Bring several cups of water to a boil in a large sauce- or soup pan. Place whole tomatoes in boiling water just long enough to split and loosen their outer skin. You may have to do this in batches. Once the skins are loose remove the tomatoes from the boiling water and drop them in a bowl of ice water. This stops the cooking process and accelerates the cooling of the tomatoes. When the tomatoes are cool enough to handle, loosen the skins with your hands. Quarter the tomatoes and remove the hard inner core.

3 In a Dutch oven, heat the olive oil over medium-high heat. Place all the tomatoes in the pot. Add ½ cup / 125 ml of water. Bring the mixture to a boil and immediately reduce the heat. Add fresh basil, cover the pot and allow the tomatoes to simmer for about 30 minutes or until they are soft. Stir the mixture occasionally. Remove from heat.

4 Place a food mill over a large bowl. Transfer cooked tomatoes to the food mill and slowly turn the handle to make a purée. Any remaining skins, seeds and other bits will not pass through the disc, and you can readily discard this. The soup will collect in the bowl. Note: If you do not own a food mill, use a hand blender, or blend in small batches in a regular blender.

5 Return the puréed soup to a saucepan and allow to simmer. Stir in the honey and lemon juice. Season with salt and pepper. Serve hot.

NUTRITIONAL VALUE PER SERVING:
Calories: 95 | Calories from Fat: 28 | Protein: 3g | Carbs: 16g
Dietary Fiber: 4g | Sugars: 10g | Fat: 3g | Sodium: 19mg

6 SERVINGS   30 MINUTES   50 MINUTES

TIP

If you would like to make your soup more nutritious, put a handful of baby spinach leaves in the bottom of each soup bowl and ladle the soup over top. By the time you eat the soup the spinach leaves will be gently wilted but still highly nutritious.

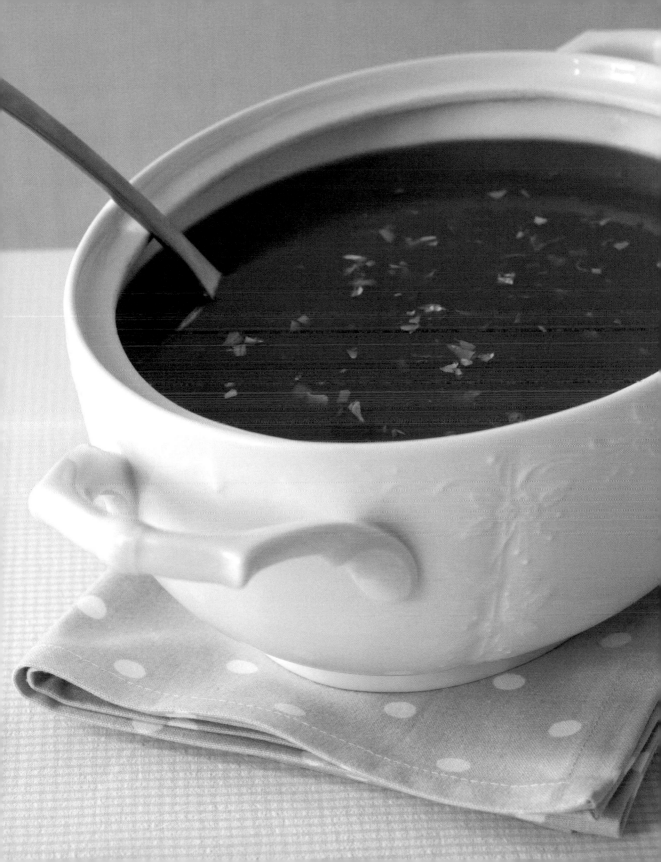

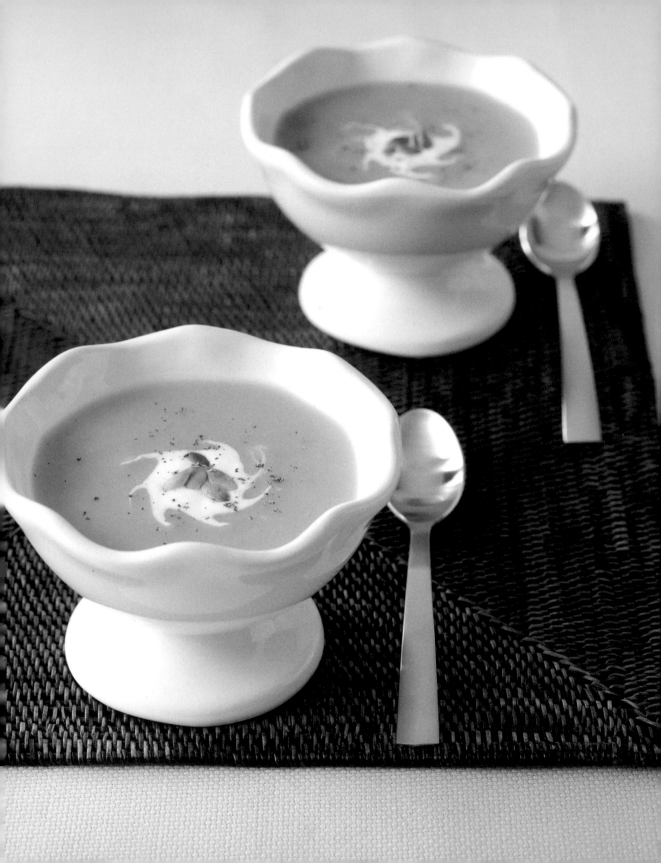

ROASTED BUTTERNUT SQUASH SOUP

I am definitely a soup fanatic. When the cooler weather rolls around I am ridiculously happy because it makes sense, once again, to fire up the stove and create beautiful soups brimming with nourishment and warmth. Butternut squash is versatile and loaded with phytonutrients. Tastes pretty good too!

INGREDIENTS:

⅓ cup / 80 ml best quality olive oil

2 large butternut squash

1 sweet onion, cut into large chunks

1 bulb garlic

½ tsp / 2.5 ml rice bran oil*

2 cups / 480 ml low-sodium, low-fat chicken or vegetable stock (gluten free if necessary)

2 Tbsp / 30 ml fresh lime juice

Sea salt and fresh black pepper to taste

Ground nutmeg

*Note: Can't find rice bran oil? Olive oil will do.

PREPARATION:

1 Preheat oven to 350°F / 177°C. Prepare a large roasting pan by pouring the oil into it, letting it coat the bottom. Cut the squash in half and remove seeds and string. Place squash in roasting pan, cut side down. Prick the skins with a sharp knife. Place onion around the squash. Using a sharp knife cut the top of the garlic bulb off and drizzle with rice bran oil. Place in the roasting pan with the other vegetables. Bake for 45 minutes to an hour or until tender. Remove and let stand.

2 Scrape baked squash into a large stock pot. Add the roasted onion and squeeze roasted garlic flesh in as well. Add chicken stock and lime juice and bring to a boil. Reduce heat and simmer for 15 minutes. Using a hand blender, purée the soup until it is evenly smooth. Ladle into soup bowls and garnish with nutmeg, salt and pepper. Serve with Ezekiel bread and High-Fiber Bean Dip (page125). Delicious and perfect for a fall family get-together.

TIP

Squash becomes plentiful during the fall. Try other squash varieties to make this soup.

NUTRITIONAL VALUE PER SERVING:

Calories: 199 | Calories from Fat: 156 | Protein: 2g | Carbs: 10g
Dietary Fiber: 1g | Sugars: 2g | Fat: 17g | Sodium: 116mg

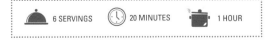

6 SERVINGS   20 MINUTES   1 HOUR

JAPANESE TOFU SOUP

All soups are delicious and this one is no exception. Beautiful vegetables swim in a golden broth, making a healthy and colorful soup.

INGREDIENTS:

6 green onions

6 cups / 1.4 L low-sodium or homemade chicken broth or vegetable broth (gluten free if necessary)

10 shiitake mushrooms, stemmed and sliced

1½ inch piece fresh ginger, minced

4 cups / 960 ml baby spinach leaves

¼ cup / 60 ml rice miso

1 cup / 240 ml edamame, shelled

12 ounces / 336 g firm tofu, cut into ½" cubes

TIP

To make this strictly vegetarian, use low-sodium vegetable stock for the soup base.

PREPARATION:

1 Peel and chop two of the six green onions into quarter-inch pieces. Set aside.

2 In a medium saucepan, place broth, mushrooms, ginger and the remaining four green onions. Cover and bring to a boil. Allow to cook for about 8 minutes. Using a fine mesh sieve, strain the resulting liquid into another pot. Pick the cooked mushrooms out of the sieve and add these to the strained liquid. Discard the rest. Add the tofu, spinach and edamame to the strained liquid and simmer until the vegetables turn bright green.

3 In a medium bowl, whip the miso with one cup of the broth. Set aside.

4 Remove the soup from the heat and blend the whipped miso into the liquid. Ladle into bowls and garnish with the green onions.

NUTRITIONAL VALUE PER SERVING:
Calories: 380 | Calories from Fat: 104 | Protein: 32g | Carbs: 48g
Dietary Fiber: 15g | Sugars: 4g | Fat: 11g | Sodium: 1857mg

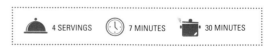

4 SERVINGS · 7 MINUTES · 30 MINUTES

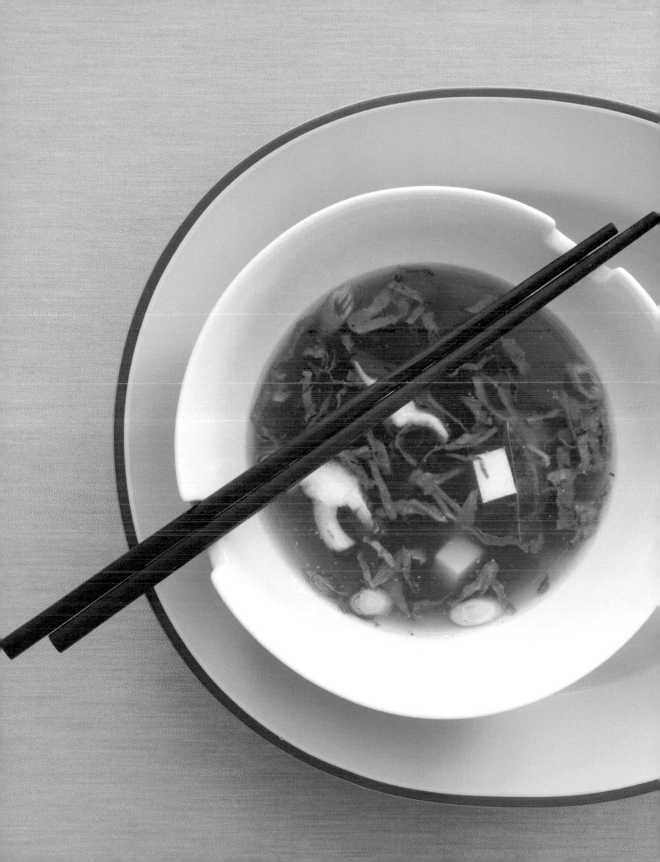

TIP

Sprouts contain abundant nutrients— use them in soups, salads and wraps.

SPROUTING INSTRUCTIONS

TO SOAK NUTS, SEEDS AND GRAINS

1 Fill a glass jar or container half way with nuts, seeds or grains.

2 Fill the container with water.

3 Each nut, seed or grain has a different soak time. Barley requires two days of soaking before it can be used in this recipe. Rinse every 12 hours.

4 After the correct soaking time has passed, dump out the water in the jar and rinse the contents several times. Drain. The soaked barley can be stored in the refrigerator for a few days, otherwise you can now begin the sprouting process.

TO SPROUT NUTS, SEEDS, AND GRAINS

1 Place the soaked grain, nut or seed in a glass jar. In this case we are using barley. Place a piece of muslin or cheesecloth over the jar and secure it with an elastic band or lid **(see note)**. This keeps dust out.

SPROUTED KALE AND BARLEY SOUP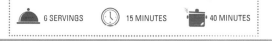

This recipe is a delicious "vehicle" for getting more highly nutritious kale into your diet. Most of us haven't got a clue what to do with these deep green leaves, but once you do know they will quickly become a favorite. Soaking and sprouting the barley (or any grain, nut or seed) enhances the nutritional value greatly, so although it is a bit time consuming it is well worth the effort. Get your kids involved with the sprouting and growing process.

INGREDIENTS:

6 cups / 1.4 L water

4 cups / 960 ml kale, finely shredded

1 large yellow onion, peeled and chopped

3 celery stalks, trimmed and chopped

1 large carrot, chopped into penny slices

1 Tbsp / 15 ml extra virgin olive oil

¾ cup / 180 ml barley, sprouted
   (see Sprouting Instructions)

¼ cup / 60 ml fresh cilantro, finely chopped

2 tsp / 10 ml dried crumbled oregano

2 tsp / 10 ml dried crumbled basil

1 tsp / 5 ml miso

PREPARATION:

1 Bring 6 cups / 1.4 L water to a boil in a medium saucepan. Once the water has boiled, turn off the heat and cover. Let it cool down until simply warm.

2 In a medium skillet, sauté onion, celery and carrot in 1 Tbsp / 15 ml olive oil until onion becomes soft.

3 Add cooked onion mixture and kale to pan along with all other ingredients except the miso. Let the mixture sit for 20 minutes. Take one cup of liquid from the pan and mix it with the miso. Return the resultant liquid to the saucepan and mix again. Remove half the soup, purée, then return to saucepan and mix with non-puréed soup. Serve immediately.

4 If you must reheat this soup, do so on low heat. Boiling it will destroy the valuable nutrients.

NUTRITIONAL VALUE PER SERVING:

Calories: 143 | Calories from Fat: 30 | Protein: 5g | Carbs: 25g
Dietary Fiber: 6g | Sugars: 2g | Fat: 3g | Sodium: 84mg

6 SERVINGS   15 MINUTES   40 MINUTES

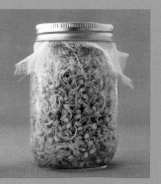

2 Put this jar in a dark place for 24 hours. Then find a sunny place and set in this area.

3 As the sprouts grow, you will have to refresh the water every four hours.

That means you need to rinse the old water out and place fresh water back in the jar. You can do this through the cheesecloth you have secured over the top of the jar. Simply dump out the old water. Fill the jar with fresh water and turn it upside down. Do this twice and then fill with fresh water for the next growing stage.

NOTE: If securing cheesecloth with a lid, do not include lid insert.

ALL-AROUND-THE-WORLD SOUP

There are so many vital ingredients in this soup you will surely eat your way to health. It seems there is a vegetable from every corner of the world alive in this soup.

INGREDIENTS:

8 purple potatoes, scrubbed and chopped

3 sweet potatoes, scrubbed and chopped

3 yams, scrubbed and chopped

8 fat carrots, scrubbed, peeled and chopped

4 stalks celery, trimmed and chopped

½ red cabbage, trimmed and shredded

½ green cabbage, trimmed and shredded

8 Brussels sprouts, trimmed and chopped

½ head cauliflower, trimmed and chopped

4 cups / 960 ml fresh spinach, trimmed and chopped

Handful shiitake mushrooms, cleaned and chopped

4 cloves garlic, peeled and chopped

1½ cups / 360 ml soaked white kidney beans

4 bay leaves

8 – 10 cups / about 2 L water

1 bunch fresh cilantro, trimmed and chopped

Sea salt and black pepper

PREPARATION:

1 Bring water to a full boil in a large stock pot. Add all ingredients except cilantro. Reduce heat, cover and allow to simmer slowly for 3 hours. You can do this in a slow cooker, too.

2 Add cilantro in the last thirty minutes of cooking. If you want a chunky soup, eat as it is. If you want more purée in the soup then remove about 2 cups / 480 ml of the soup mixture, including vegetables, and purée. Return it to the soup pot and mix.

TIP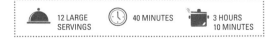

Did I forget a vegetable? Throw in one of your favorites to make it your own.

NUTRITIONAL VALUE PER SERVING:

Calories: 224 | Calories from Fat: 6 | Protein: 7g | Carbs: 47g
Dietary Fiber: 10g | Sugars: 8g | Fat: 0.6g | Sodium: 189mg

12 LARGE SERVINGS   40 MINUTES   3 HOURS 10 MINUTES

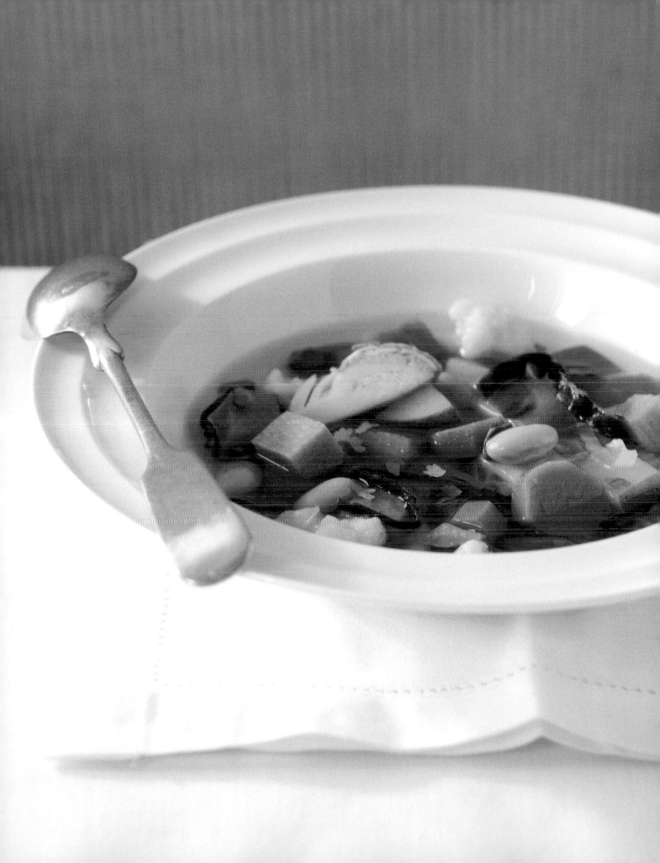

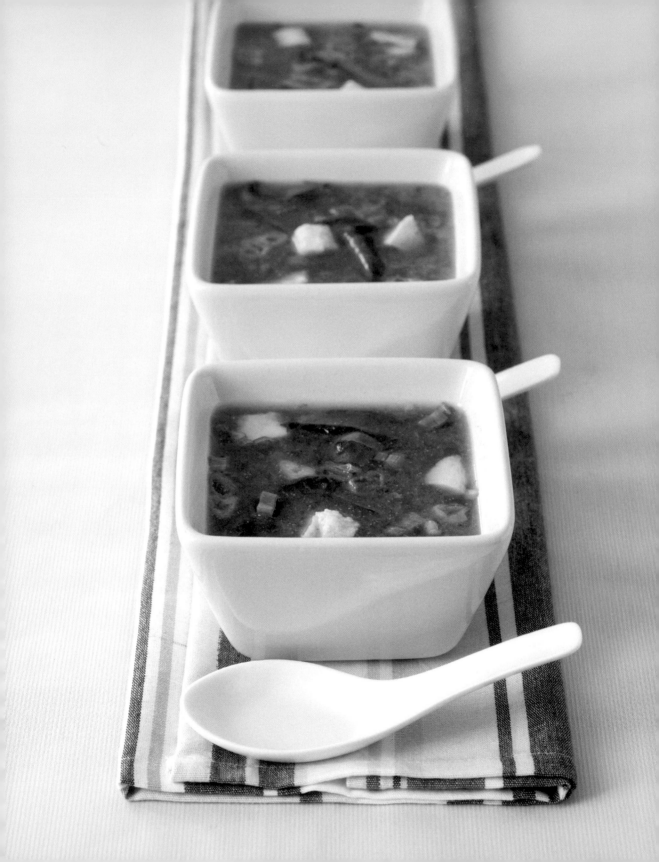

MISO, CHICKEN AND GREEN ONION SOUP

Miso is fermented soy, hailing primarily from Japan. It has traveled all the way to your kitchen in order to provide you with an immensity of protein, vitamins and minerals. Offering miso paired with portobello mushrooms, the flavor of this soup just may entice you to sojourn in miso's home country!

INGREDIENTS:

2 cups / 480 ml cooked lean chicken breast, cut in ½" cubes

OR

cooked lean turkey breast, cut in ½" cubes

OR

firm tofu, cut in ½" cubes

1 cooking onion, peeled and chopped

5 green onions, trimmed and chopped

1½ cups / 360 ml portobello mushrooms, peeled and sliced

8 cups / 1.9 L low-sodium chicken or vegetable broth

2 Tbsp / 30 ml miso

Sea salt and black pepper

PREPARATION:

1 In a large skillet, sauté onions until just golden. Add sliced mushrooms and cook 5 minutes more. Use ½ cup / 120 ml of cooking liquid – vegetable or chicken broth – to continue cooking onions and mushrooms. Let liquid almost disappear.

2 In small bowl whisk miso paste with 2 Tbsp / 30 ml broth. Pour into skillet and cook. Season with sea salt and pepper. Add remaining broth and cooked chicken, turkey breast or tofu. Cook for 30 minutes more over low heat.

VEGETARIAN OPTION: Make it vegan by substituting firm tofu for the chicken.

TIP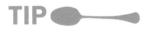

Miso improves both the nutritional value and flavor of this soup. Try it in other foods as well.

NUTRITIONAL VALUE PER SERVING:

Calories: 136 | Calories from Fat: 17 | Protein: 23g | Carbs: 6g
Dietary Fiber: 1g | Sugars: 3g | Fat: 1g | Sodium: 1383mg

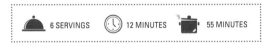

6 SERVINGS   12 MINUTES   55 MINUTES

THE SECRET TO A
BETTER BODY

Eighty percent of the answer to achieving a more beautiful physique lies on your plate. Everything you put in your mouth shapes what you look like. If you eat loads of sugary doughnuts and greasy fried foods you will probably look a lot like that – doughy and heavy. If you eat fresh fruits and vegetables along with other wholesome foods you will look healthy, fresh and vibrant. The choice is yours, but why wouldn't you want to look and feel your best?

"Everything you put in your mouth shapes what you look like."

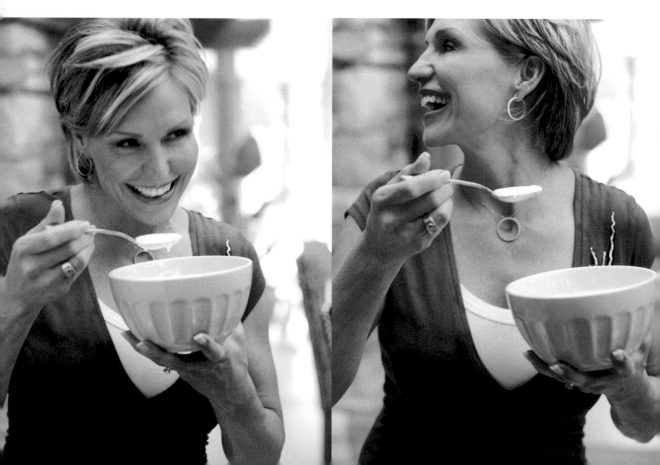

It is possible that you are among the many who believe that the more you work out the fitter and healthier you will be? This is not entirely true. I know a man who trains every day, whether it is playing hockey, lifting weights, running or dragon boating. But at the end of a workout he sits on the couch clutching a bag of potato chips, the biggest he can find, and munches until the bag is empty. If there are no chips in the cupboard, then he eats ice cream, the whole container. He is definitely not in shape, although at first glance you might think so. He is at least 25 pounds overweight and has a flabby belly to prove it. I can't imagine his blood work would reveal ideal numbers either. How "in shape" are you?

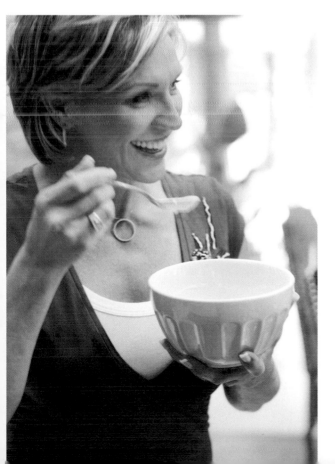

Don't be misled by the same notion that working out offsets the need to eat properly. It definitely does not. The only way to accomplish the physique of your dreams along with excellent health is to put nutritious clean foods on your plate, eat them regularly and follow the Clean-Eating principles. That's how it's done.

Some of us just don't know what to eat because we have relied on manufacturers and grocery stores to "tell" us what food is. We believe that when we enter the grocery store we will find wholesome foods to sustain us and our loved ones. Perhaps we are a little too trusting. Perhaps food companies have taken advantage of that trust. Not everything you find on the shelves is actually nourishing food. The overwhelming variety of packaged, processed foods should prove that. Have a close look at their labels. There are too many decidedly Not-Clean ingredients in these Not-Clean "foods."

Rely only on wholesome foods to form the backbone of your Clean-Eating meals. It won't take long to see results, the results you have been chasing for a long time. Remember it takes 80 percent clean nutrition to build your ideal physique. Still another 10 percent devoted to resistance training and cardiovascular exercise will give your body striking definition. The remaining 10 percent is given to you courtesy of your parents. Your genetic package is virtually unchangeable, so try to enjoy your dimples and freckles. Thanks Mom and Dad!

SQUASH AND FLAX SOUP

It's hard to believe you would include flax seed or sprouts in this delightfully colored soup, but they are subtle additions that add powerful nutritional value. I urge you to try them. The flax and sunflower seeds get a good soaking before they are used, to make them soft.

INGREDIENTS:

2 Tbsp / 30 ml flax seed, soaked

¼ cup / 60 ml sunflower seeds, soaked

1½ Tbsp / 23 ml extra virgin olive oil

1 medium yellow onion, chopped

2 cloves garlic, passed through a garlic press

2 ribs celery, trimmed and chopped

2 large carrots, peeled and chopped

1 medium butternut squash, cooked

4 cups / 960 ml low-sodium vegetable stock or
    water (gluten-free if necessary)

1 cup / 240 ml sprouts – use your favorite sprouts

2 Tbsp / 30 ml organic apple cider vinegar

1 tsp / 5 ml dried crumbled basil

1 tsp / 5 ml dried crumbled oregano

Sea salt and fresh ground black pepper

PREPARATION:

1 Soak the flax seed in one bowl of water and the sunflower seeds in another bowl of water, for 1 hour.

2 Heat olive oil in a medium skillet over medium high heat. Sauté onions, garlic, celery and carrots until onions become soft.

3 Scoop flesh out of cooked squash into a large saucepan or Dutch oven. Add cooked onion, celery, garlic and carrot. Add 4 cups / 960 ml liquid and set over medium heat. Bring to a gentle boil. Purée these ingredients right in the pan with a hand blender. Blend until smooth. Remove from heat. Add all remaining ingredients including the soaked seeds, and purée until smooth. Add sea salt and fresh ground black pepper. If the soup is still too thick add some water and purée again. Serve immediately.

NOTE: Do not heat this soup over high heat, as doing so would destroy the valuable and volatile nutrients in the flax and sunflower seeds. If you need to reheat it, do so over a gentle, slow heat.

TIP

Everyone knows how much I love flax seed. Putting it in this soup helps you increase your daily intake.

NUTRITIONAL VALUE PER SERVING:

Calories: 156 | Calories from Fat: 80 | Protein: 3g | Carbs: 16g
Dietary Fiber: 4g | Sugars: 7g | Fat: 85g | Sodium: 434mg

6 SERVINGS   1 HOUR 25 MINUTES   30 MINUTES

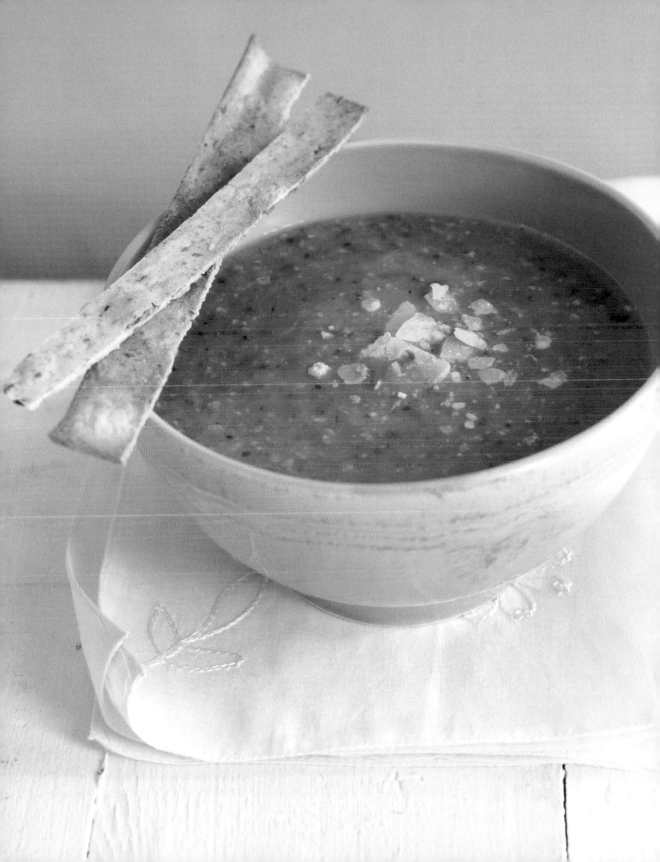

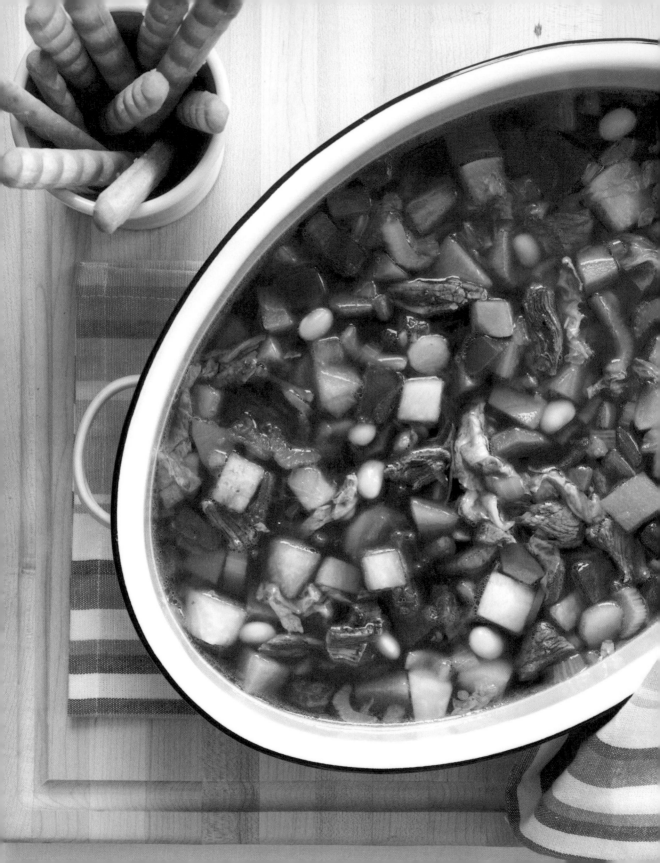

COUNTRY STYLE BEEF SOUP

The French version of this soup, called pot au feu, literally means "pot over the fire." We can dispense with the fire, but my adaptation of this hearty soup is perfect for Clean Eating. The best idea is to prepare the stock ahead of time and refrigerate it so you can "de-fat" the soup by skimming off the congealed fat.

INGREDIENTS:

2 pounds / 908g beef soup bones, such as short ribs. No fat!

8 cups / 1.9 L water

2 cups / 480 ml low-sodium beef stock (gluten free if necessary)

2 sprigs thyme

3 bay leaves

2 Tbsp / 30 ml extra virgin olive oil

2 onions, peeled and chopped

4 ribs celery, trimmed and chopped

2 cloves garlic, passed through a garlic press

2 cups / 480 ml chopped fresh tomatoes

2 Tbsp / 30 ml tomato paste

2 large carrots, peeled and chopped

2 sweet potatoes, peeled and chopped

2 parsnips, peeled and chopped

2 cups / 480 ml shredded nappa cabbage

2 cups / 480 ml turnip, peeled and chopped

1 cup / 240 ml frozen edamame

1 cup / 240 ml butternut squash, peeled and cubed

PREPARATION:

1 In a large stock pot, place ribs, water, beef stock, thyme and bay leaves. Bring to a boil and reduce heat. Cover and simmer for 1 to 2 hours.

2 Remove the pan from heat and let cool. Strain the stock into a large bowl through a sieve. Take any meat from the bones, shred it and return it to the soup. Discard the bones and other cooked ingredients.

3 In a Dutch oven heat olive oil over medium heat. Add onions, celery and garlic. Sauté until onions become soft and translucent – about 8 minutes. Add cooked beef and broth, tomatoes, tomato paste, carrots and other vegetables. Bring mixture to a boil. Reduce heat and let simmer, covered, for 30 minutes. Serve hot.

TIP

If your soup bones are substantial, you will derive a load of nutrition from the marrow. Don't throw it out. Blend it into your soup.

NUTRITIONAL VALUE PER SERVING:

Calories: 140 | Calories from Fat: 33 | Protein: 4g | Carbs: 22g
Dietary Fiber: 5g | Sugars: 2g | Fat: 3g | Sodium: 339mg

10 SERVINGS   35 MINUTES   2 HOURS 50 MINUTES

SPLIT PEA AND ROOT VEGETABLE SOUP

This hearty soup will warm you after a day spent skiing or skating. If you make it ahead of time the flavors develop beautifully and all you have to do is heat it when you come in the door. There are so many vegetables in this soup it is a nutritional wonder. Get ready to enjoy!

INGREDIENTS:

6 Tbsp / 90 ml best-quality olive oil or rice bran oil

3 medium carrots, peeled and chopped

2 large parsnips, peeled and chopped

2 medium leeks, white and lightest green parts only, well washed and chopped

½ cup / 120 ml fresh parsley or cilantro, chopped

2½ tsp / 12 ml dried thyme

2 tsp / 10 ml dried marjoram

3 bay leaves

11 cups / 2.6 L low-fat, low-sodium chicken stock (gluten free if necessary)

3 cups / 720 ml dried split peas

1½ lbs / 680 g roasted turkey breast, bone in

PREPARATION:

1 Heat olive oil in heavy stockpot over low heat. Add root vegetables and dried herbs. Cover and cook until all vegetables are soft, about 20 minutes.

2 Add all the chicken stock, peas and roasted meat. Bring to a simmer, cover partially and cook until peas are tender and the soup begins to thicken a little. This takes about 45 minutes.

3 Remove turkey and cut meat into one-inch cubes. Discard the bone. Remove bay leaves. Return meat to soup and serve.

TIP

I always have this soup ready to go after a day spent watching the Christmas parade, or going out with the family to find the perfect festive tree.

NUTRITIONAL VALUE PER SERVING:
Calories: 522 | Calories from Fat: 103 | Protein: 42g | Carbs: 62g
Dietary Fiber: 0.70g | Sugars: 6g | Fat: 11g | Sodium: 784mg

8 SERVINGS   18 MINUTES   65 MINUTES

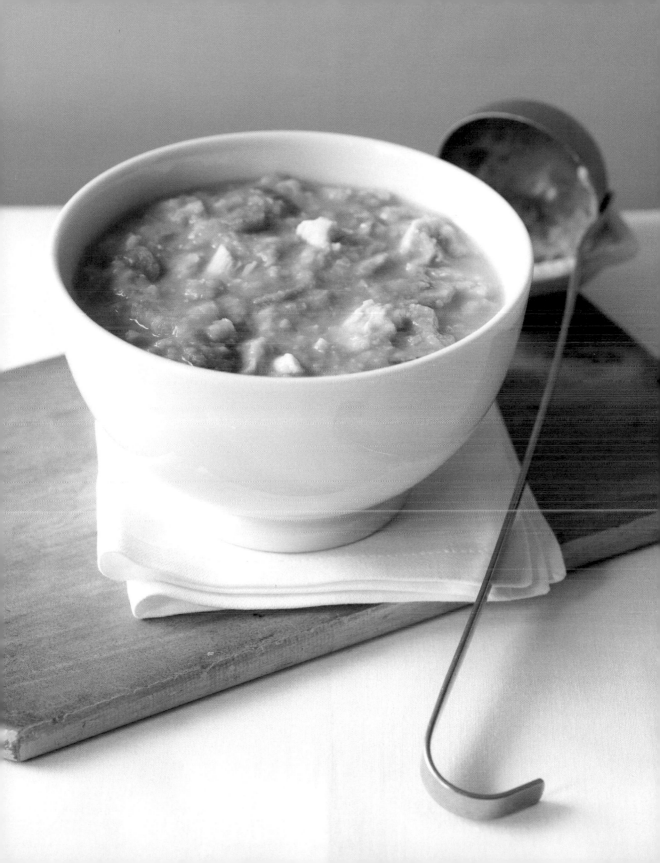

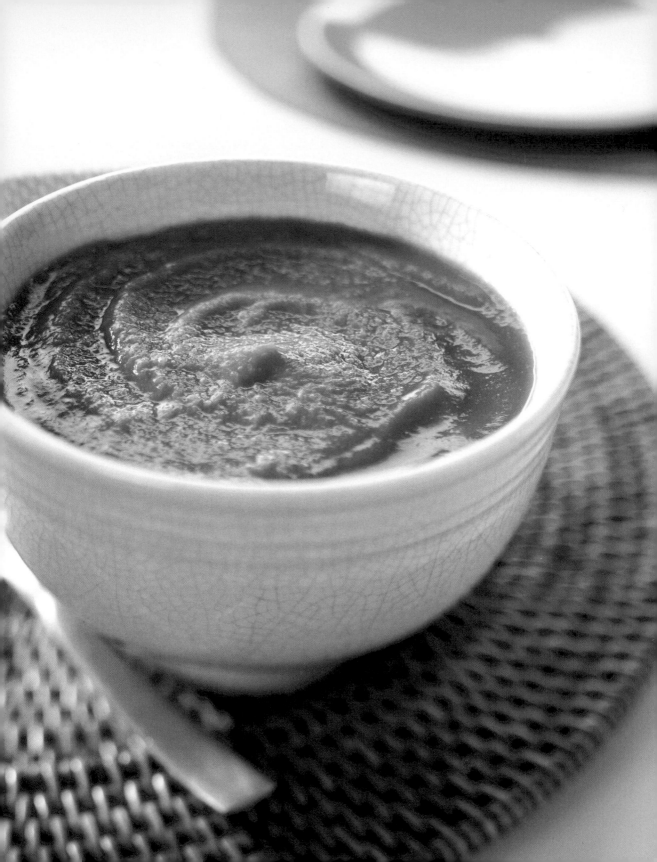

CREAMY PUMPKIN TOFU SOUP

Who would think that the combination of pumpkin and tofu could taste so good? This is a delicious and beautifully colored soup that would satisfy any hungry tummy. Pumpkin is loaded with nutrients and antioxidants, while tofu comes with its own set of nourishing qualities. These are both superfoods.

INGREDIENTS:

2 Tbsp / 30 ml best-quality olive oil

1 cup / 240 ml leeks, whites only, thinly sliced and well washed

4 cups / 1.4 L low-sodium chicken or vegetable broth (gluten free if necessary)

1 cup / 240 ml fresh pumpkin, peeled and seeded, cut into 1" cubes

2 cloves garlic, minced or passed through a garlic press

1 tsp / 5 ml freshly grated ginger root *(optional)*

½ cup / 125 ml silken tofu

Sea salt to taste

PREPARATION:

1 Add oil to a small frying pan and sauté leeks until softened. In a large saucepan add the broth, leeks and pumpkin. Bring to a boil. Reduce heat and cook for 30 minutes.

2 Add garlic, ginger (if using) and tofu. Simmer for another 15 minutes. Using a hand blender, purée soup mixture until uniformly smooth. Add sea salt as desired. Serve hot!

TIP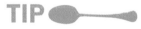

If you find the soup too thick, thin it with a little broth. You can adjust the consistency any way you like.

NUTRITIONAL VALUE PER SERVING:

Calories: 191 | Calories from Fat: 129 | Protein: 4g | Carbs: 11g
Dietary Fiber: 1g | Sugars: 2g | Fat: 14g | Sodium: 927mg

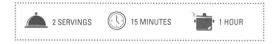

2 SERVINGS   15 MINUTES   1 HOUR

MAUI BLACK BEAN SOUP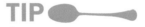

The first time I tasted this marvelous soup I was in Maui for my recent wedding. It was a glorious evening and I was celebrating with my family at an outdoor restaurant. This soup became everyone's favorite in a hurry. I got the recipe and played with it to make it Clean-Eating friendly. Hope you like it too!

INGREDIENTS:

2 Tbsp / 30 ml extra virgin olive oil

2 ribs celery, trimmed and coarsely chopped

1 fat carrot, peeled and chopped

1 small purple onion, peeled and chopped

1 red pepper, seeded and de-veined, chopped

1 green pepper, seeded and de-veined, chopped

2 cloves garlic passed through a garlic press

1 tsp / 5 ml dried cumin

1 tsp / 5 ml dried oregano

1 tsp / 5 ml dried basil

1 tsp / 5 ml chili powder

4 cups / 960 ml low-sodium chicken or vegetable
stock (gluten free if necessary)

2 x 15 oz / 420 ml cans black beans

1 x 15 oz / 420 ml canned diced tomatoes

1 cup / 240 ml fresh corn kernels

Sea salt and fresh ground black pepper

PREPARATION:

1 In large skillet, heat olive oil over medium heat. Add celery, carrot, onion and bell peppers. Sauté until onion becomes translucent, about 8 minutes. Add garlic and spices. Cook another 2 minutes.

2 Add stock or cooking liquid of your choice, beans and tomatoes. Bring mixture to a boil and then reduce heat. Cover and let simmer for about 20 minutes. Using a hand-held blender, purée soup to desired consistency. Add corn and let simmer for 5 minutes. Season with salt and pepper. Serve hot.

TIP

When puréeing the soup, allow some of the ingredients to remain coarse. I prefer it slightly coarse to completely puréed.

NUTRITIONAL VALUE PER SERVING:

Calories: 178 | Calories from Fat: 38 | Protein: 9g | Carbs: 26g
Dietary Fiber: 8g | Sugars: 6g | Fat: 4g | Sodium: 597mg

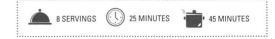

8 SERVINGS   25 MINUTES   45 MINUTES

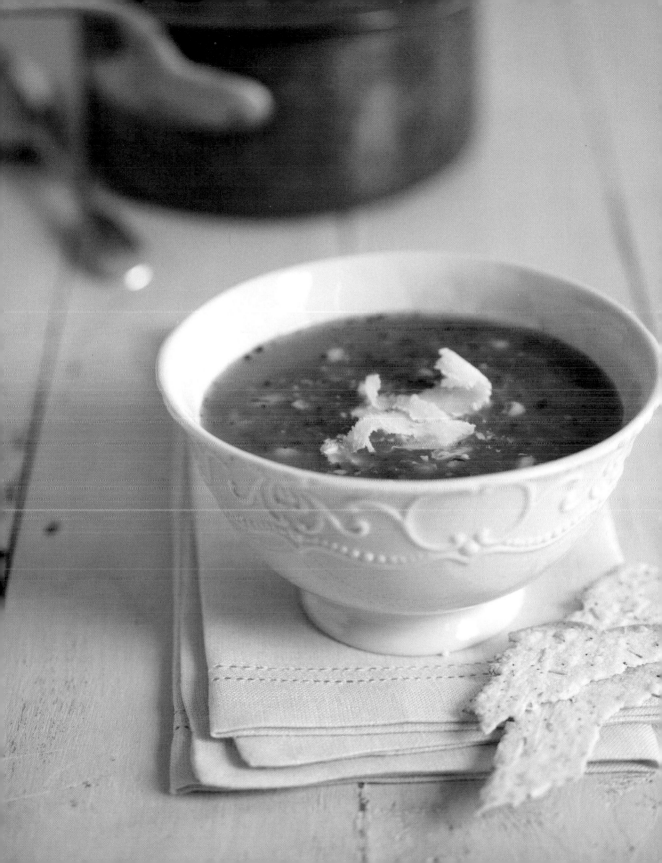

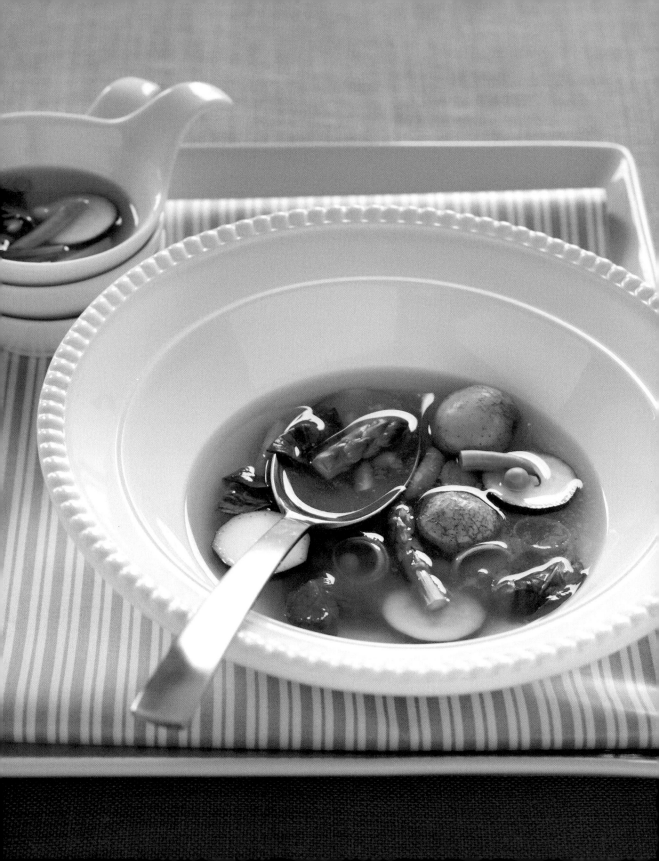

SPRING IN A BOWL

Homemade soup is such a restorative meal. Can there be anything better than a nourishing soup? When it is loaded with delightfully colored fresh vegetables in every shade of green the goodness of spring just begs to be eaten!

INGREDIENTS FOR BROTH:

2 medium onions, peeled and chopped

1 fat carrot, peeled and chopped

2 ribs celery, trimmed and chopped

1 leek, well washed and trimmed, white parts only, chopped

1 bulb fennel, trimmed and chopped

2 parsnips, peeled and chopped

4 cloves garlic, flattened with a knife but not chopped

2 Tbsp / 30 ml extra virgin olive oil

Sea salt

8 cups / 1.9 L water or low-sodium chicken or vegetable stock (gluten free if necessary)

PREPARATION FOR BROTH:

1 Place all ingredients except liquid in large stock pot or Dutch oven. Cover and cook over low heat for 10 minutes. Let vegetables become soft. Add 8 cups / 1.9 L liquid. Bring mixture to a boil and reduce to low again. Simmer for 20 minutes. Remove from heat and strain broth through a fine-mesh sieve into a large container.

NUTRITIONAL VALUE PER SERVING:

Calories: 302 | Calories from Fat: 62 | Protein: 12g | Carbs: 50g
Dietary Fiber: 8g | Sugars: 9g | Fat: 6g | Sodium: 392mg

8 SERVINGS   45 MINUTES   45 MINUTES

INGREDIENTS FOR SOUP:

12 baby potatoes (tiniest possible)

2 large leeks, whites only, well washed and chopped into rings

10 stalks asparagus (not too skinny), trimmed and cut into 1" pieces

Handful green beans, trimmed and cut into 1" pieces

2 – 3 cups (about 600 ml) baby spinach leaves

2 small zucchini, cut into rounds

Green onions, chopped for garnish

1 cup / 240 ml fresh green peas

Parsley and thyme, 1 Tbsp each, fresh

Sea salt and fresh ground black pepper

PREPARATION FOR SOUP:

1 Bring the prepared broth to a simmer in a large stock pot. Add the potatoes and leeks and simmer for a few minutes. Add all other vegetables and let simmer 10 more minutes. Add sea salt, black pepper and herbs. Ladle into soup bowls and garnish with chopped green onion.

TIP

Many spring vegetables require very little cooking time. Don't allow them to overcook in the soup. This is one soup I don't make too much of since it soon becomes mushy.

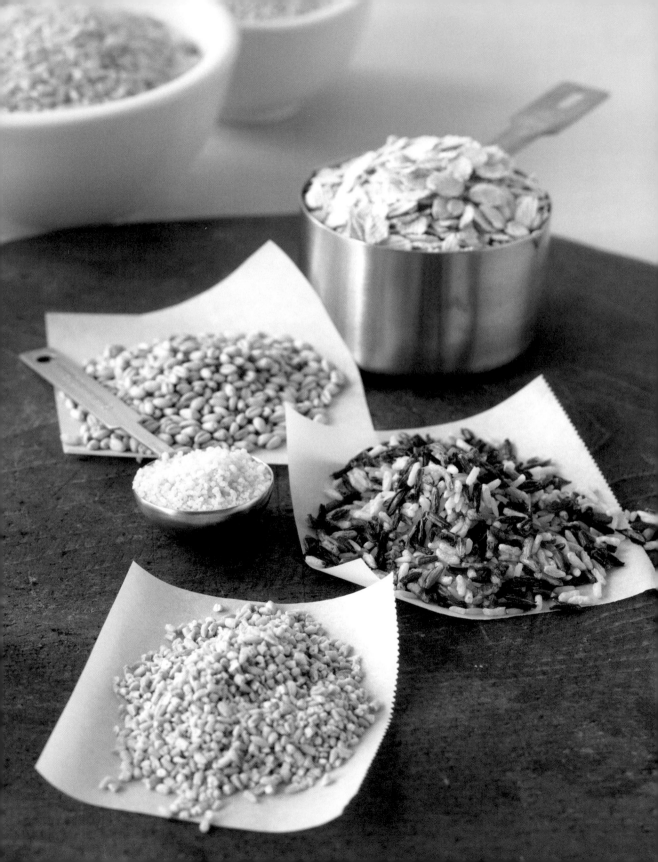

Grains

In some countries, grains sustain an entire nation. The Maya, for example, based much of their civilization on the superfood quinoa – in their language quinoa means "mother grain." Asians have long subsisted on rice as a staple grain. More and more balanced diets are embracing the powerful nutrition of whole grains, valued for an array of complex carbohydrates, protein, vitamins and antioxidant power. Today we enjoy wheat berries, rye, barley and oats like never before.

Enjoy whole grains either sweet or savory, but do make them part of your Clean-Eating nutrition today!

QUINOA WITH SUNDRIED TOMATOES

Quinoa is one of my favorite grains. It is a superfood loaded with nutrients. Quinoa is not really a cereal grain but the small spherical fruit of an herb plant. Quinoa is rapidly gaining popularity on the North American dinner table. That's probably because it is so nourishing and tasty. I urge you to try it. It can be cooked as a hot cereal or as a dinner side dish. Eat it cold for lunch or as a salad.

INGREDIENTS:

1 tsp / 5 ml best-quality olive oil

8 sundried tomatoes, not packed in oil

2 minced shallots

1 clove garlic minced

2 cups / 480 ml low-sodium, low-fat chicken or
   vegetable stock (gluten free if necessary)

1 cup / 240 ml dry quinoa grains

Pinch cayenne pepper

2 Tbsp / 30 ml fresh chopped cilantro

1 tsp / 5 ml sea salt

Fresh ground black pepper

PREPARATION:

1 Place quinoa in fine mesh sieve. Rinse well under lukewarm running water for about 1 minute. Set aside.

2 Heat oil in large saucepan. Add tomatoes, shallots and garlic and sauté for 3 to 5 minutes or until shallots are softened. Add stock or water and bring to a boil. Stir in quinoa grains and cayenne pepper. Return to a boil. Reduce heat and simmer for 30 minutes or until liquid is absorbed. Let stand for 5 minutes. Fluff with fork to separate grains. Stir in seasonings.

TIP

You must remember to rinse quinoa grains well before cooking to remove the bitter saponin covering. Rinse until the water runs clear.

NUTRITIONAL VALUE PER SERVING:

Calories: 128 | Calories from Fat: 23 | Protein: 5g | Carbs: 23g
Dietary Fiber: 2g | Sugars: 1g | Fat: 3g | Sodium: 211mg

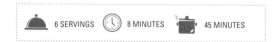

6 SERVINGS   8 MINUTES   45 MINUTES

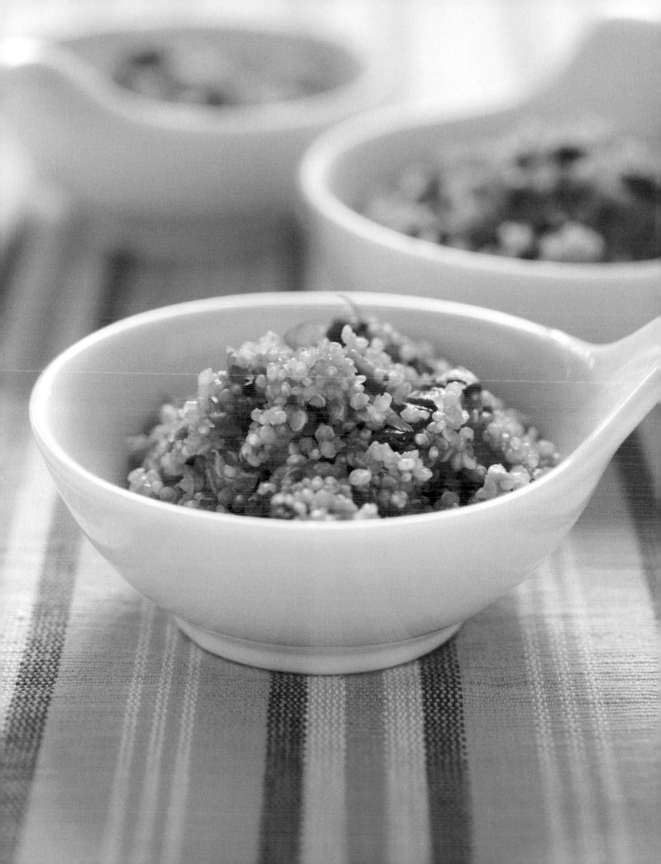

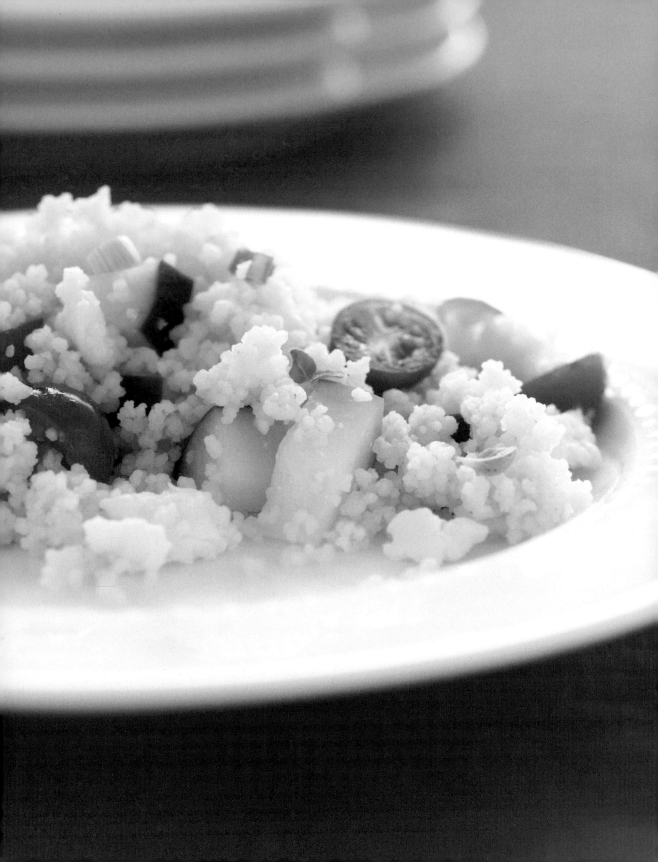

COUSCOUS SALAD GREEK STYLE

This recipe is a variation of Greek Salad. I have just added the couscous to up the nutritional quality of the dish. It's a wonderful salad to have on hand during the hot summer months— especially when cucumbers and tomatoes are in season and taste so brilliant.

INGREDIENTS:

1 cup / 240 ml dry whole-wheat couscous

¾ cup / 180 ml low-fat, low-sodium chicken or
    vegetable stock

¾ cup / 180 ml fresh squeezed orange juice

2 Tbsp / 30 ml best-quality olive oil

1 Tbsp / 15 ml lime juice – that's the juice in one lime

½ cup / 120 ml grape tomatoes, cut in half

¼ cup / 60 ml green onions, chopped

1 cup / 240 ml cucumber, chopped and seeded

¼ cup / 60 ml chopped fresh oregano

½ cup / 120 ml goat cheese or feta cheese

Sea salt and black pepper to taste

PREPARATION:

1 Bring stock and orange juice to a boil. Add couscous and stir. Then turn off heat and cover pot tightly. Don't peek. Let stand.

2 Make dressing by combining olive oil and lime juice. Whisk and set aside.

3 Back to the couscous. Remove lid and fluff grains with a fork. Add chopped vegetables and drizzle with dressing. Add oregano and season with sea salt and ground black pepper.

TIP

This salad is ideal for serving poolside. While everyone is getting ready to lounge by the pool, I quickly whip up this salad – it takes no time at all.

NUTRITIONAL VALUE PER SERVING:
Calories: 233 | Calories from Fat: 77 | Protein: 7g | Carbs: 33g
Dietary Fiber: 6g | Sugars: 4g | Fat: 8g | Sodium: 222mg

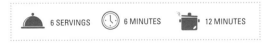

6 SERVINGS   6 MINUTES   12 MINUTES

ORZO PRIMAVERA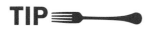

Orzo is a delicious and versatile grain that isn't really a grain at all. Orzo is the Italian word for barley, but cooks know it as pasta in the shape of rice. It is a versatile "grain" often used in soups and salads. It cooks easily and can readily be made in advance. This version adds more healthy complex carbohydrates from fresh vegetables. Using edamame boosts the protein content of the salad. Remember, extras make for a great meal the next day.

INGREDIENTS:

1 cup / 240 ml whole-wheat orzo, dry

1 tsp / 5 ml sea salt

1 cup / 240 ml frozen baby peas and/or edamame, thawed

1 small red pepper, seeded and diced

1 Tbsp / 15 ml chopped fresh dill

1 – 2 Tbsp (about 20 ml) fresh lemon juice

1 tsp / 5 ml best-quality olive oil

Fresh ground black pepper

PREPARATION:

1 Bring a large pot of water to a rolling boil. Stir in orzo and salt. Return to a boil. Cook for 5 to 6 minutes, stirring occasionally to keep orzo from sticking. Grains should be tender yet firm when done.

2 Drain and transfer to a colorful serving bowl. Add all remaining ingredients and mix well. Season with salt and pepper.

TIP

This is one "grain" kids really love. You can convince them to eat just about anything when this pasta grain is mixed into it.

NUTRITIONAL VALUE PER SERVING:

Calories: 207 | Calories from Fat: 37 | Protein: 10g | Carbs: 34g
Dietary Fiber: 3g | Sugars: 1g | Fat: 4g | Sodium: 383mg

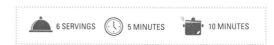 6 SERVINGS 5 MINUTES 10 MINUTES

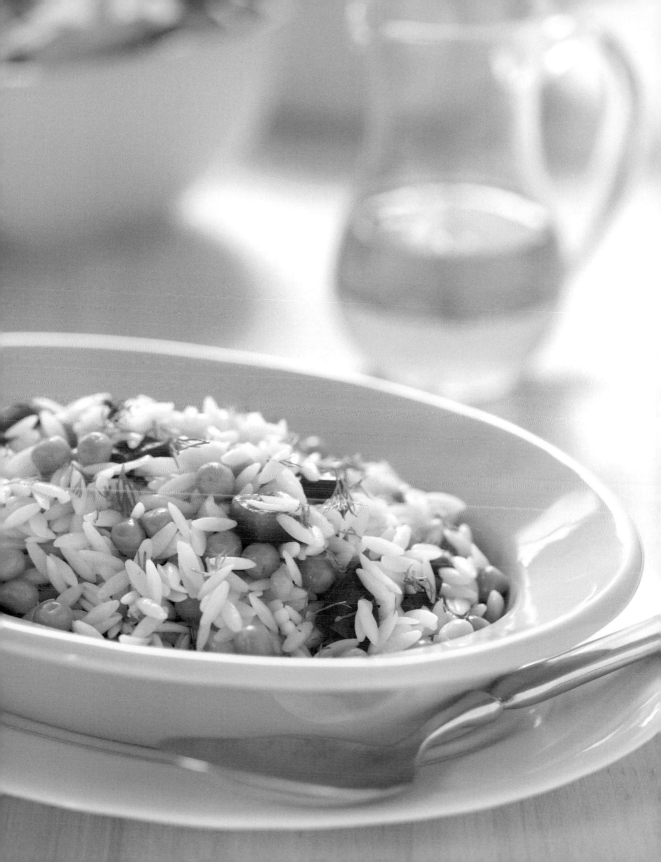

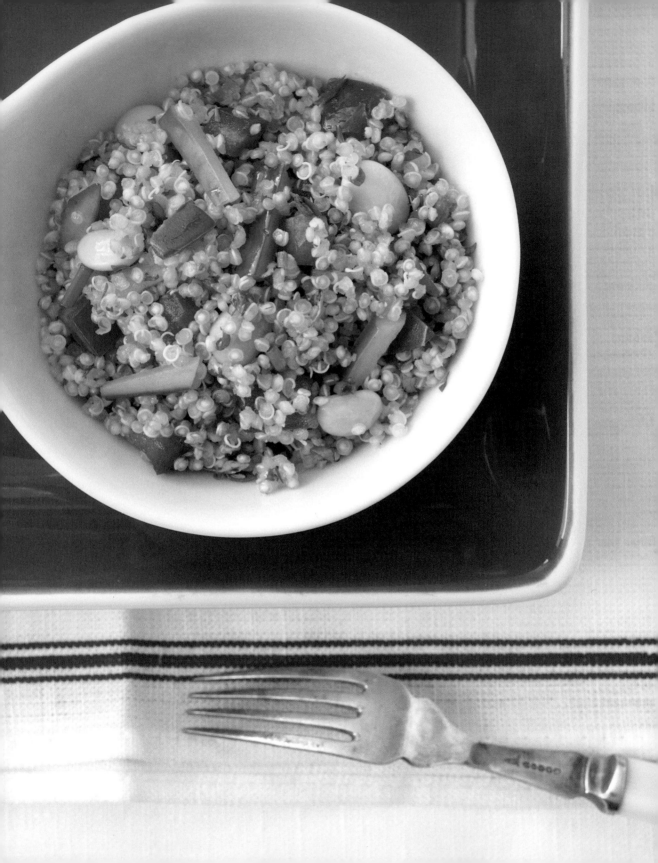

QUINOA TABBOULEH

Tabbouleh is a Mediterranean salad dish made with bulgur and a variety of herbs and chopped vegetables. This version makes use of the super grain quinoa and is a must-try. I make this salad early in the morning on a hot summer day and have it ready to go for dinner or lunch.

INGREDIENTS:

1 cup / 240 ml quinoa, well rinsed and drained

2 cups / 480 ml water

Sea salt

½ cup / 125 ml edamame, frozen

1 fresh tomato, chopped

½ cucumber, unpeeled, chopped

1 Tbsp / 15 ml fresh lime juice

1 Tbsp / 15 ml fresh lemon juice

1 Tbsp / 15 ml low-sodium soy sauce (gluten-free if necessary)

Fresh chives, minced

Fresh parsley, minced

Fresh thyme, minced

PREPARATION:

1 Remember to rinse the quinoa well before using. Combine quinoa with water and salt in a medium saucepan. Bring to a boil and then reduce. Let simmer for 20 minutes.

2 Remove from heat. Place edamame on top of quinoa and let sit for 5 minutes. Fluff with a fork. Put all ingredients in a glass serving bowl and toss. Add herbs, citrus juices and soy sauce and toss again.

TIP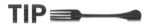

I prefer this salad served at room temperature. This promotes the juices of the fresh tomatoes to slowly infuse into the salad.

NUTRITIONAL VALUE PER SERVING:
Calories: 213 | Calories from Fat: 42 | Protein: 10g | Carbs: 34g
Dietary Fiber: 4g | Sugars: 0.75g | Fat: 4.5g | Sodium: 165mg

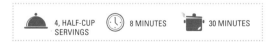

4, HALF-CUP SERVINGS   8 MINUTES   30 MINUTES

ERICA'S COUSCOUS SLAW

This recipe comes from my good friend Erica, a Dutch girl who knows how to Eat Clean! Try this salad and enjoy the little twist that comes from cinnamon.

INGREDIENTS:

1½ cups / 360 ml low-sodium chicken or vegetable stock

1 Tbsp / 15 ml extra virgin olive oil

¼ tsp / 1.25 ml powdered saffron

1½ cups / 360 ml whole-wheat couscous

½ cup / 360 ml diced celery

⅔ cup / 160 ml dried currants (soaked in water)

⅓ cup / 80 ml thinly sliced scallions

⅓ cup / 80 ml pine nuts, lightly toasted

¼ cup / 60 ml fresh minced parsley

¼ cup / 60 ml fresh lemon juice

¼ tsp / 1.25 ml cinnamon

1 - 2 Tbsp (about 20 ml) extra virgin olive oil

PREPARATION:

1 In a medium saucepan, place chicken or vegetable stock, olive oil and saffron. Bring to a boil. Add couscous to the boiling water. Cover and remove from heat. Let stand covered for 4 minutes.

2 Transfer couscous to a decorative serving bowl. Add remaining ingredients and toss until well combined. Serve immediately as a Clean-Eating accompaniment to any lean protein.

TIP

Erica and I met in the gym when my physique transformation was just beginning. That was eight years ago. Today we both Eat Clean and keep our health and figures as tight as our friendship.

NUTRITIONAL VALUE PER SERVING:

Calories: 300 | Calories from Fat: 81 | Protein: 7g | Carbs: 47g
Dietary Fiber: 3g | Sugars: 110g | Fat: 9g | Sodium: 159mg

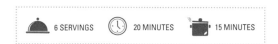

6 SERVINGS   20 MINUTES   15 MINUTES

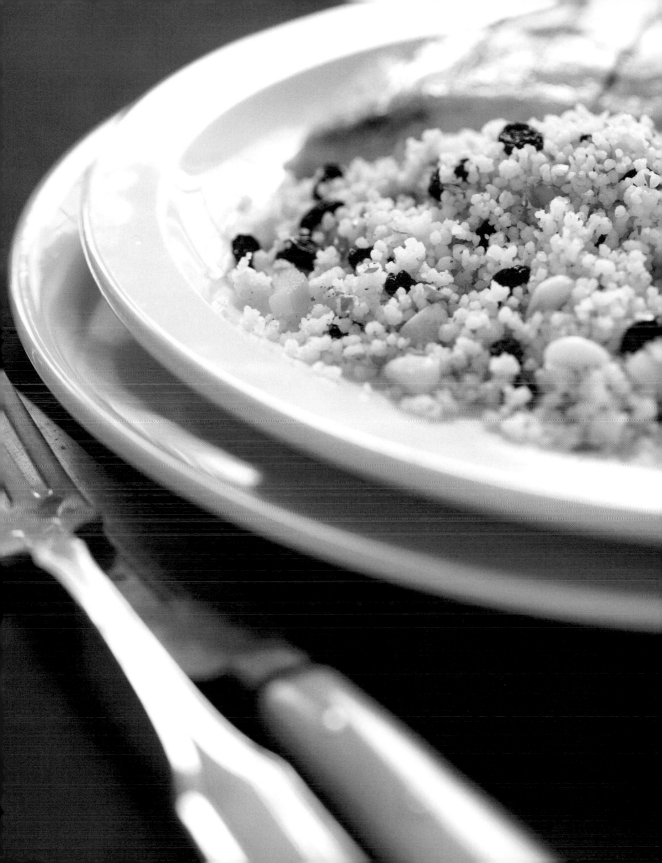

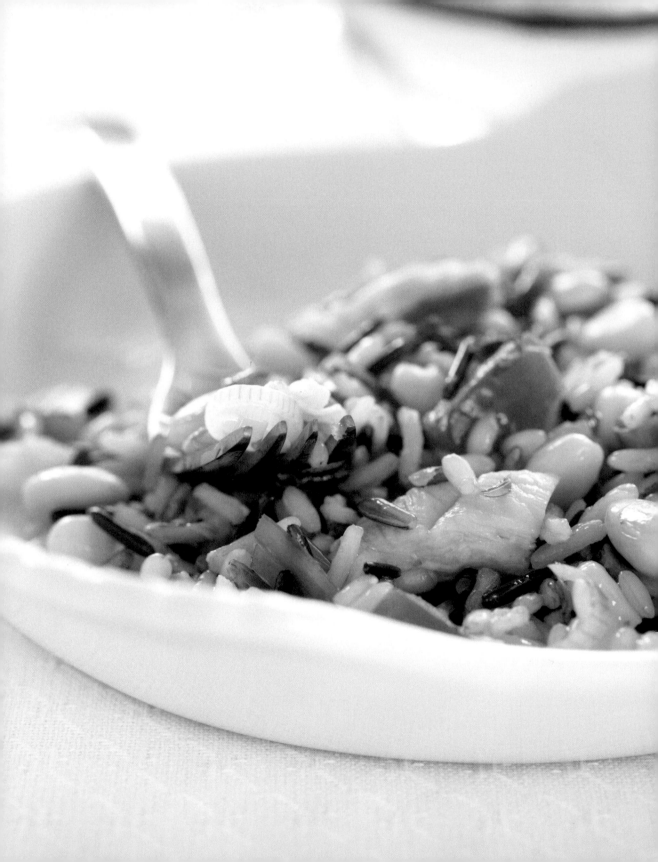

WILD RICE SUMMER SALAD

Enjoy the nutty, slightly chewy texture of this wild-rice-based salad. Loaded with chicken, fresh summer vegetables and wonderful flavor, this is the perfect summertime meal, and superb Clean Eating. The colors look pretty alongside grilled meats and fish.

INGREDIENTS:

1 cup / 240 ml wild rice or wild rice blend

4 Tbsp / 60 ml rice vinegar

1 Tbsp / 15 ml toasted sesame oil

1 clove garlic, passed through a garlic press

1 cup / 240 ml cooked boneless, skinless chicken or
  turkey breast, cubed (optional)

1 medium tomato, seeded and diced

1 bunch scallions, trimmed and chopped

⅓ cup / 80 ml cooked edamame

½ cup / 120 ml fresh corn kernels, cooked

½ tsp / 2.5 ml tarragon, minced

¼ cup / 60 ml fresh basil leaves, chopped

½ tsp / 2.5 ml sea salt

½ tsp / 2.5 ml black pepper

PREPARATION:

1 Cook rice according to package instructions. Set aside to cool.

2 In small bowl, combine rice vinegar, sesame oil and garlic to make the dressing. Whisk.

3 In medium decorative serving bowl, combine cooked rice with remaining ingredients. Toss until vegetables, salt, pepper and herbs are well blended. Pour dressing over salad, mix again and serve.

TIP

I like to make a double batch of the rice the night before. Then I can turn it into this salad in a flash the next day.

NUTRITIONAL VALUE PER SERVING:

Calories: 202 | Calories from Fat: 39 | Protein: 8g | Carbs: 32g
Dietary Fiber: 2g | Sugars: 5g | Fat: 0.1g | Sodium: 467mg

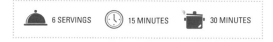 6 SERVINGS   15 MINUTES   30 MINUTES

QUINOA WITH OATS

Quinoa will be your new best friend after you incorporate it into this breakfast treat. And what a great way to wake up your everyday oatmeal. To sweeten don't reach for the sugar bowl; try fresh fruit, unsweetened applesauce or even pumpkin!

INGREDIENTS:

1 cup / 240 ml quinoa, soaked for 2 hours

1 cup / 240 ml steel-cut oats (uncontaminated if necessary)

¼ tsp / 1.25 ml sea salt

3 cups / 720 ml water

1 tsp / 5 ml cinnamon

1 tsp / 5 ml vanilla

¼ cup / 60 ml organic raisins

PREPARATION:

1 In a medium saucepan with a lid, place soaked quinoa, steel-cut oats, sea salt and water. Bring the mixture to a boil and reduce heat. Cover and let simmer for 30 minutes. Remove from heat, stir in cinnamon, vanilla and raisins and let sit for several minutes. Serve hot.

TIP

To sweeten don't reach for the sugar bowl; try fresh fruit, unsweetened applesauce or pumpkin.

NUTRITIONAL VALUE PER SERVING:

Calories: 187 | Calories from Fat: 24 | Protein: 6g | Carbs: 37g
Dietary Fiber: 1g | Sugars: 8g | Fat: 3g | Sodium: 6mg

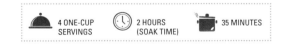

4 ONE-CUP SERVINGS   2 HOURS (SOAK TIME)   35 MINUTES

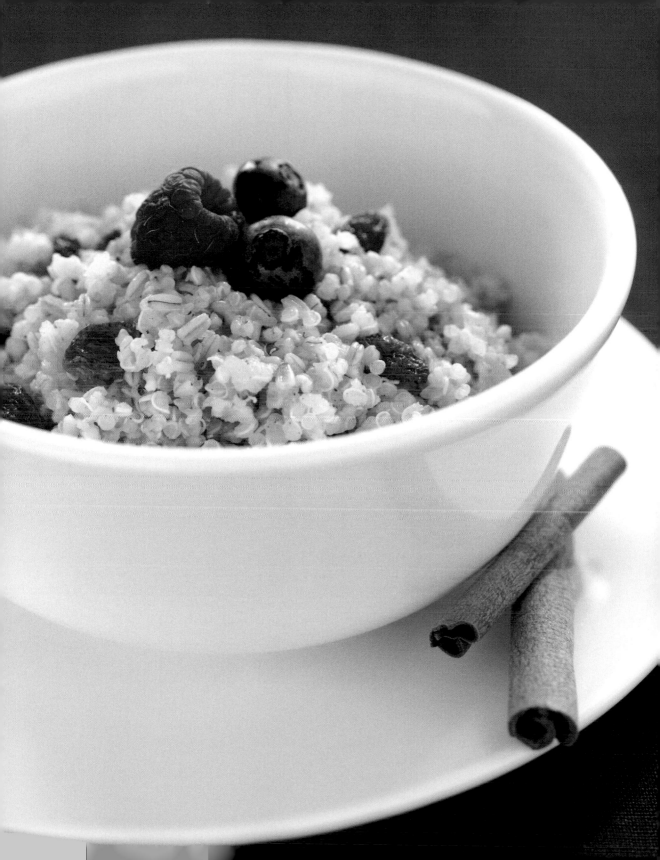

OATS, GROATS, INSTANT AND MINUTE

Confused about oats? You know they are good for you, but which ones are best and what should you be eating? *The Eat-Clean Diet* book recommends eating oats and eating a lot of them! I'd like to clear up the confusion about oats and oatmeal. Consider this your oatmeal primer.

OATS

Oats are a highly nutritious and valued food. Their cholesterol-fighting fiber helps fight heart disease but their slightly nutty flavor makes them easy to eat both sweet and savory.

GROATS

What? Never heard of groats? Groats are minimally processed whole oats with just the outer hull removed. They are quite chewy and need a good soaking before use. Groats also require lengthy cooking times. However don't overlook these. They are loaded with nutrients. Try cooking them in the crock pot.

INSTANT OATS

If you are used to eating the pre-packaged instant oats then you know the drill. These oats are thin because they have been rolled to look that way. Their thinness makes them easier to cook – hence their "instant" nature. Be careful if you are serious about Eating Clean! These oats may be convenient but they are often loaded with unnecessary salts and sugars and in some cases flavorings. These are the chemical calories I often warn you about.

PINHEAD OATS

This is a variety of oatmeal that has been slivered or flaked so the cooking time is hastened. This may be a good choice for baking; however the rolled oat is superior.

ROLLED OATS

Remember the groat? Rolled oats are simply oat groats that have been steamed, rolled and flaked so they cook more quickly. This is the most common type of breakfast oatmeal or muesli. Rolled oats usually take about 3 to 5 minutes to cook. Instant rolled oats cook more quickly.

STEEL-CUT OATS OR SCOTCH OATS

Oprah loves these and so do I! These are oat groats (they keep popping up don't they?) that have been, as the name implies, chopped into smaller pieces. The steel cut oat is the chewiest form of oatmeal and provides the most textural experience. They do well in the slow cooker and even better in your tummy.

OAT FACTS
Did you know?

Oatmeal is not just for breakfast. This grain formerly considered animal feed pops up in alcoholic beverages, cosmetics, soap, as a thickening agent in some canned products, medications for the skin, and animal food.

. . . .

The Queen loves oatmeal! She enjoys Hamlyns of Scotland steel-cut oats for breakfast. This same company hosts the World Porridge Making Championships each year.

. . . .

Black pudding and oatmeal go together. Oatmeal is mixed with sheep's blood, salt and pepper to make this "gotta develop a taste for" bread accompaniment. Who thought of this?

. . . .

Vermonters lead the continent in oatmeal consumption, having a long history of oat farming. The standard dish of steel-cut oats begins the night before by soaking oats in water, salt and maple syrup. In the morning nutmeg, ginger and cinnamon are added. Then the oats are boiled and served hot!!

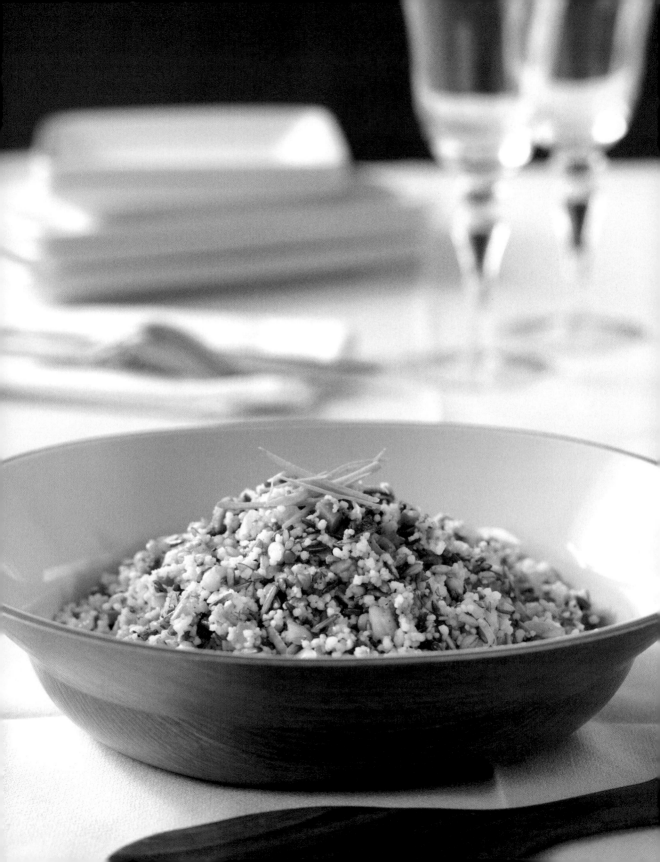

WILD-GRAINS RICE PILAF

This dish can be made as a separate complex carbohydrate dish or as a complete meal by adding previously cooked chicken, turkey, tofu or legumes. Don't forget to use leftovers in wraps for breakfast or lunch! Make the job of cooking the grains easier by preparing them as early as two days in advance. This dish can be eaten hot or cold.

INGREDIENTS:

1 cup / 240 ml brown, wild or Wehani rice
2 cups / 480 ml water
Pinch sea salt

¼ cup / 60 ml wheat berries
1 cup / 240 ml water
Pinch sea salt

1 cup / 240 ml whole-wheat couscous
1½ cups / 360 ml boiling water
Pinch sea salt
2 Tbsp / 30 ml avocado oil

3 Tbsp / 45 ml extra virgin olive oil
1 Vidalia onion, chopped fine
2 ribs celery, chopped
2 large sweet carrots, peeled and chopped fine
4 cloves garlic, passed through a garlic press
¼ cup / 60 ml low-sodium black bean sauce mixed
    with 1 Tbsp water
4 green onions with light green leaves, chopped
½ cup / 120 ml fresh cilantro, finely chopped
½ cup / 120 ml pine nuts, toasted
Sea salt and black pepper

PREPARATION:

1 Cook all grains **separately** according to package directions. Let each grain cool.

2 In a large nonstick skillet, heat olive oil. Sauté onions, celery, carrots and garlic until the vegetables just turn golden. Do not over brown. Add the cooked grains while stirring to distribute the vegetables. Add diluted black bean sauce, green onions, cilantro and toasted pine nuts. Toss lightly. Season with sea salt and black pepper. Serve.

TIP

You could eat this dish as a complete meal any day of the week. I like it cold too. Wheat berries are a personal favorite because they are so crunchy.

NUTRITIONAL VALUE PER SERVING:

Calories: 367 | Calories from Fat: 153 | Protein: 6g | Carbs: 45g
Dietary Fiber: 4g | Sugars: 2g | Fat: 17g | Sodium: 565mg

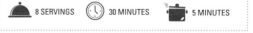

8 SERVINGS   30 MINUTES   5 MINUTES

GARLICKY COUSCOUS
with Roasted Peppers

The new food guide recommends getting plenty of whole grains each day. Couscous is a delicious and versatile wheat product similar to a grain. It is easy to cook and prepare especially if you are in a hurry – it cooks in 5 minutes. It is excellent as a potato alternative and can be eaten hot or cold for a Clean-Eating lunch the next day.

INGREDIENTS:

1¼ cups / 300 ml water

1 Tbsp / 15 ml best-quality olive oil

½ tsp / 2.5 ml sea salt

2 large cloves garlic, peeled and crushed

1 cup / 240 ml whole-wheat couscous grains

1 small red pepper roasted or one 6-ounce jar
    roasted peppers, drained and diced

2 Tbsp / 30 ml fresh basil, chopped

Fresh ground black pepper

PREPARATION:

1 In a medium saucepan combine 1¼ cup / 300 ml water, oil, salt and garlic. Bring to a boil. Stir in couscous. Remove from heat. Cover and let stand for 5 minutes. (I told you it was easy!) Fluff with a fork. Remove garlic cloves and stir in red peppers and fresh basil. Season with pepper and serve with any meat.

NUTRITIONAL VALUE PER SERVING:
Calories: 205 | Calories from Fat: 34 | Protein: 5g | Carbs: 37g
Dietary Fiber: 3g | Sugars: 0.05g | Fat: 3g | Sodium: 32mg

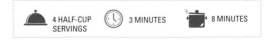

4 HALF-CUP SERVINGS   3 MINUTES   8 MINUTES

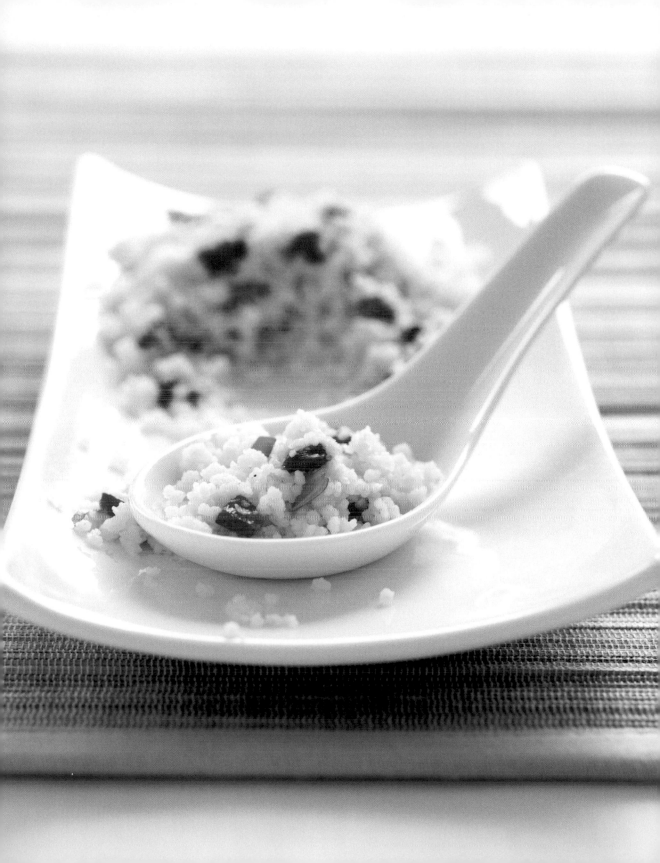

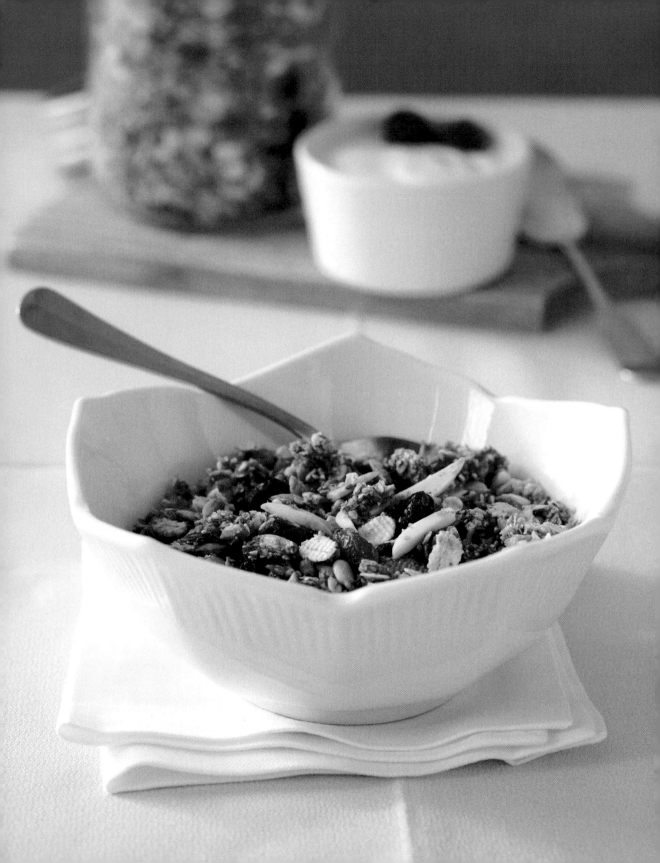

GRANOLA – *The Eat-Clean Way*

What tastes better than granola? Eat it as a cereal, in yogurt or just plain out of your hand. It is good Clean-Eating food. But is it? Many commercial brands contain ingredients you don't want, including high levels of sugar, sugar substitutes, sweeteners, sodium, preservatives and more. Why not make your own? It's easy and satisfying.

DRY INGREDIENTS:

1 cup / 240 ml organic rye flakes

1 cup / 240 ml organic oat flakes (rolled oats)

1 cup / 240 ml organic kamut flakes

1 cup / 240 ml organic wheat flakes

1 cup / 240 ml raw, sliced, unsalted almonds

½ cup / 120 ml unsalted sunflower seeds

¼ cup / 60 ml sesame seeds

COATING MIXTURE INGREDIENTS:

½ cup / 120 ml Sucanat or Rapadura sugar

Pinch sea salt

½ tsp / 2.5 ml cinnamon

¼ cup / 60 ml olive, safflower, canola or avocado oil

1 tsp / 5 ml best-quality vanilla

¼ cup / 60 ml organic honey

AT THE END:

½ cup / 120 ml Sultana raisins

½ cup / 120 ml dried cranberries

Call the kids! This is a fun and easy recipe for kids to get involved in. Let them measure and mix with you. They can help decide what goes into the mix. What a sense of accomplishment when they get to eat the delicious finished product.

NUTRITIONAL VALUE PER ONE-CUP SERVING:

Calories: 340 | Calories from Fat: 140 | Protein: 12g | Carbs: 41g
Dietary Fiber: 8g | Sugars: 1g | Fat: 15g | Sodium: 14mg

PREPARATION:

1 Preheat oven to 300°F / 150°C. In a large bowl mix all dry ingredients until evenly distributed. Set aside.

2 Meanwhile, in a small saucepan, place all coating mixture ingredients. Gently warm contents and stir until honey is dissolved.

3 Pour liquid coating mixture over dry ingredients in mixing bowl. Using a large wooden spoon or clean bare hands mix well until all ingredients are coated.

4 Spread granola onto a large cookie sheet lined with parchment paper.

5 Baking time is 40 minutes, but you can't walk away from the oven. You need to stir the granola every so often with a wooden spoon so everything gets nicely toasted.

6 Transfer baked granola to a cooling rack and sprinkle with raisins and cranberries (or other dried fruit). Let cool completely. When cool, transfer to an airtight container. Keeps in your cereal cupboard for one week. You can freeze it too!

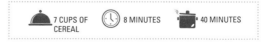

7 CUPS OF CEREAL | 8 MINUTES | 40 MINUTES

BLACK BEAN AND RICE SALAD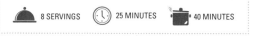

Rice and black beans come together in this delicious salad that will become a family favorite during hot summer weather and year-round. Enjoy it as a meal when it's just too hot to cook.

INGREDIENTS:

¾ cup / 180 ml fresh lemon juice

2 Tbsp / 10 ml avocado oil

1½ cups / 360 ml fresh corn kernels

1½ cups / 360 ml canned black beans, rinsed and
    drained

2 medium ripe tomatoes, chopped

1 large red bell pepper, seeded and chopped

1 medium green zucchini, chopped

½ cup /120 ml chopped green onions

3 cloves garlic passed through garlic press

½ cup / 120 ml fresh cilantro, chopped

Pinch red pepper flakes

3 cups / 720 ml cooked brown rice

Sea salt and black pepper to taste

PREPARATION:

1 In small bowl combine lemon juice and oil. This will be the salad dressing.

2 In large decorative serving bowl combine all remaining ingredients. Toss lightly to distribute ingredients. Pour dressing over salad. Toss again. Serve.

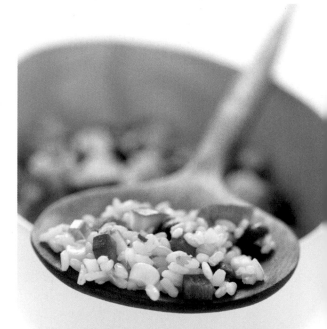

NUTRITIONAL VALUE PER SERVING:

Calories: 193 | Calories from Fat: 43 | Protein: 5g | Carbs: 34g
Dietary Fiber: 4g | Sugars: 4g | Fat: 4g | Sodium: 207mg

8 SERVINGS   25 MINUTES   40 MINUTES

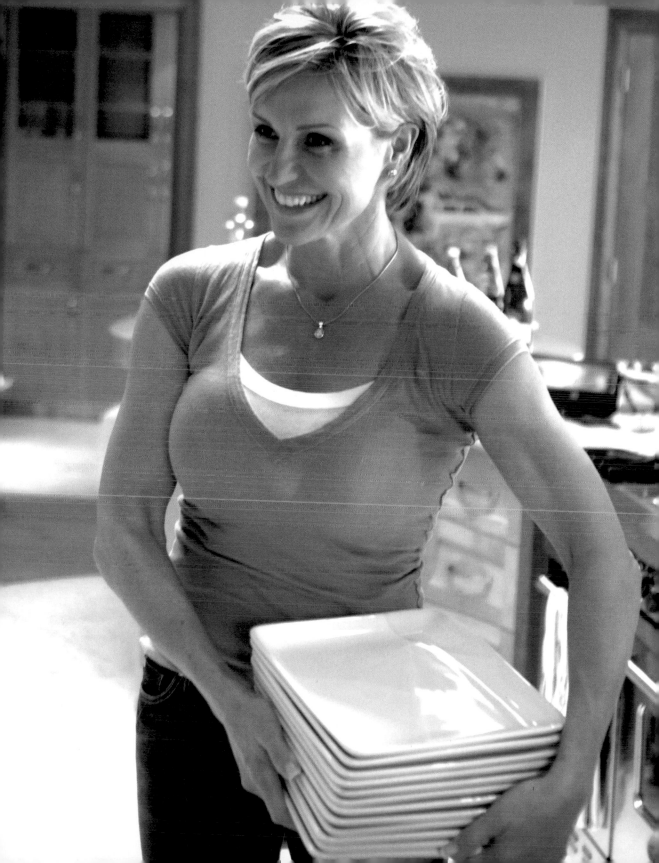

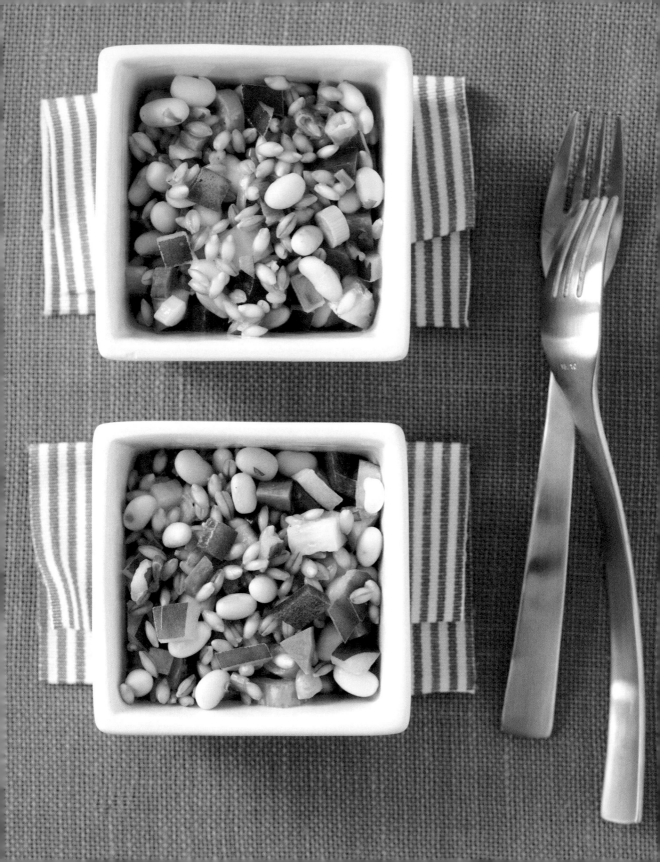

WHEAT BERRY SALAD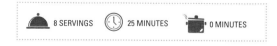

The wheat berry is a wonderful grain; it is nutrient dense and delightfully flavored. Combined with legumes, wheat berries form a complete protein so this is an ideal alternative for vegetarians and non-vegetarians alike.

INGREDIENTS:

1 cup / 240 ml raw soybeans, soaked for 4 hours, cooked till soft, and cooled

1 cup / 240 ml raw wheat berries, soaked for 1 hour, cooked till soft, and cooled

1 bunch fresh green onions, trimmed and chopped

1 large sweet carrot, peeled and chopped fine

1 English cucumber, chopped

1 medium purple onion, peeled and chopped

1 red bell pepper, seeded and deveined, chopped fine

2 stalks celery, trimmed and chopped fine

½ cup / 120 ml fresh basil, chopped

DRESSING INGREDIENTS:

Sea salt and black pepper

¼ tsp / 60 ml dry mustard

½ cup / 120 ml plain, nonfat yogurt

2 Tbsp / 30 ml fresh lime juice

¼ cup / 60 ml chopped fresh basil

½ cup / 120 ml rice wine vinegar

3 cloves garlic, passed through garlic press

PREPARATION:

1 In small bowl whisk together dressing ingredients. Set aside.

2 Place cooked, cooled beans and wheat berries in large decorative serving bowl. Add diced vegetables and herbs. Toss well. Pour dressing over salad and toss again. Season with sea salt and black pepper. Serve immediately or chill and serve later.

TIP 🍴

Soaking the wheat berries in advance will speed up the cooking time.

NUTRITIONAL VALUE PER SERVING:

Calories: 170 | Calories from Fat: 19 | Protein: 8g | Carbs: 30g
Dietary Fiber: 6g | Sugars: 6g | Fat: 2g | Sodium: 283mg

8 SERVINGS   25 MINUTES   0 MINUTES

BROWN RICE PILAF

I haven't eaten white rice since I learned the nutritional benefits of brown rice. I get so creative with rice now I even love the taste of black, wild and mahogany rice. I urge you to try these many varieties. I always make extra rice so I can stuff it into a wrap the next day for a delicious Clean-Eating wrap. You'll never eat white rice again.

INGREDIENTS:

¼ cup / 60 ml chopped mushrooms

¼ cup / 60 ml chopped celery

¼ cup / 60 ml chopped green onions

¼ cup / 60 ml chopped red pepper

1 cup / 240 ml dry brown rice

2½ cups / 600 ml water

Cooking spray

NUTRITIONAL VALUE PER SERVING:

Calories: 181 | Calories from Fat: 12 | Protein: 4g | Carbs: 37g
Dietary Fiber: 2g | Sugars: 1g | Fat: 1g | Sodium: 15mg

PREPARATION:

1 Preheat oven to 350°F / 177°C. Coat a large 3-quart (about 3 L) casserole dish with cooking spray.

2 Briefly sauté vegetables in small fry pan until translucent or soft but not mushy. Place all ingredients in casserole dish and cover. Put in the oven and bake for 45 minutes or until all liquid is absorbed. Serve as a delicious accompaniment to meats and seasonal vegetables.

4 SERVINGS   10 MINUTES   45 MINUTES

RICE IS NOT JUST WHITE!

The recently revamped Food Guide suggests consuming at least 10 servings of whole grains each day. This is not an easy task when you consider the plethora of over-processed and refined foods available. Most of these have been stripped of their nutritional value. White rice is one of these and I encourage you, as a Clean Eater, to consider switching your regular white rice to brown rice. Once you have developed a taste for it, which won't take long since brown rice has a gorgeous nutty flavor and slightly chewy texture, you can reach for the many varieties of black, mahogany and wild rice.

Try such exciting varieties as China black, originally reserved for Chinese emperors, Bhutanese red, which possesses an earthy flavor that pairs beautifully with bison and other game, or kalijira or miniature basmati. Once you get started with these multifaceted whole grains it will be a challenge to go back to the Wonderbread of rice, white! I promise.

These exotic-sounding names for an age-old grain belie their versatility in the kitchen. Don't be afraid! These types are just as easy to cook as regular rice and I have a tip for making it even easier. Of course if you own a rice cooker making rice is supremely simple. Otherwise preheat your oven to 350°F / 177°C. Spray a covered casserole dish with a light coating of cooking spray. Measure the desired quantity of rice and water. Cover and place in the oven. Let bake until all water is absorbed. This is the simplest, no-fuss method of making rice, in my opinion. I like to do it this way because I don't have to mess around with it. I often roast a whole turkey breast or several chicken breasts and an assortment of fresh vegetables alongside so that the rice and the rest of the meal are ready at the same time.

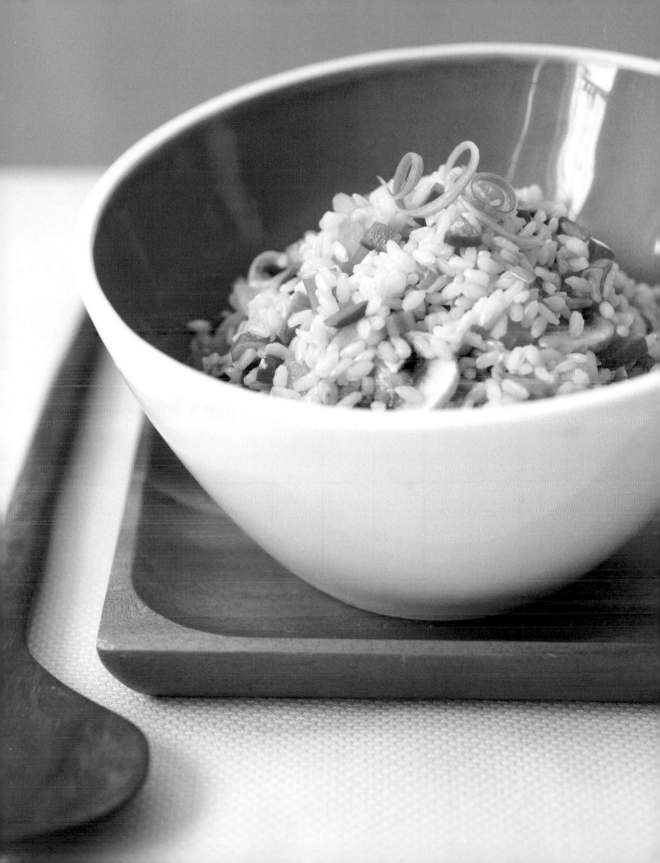

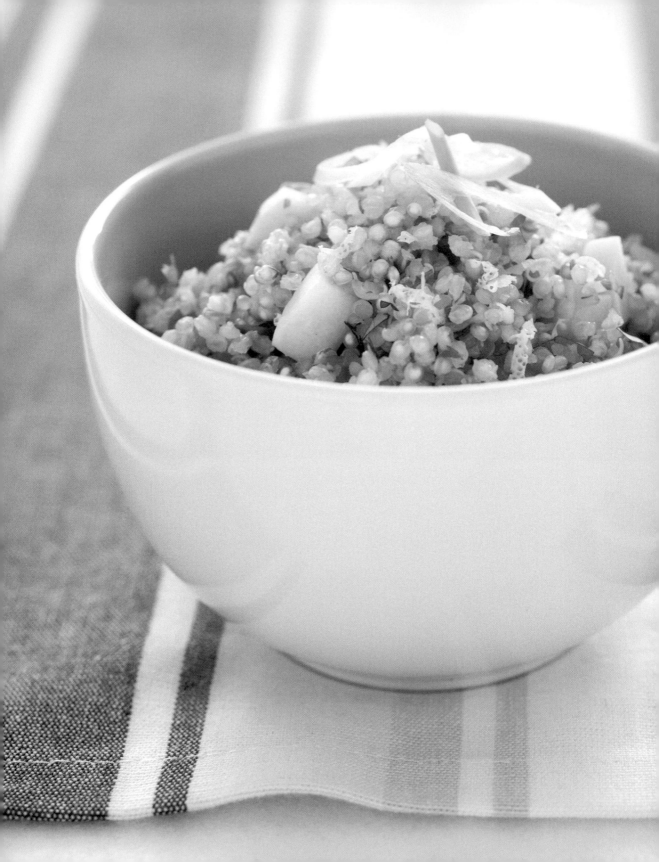

QUINOA PILAF

I am doing my best to reintroduce quinoa into our collective diet. This multitalented grain can be used sweet or savory. It is an important grain to include in any nutrition plan, but particularly for those of you who are vegetarian, since the protein in quinoa is complete. Quinoa is actually the seed of the goosefoot plant but it is generally referred to as a grain.

INGREDIENTS:

1 tsp / 5 ml extra virgin olive oil

1 medium onion, peeled and chopped

2 cups / 480 ml red or white quinoa, well rinsed and drained (remember, quinoa has a bitter coating that must be rinsed off before you cook it)

1¾ cups / 420 ml low-sodium chicken or vegetable stock (gluten free if necessary)

1 tsp / 5 ml freshly grated lemon zest

1 small, yellow zucchini, diced

2 tsp / 10 ml fresh cilantro, chopped

2 tsp / 10 ml fresh parsley, chopped

1 tsp / 5 ml fresh lemon juice

1 tsp / 5 ml fresh lime juice

Sea salt and freshly ground black pepper

4 scallions, trimmed and chopped for garnish

PREPARATION:

1 Place olive oil in a large skillet, and heat over medium heat. Add onion and cook until translucent. Now add rinsed and drained quinoa and cook for 5 minutes. The grains should become lightly browned. Toasting the quinoa before cooking further develops the flavor of the grain. Add stock, lemon zest and zucchini. Bring to a boil. Reduce heat and let cook, covered, for 20 minutes until quinoa becomes translucent. That's when you know it's done.

2 Remove the pan from the heat and let stand for 10 minutes. Fluff with a fork and add cilantro, parsley and citrus juices. Season with sea salt and pepper. Serve immediately. Garnish each serving with chopped green onion.

NUTRITIONAL VALUE PER SERVING:

Calories: 186 | Calories from Fat: 28 | Protein: 8g | Carbs: 33g
Dietary Fiber: 4g | Sugars: 2g | Fat: 3g | Sodium: 86mg

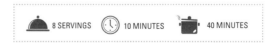

8 SERVINGS   10 MINUTES   40 MINUTES

BROWN RICE MEATLOAF

This is an interesting variation of a family favorite. Many of the unnecessary calories and fats have been whisked out of the standard version. Yogurt cheese does a superb job of holding the loaf together while adding valuable protein and a tangy flavor. Adding brown rice ups the nutrition profile substantially. You will be able to use leftovers for a few more Clean-Eating meals. Try it cold on lunch wraps or pitas. Better still, double the recipe – planned leftovers make your job of being a Clean-Eating cook much easier.

INGREDIENTS:

1 pound / 454 g lean ground turkey or chicken or
    ground bison
1 cup / 240 ml cooked brown rice (any color of
    brown rice will do)
1 egg
¾ cup / 180 ml plain, low-fat yogurt cheese
    (see recipe on page 141)
½ cup / 120 ml finely chopped onion
½ cup / 120 ml finely chopped red, green or yellow
    bell pepper
½ cup / 120 ml finely chopped celery
1 Tbsp / 15 ml low-sodium soy sauce or tamari
    (Tamari is usually gluten-free – make sure
    to check the ingredients.)
1 tsp / 5 ml sea salt
Fresh ground black pepper
1 tsp / 5 ml crumbled dried oregano
1 tsp / 5 ml crumbled dried basil
Cooking spray

PREPARATION:

1 Preheat oven to 350°F / 177°C.

2 In a large mixing bowl combine all ingredients with a pair of clean hands. Place in a loaf pan that has been prepared with a light coating of nonstick cooking spray. Bake for about an hour. Remove from oven and let stand for 10 minutes before cutting.

NUTRITIONAL VALUE PER SERVING:

Calories: 149 | Calories from Fat: 15 | Protein: 20g | Carbs: 12g
Dietary Fiber: 1g | Sugars: 3g | Fat: 1g | Sodium: 285mg

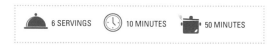
6 SERVINGS   10 MINUTES   50 MINUTES

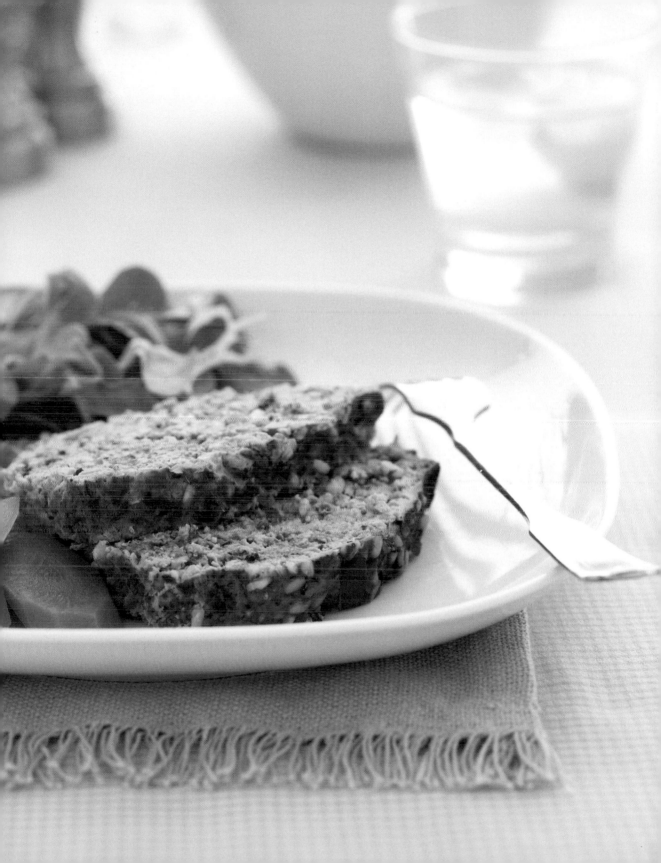

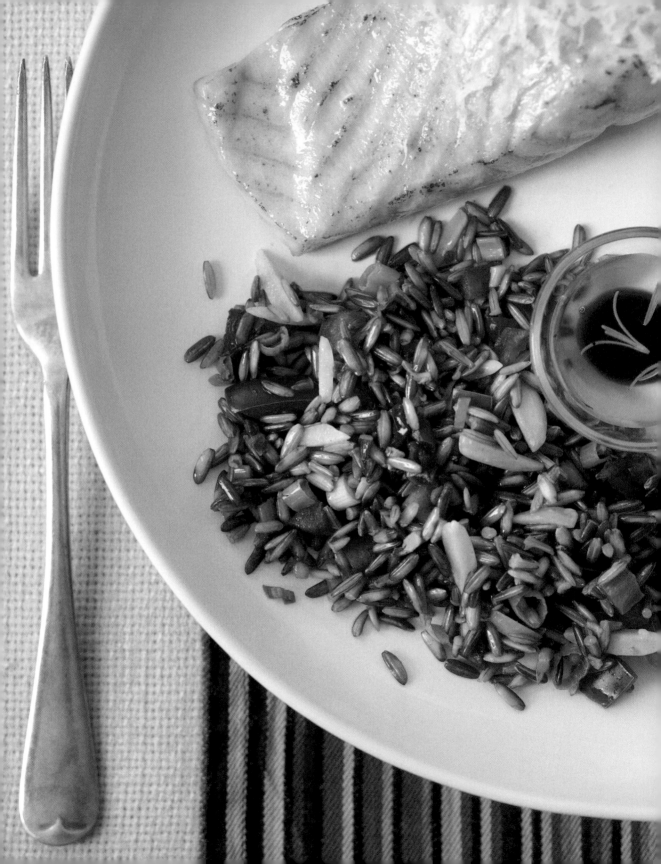

WEHANI RICE SALAD

Wehani rice is delicious popcorn-flavored rice loaded with nutritious complex carbohydrates. Try it in this salad or next time you want rice for dinner.

INGREDIENTS:

3 cups / 720 ml hot cooked Wehani rice

2 Tbsp / 30 ml best-quality olive oil

Juice of half of one fresh lemon

2 Tbsp / 30 ml balsamic vinegar

2 cloves garlic, passed through a garlic press

½ tsp / 2.5 ml dried rosemary

½ tsp / 2.5 ml fresh ground black pepper

½ cup / 120 ml lightly toasted almond slivers

1 cup / 240 ml fresh basil, finely chopped

2 red bell peppers, seeded and chopped

¾ cup / 180 ml sundried tomatoes, chopped

5 scallions, trimmed and chopped

PREPARATION:

1 Place rice in large decorative serving bowl. Combine oil, lemon juice, vinegar, garlic, rosemary and black pepper in a jar or container with tight-fitting lid. Shake well. Pour over rice and toss gently. Add remaining ingredients and toss again. Serve immediately or refrigerate.

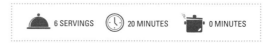

Make it a Clean-Eating meal by adding a source of lean protein.

TIP

This is a kid-friendly dish because they love the popcorn flavor of the rice.

NUTRITIONAL VALUE PER SERVING:
Calories: 241 | Calories from Fat: 90 | Protein: 6g | Carbs: 34g
Dietary Fiber: 6g | Sugars: 3g | Fat: 9g | Sodium: 103mg

6 SERVINGS   20 MINUTES   0 MINUTES

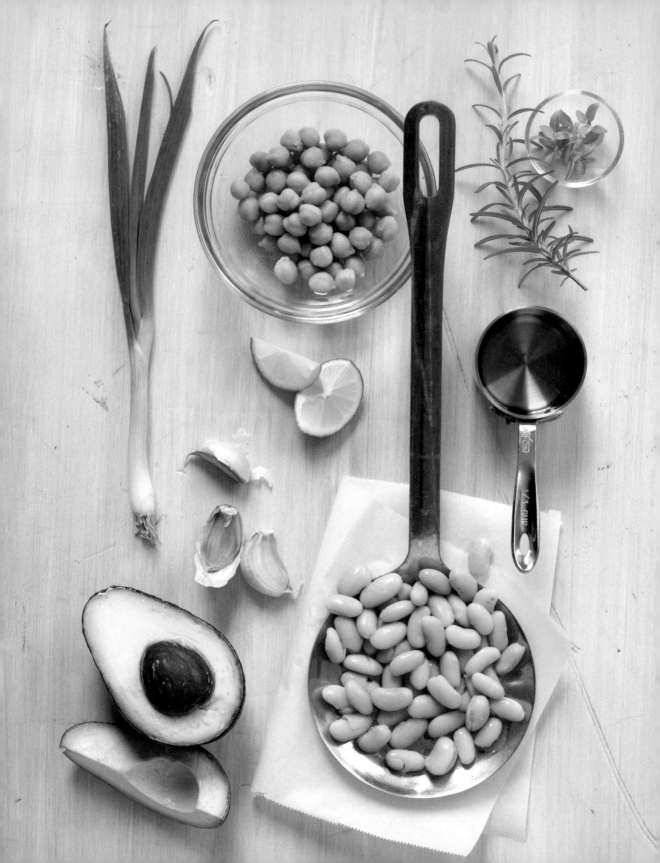

Sauces, Spreads & Salsas

What would those chips be without the dip? And for that matter the tortillas without the salsa? With the proliferation of industrialized foods, however, there is a tendency to over-indulge in chemical calories and junk.

Here's your chance to get creative in your kitchen. Sauces, spreads and salsas are like the tie on a three-piece suit, or the scarf around a woman's neck – the final pleasing stroke of brilliance to jazz things up. Rather than drowning foods in gravy and creamed sauce, "accessorize" your Clean-Eating food with this delicious array of accompaniments. You'll never be bored again.

CLEAN-EATING GUACAMOLE

Guacamole is often overlooked as a viable Clean-Eating option since it is loaded with ingredients that make it fatty – mayonnaise or sour cream. You can enjoy this delicious and nutritious food by making a few low-fat changes and voilà! Guacamole is suddenly off the AVOID list. Try it on breads, chicken or virtually anything else you can think of.

INGREDIENTS:

3 ripe avocados

Juice of ½ fresh lime

1 Tbsp / 15 ml chopped cilantro

½ red or purple onion, minced well

1 clove garlic passed through a garlic press

Sea salt and fresh ground black pepper to taste

PREPARATION:

1 Cut avocados in half. Discard pit and scoop flesh into bowl. Place all ingredients in medium bowl and mix until just combined. Don't overmix.

TIP

Guess what? Eating guacamole is good for your face too. Avocados are loaded with skin-enhancing nutrients.

NUTRITIONAL VALUE PER SERVING:
Calories: 166 | Calories from Fat: 132 | Protein: 2g | Carbs: 10g
Dietary Fiber: 6g | Sugars: 1g | Fat: 14g | Sodium: 8mg

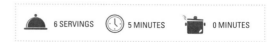

6 SERVINGS   5 MINUTES   0 MINUTES

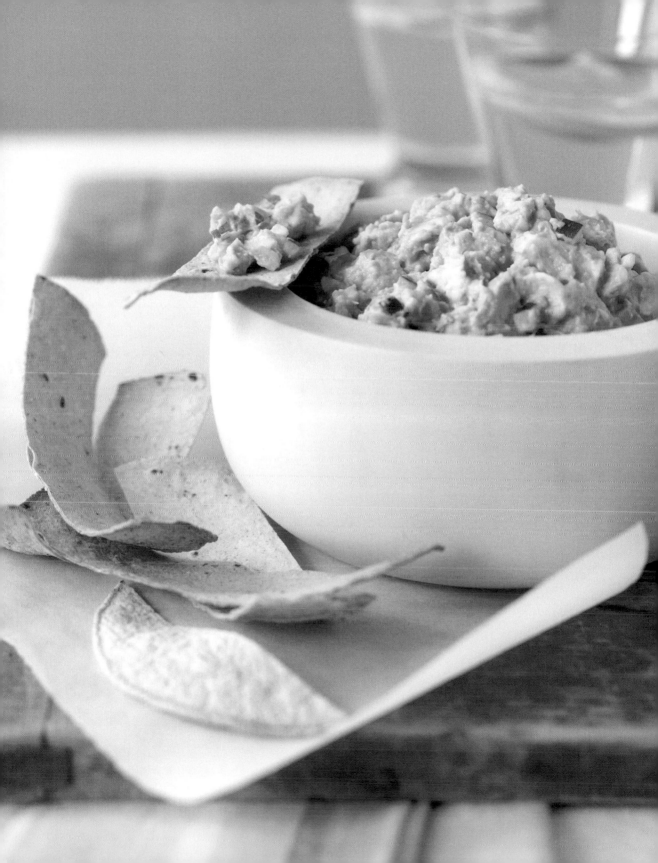

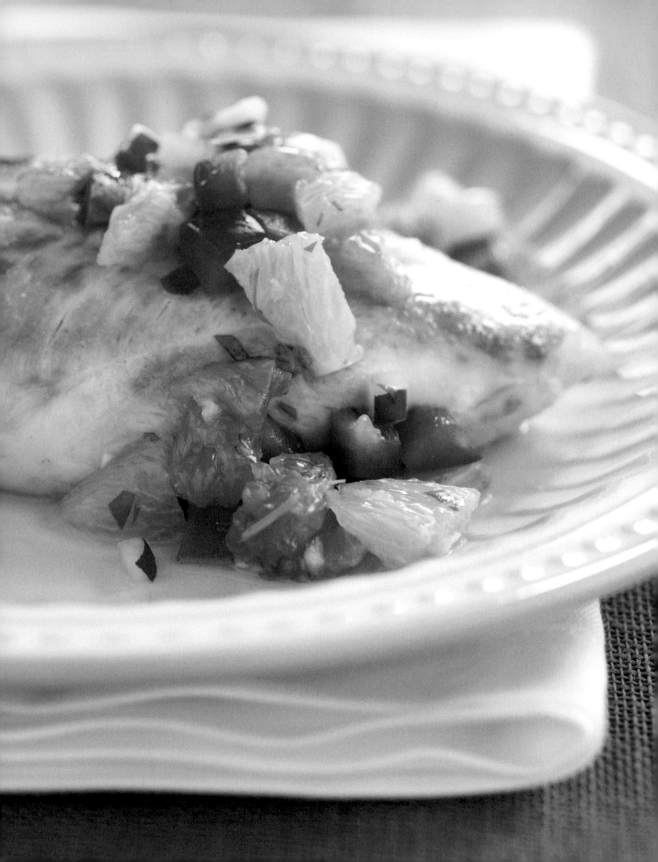

GRAPEFRUIT SALSA

This is a beautiful side dish to serve with grilled fish, egg dishes and poultry. Serving a salsa like this, or another of your choice, helps make drier foods taste so much better. You'll be eating this every day!

INGREDIENTS:

1 sweet, red, large grapefruit

1 medium navel orange

½ cup / 120 ml purple onion, chopped fine

1 small red bell pepper, seeded and deveined, chopped fine

1 clove garlic, passed through a garlic press

Juice of one fresh lime

¼ cup / 60 ml fresh cilantro, chopped fine

Sea salt and fresh ground black pepper to taste

PREPARATION:

1 Using a sharp knife, pare the grapefruit and orange. Hold the fruit over a glass bowl to catch any dripping juices. Remove skin, pith and tougher membranes. Place the fruit in a glass serving bowl, along with the juices. Squeeze any remaining juice out of the remnants. Add remaining ingredients and toss to distribute.

2 Refrigerate if not using right away. Otherwise, serve cold or at room temperature. When I am serving this with cooked meats I like to have it at room temperature.

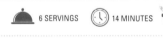

6 SERVINGS   14 MINUTES   0 MINUTES

NUTRITIONAL VALUE PER SERVING:

Calories: 50 | Calories from Fat: 2 | Protein: 1g | Carbs: 13g
Dietary Fiber: 2g | Sugars: 4g | Fat: 0.21g | Sodium: 2mg

SUPER EASY MANGO SALSA

Why not create your own "Clean Eating" salsa rather than opting for your typical store-bought version? The mango hits that sweet spot, while the lime juice adds just enough tartness. Enjoy!

INGREDIENTS:

1 **firm mango** (not too ripe), chopped fine

1 quarter of a **purple onion**, chopped fine

½ **red pepper,** seeded and deveined, chopped fine

½ cup / 120 ml **fresh cilantro**, chopped fine

1 clove **garlic**, passed through garlic press

1 tsp / 5 ml **sea salt**

Freshly ground black pepper

1 Tbsp / 15 ml **fresh lime juice**

PREPARATION:

1 Toss all ingredients together. Rather than dicing up the mango, onion, red pepper, and cilantro by hand, try using a food processor and pulsing until the ingredients resemble salsa consistency. Keep refrigerated until ready to use.

7 SERVINGS OF 4 TBSP EACH   10 MINUTES   0 MINUTES

NUTRITIONAL VALUE PER SERVING:

Calories: 24 | Calories from fat: 1 | Protein: 0.3g | Carbs: 6g
Dietary Fiber: 1g | Sugars: 0.8g | Fat: 0g | Sodium: 1mg

DO-IT-YOURSELF OLIVE BUTTER SPREAD 🍃 Ⓝ

Making your own olive oil-based spread has many advantages. Besides the obvious freshness and lack of chemical calories, you will find it tastes much better. My famous Grandmother's Favorite Oatmeal Cookies (recipe in *The Eat-Clean Diet* book) also calls for an olive oil-based margarine, which many people don't have access to. You can use this as a substitute.

INGREDIENTS:

½ cup / 120 ml low-salt butter at room temperature

½ cup / 120 ml olive oil

PREPARATION:

1 Place both ingredients in a food processor. Process until well combined. The mixture should resemble thick yogurt. Transfer into a serving bowl, preferably ceramic, glass or porcelain. Cover with plastic wrap and refrigerate.

OPTIONS

Add any herbs of your liking to this mix or try minced garlic — even grated citrus peels.

NUTRITIONAL VALUE PER ONE-TBSP SERVING:

Calories: 110 | Calories from Fat: 110 | Protein: 0g | Carbs: 0g
Dietary Fiber: 0g | Sugars: 0g | Fat: 12g | Sodium: 40mg

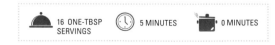

16 ONE-TBSP SERVINGS   5 MINUTES   0 MINUTES

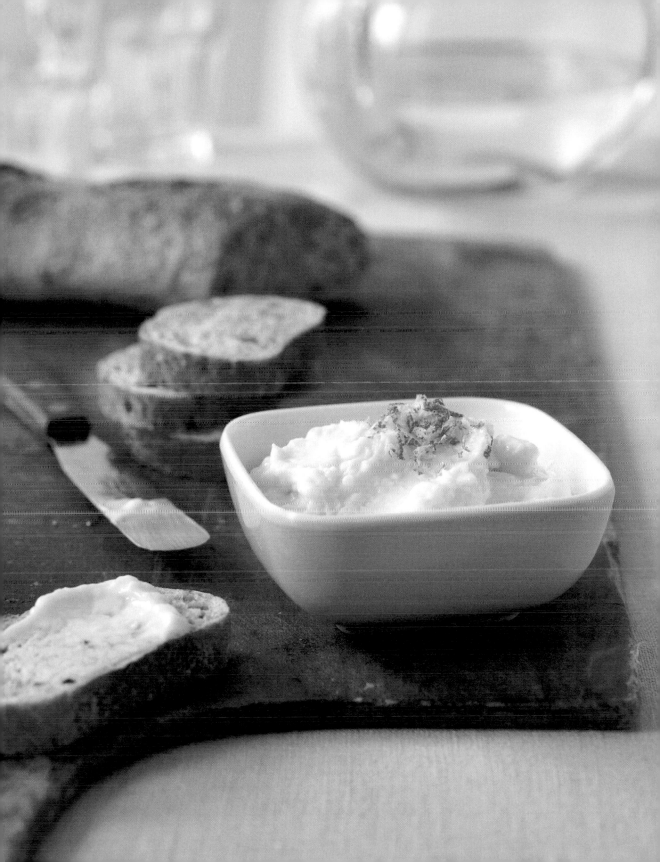

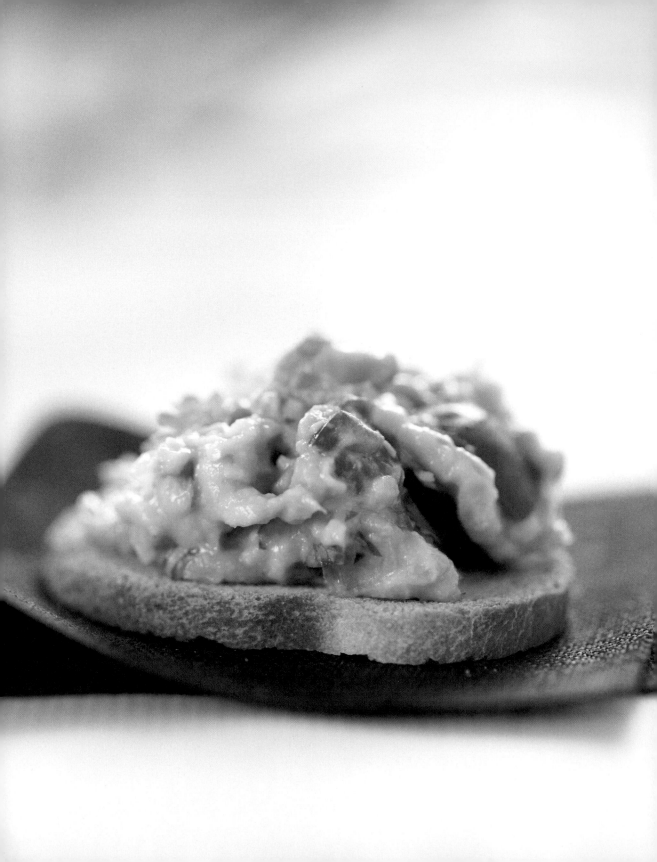

GUACAMOLE – *A New Way*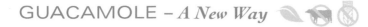

Try this interesting variation on guacamole. You will discover that frozen peas are useful for more than just icing a bruised body part!

INGREDIENTS:

2 small ripe avocados

5 oz / 140 g frozen peas, lightly cooked, rinsed and drained

½ cup / 120 ml cilantro, trimmed and chopped

1 ripe plum tomato, chopped

⅓ cup / 80 ml chopped green onion, whites only

Juice of one lime

PREPARATION:

1 Combine all ingredients in a food processor and pulse until just combined. Transfer to a serving bowl and cover with plastic wrap. Refrigerate. Enjoy this spread anywhere you might use regular guacamole.

NUTRITIONAL VALUE PER SERVING:
Calories: 130 | Calories from fat: 89 | Protein: 2g | Carbs: 10g
Dietary Fiber: 6g | Sugars: 1g | Fat: 9g | Sodium: 25mg

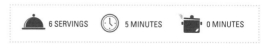
6 SERVINGS   5 MINUTES   0 MINUTES

NO-COOK BEST-EVER APPLESAUCE

The Dutch often use applesauce as an accompaniment. My own Dutch background finds me doing the same, and I love fresh applesauce best. I can my own sauce when the fall harvest brings in a bounty of gorgeous, blushing apples. When I want the flavor of fresh, but don't have the time to bother with peeling and cooking, I use this amazing trick. When apples freeze they become soft and mushy, making it a snap to peel and mush them. Get your kids to help with the peeling job – it's fun and messy. What child wouldn't love that?

INGREDIENTS:

4 – 6 medium apples, unpeeled, washed, cored and
    quartered
1 tsp / 5 ml ground cinnamon
¼ tsp / 1.25 ml ground nutmeg
2 Tbsp / 30 ml fresh lemon juice

PREPARATION:

1 Place all ingredients in a large Ziploc bag. Toss well to distribute evenly. Place in freezer for at least 4 hours. Remove from freezer and allow to thaw for an hour or more. Gently rub skin from frozen apples and place apple pulp into a glass serving bowl. Mash with a fork or potato masher. Serve cold.

A note about sugar

The temptation will be great to sweeten the applesauce with some form of sugar. I suggest you prepare the applesauce first and then taste it. The apples are so sweet on their own I don't ever add sugar myself, but if you feel the need to you can mix in about ¼ cup / 60 ml of Sucanat or organic brown sugar.

NUTRITIONAL VALUE PER SERVING:
Calories: 54 | Calories from Fat: 1 | Protein: 0.25g | Carbs: 14g
Dietary Fiber: 2.5g | Sugars: 10g | Fat: 0.14g | Sodium: 1mg

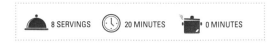

8 SERVINGS   20 MINUTES   0 MINUTES

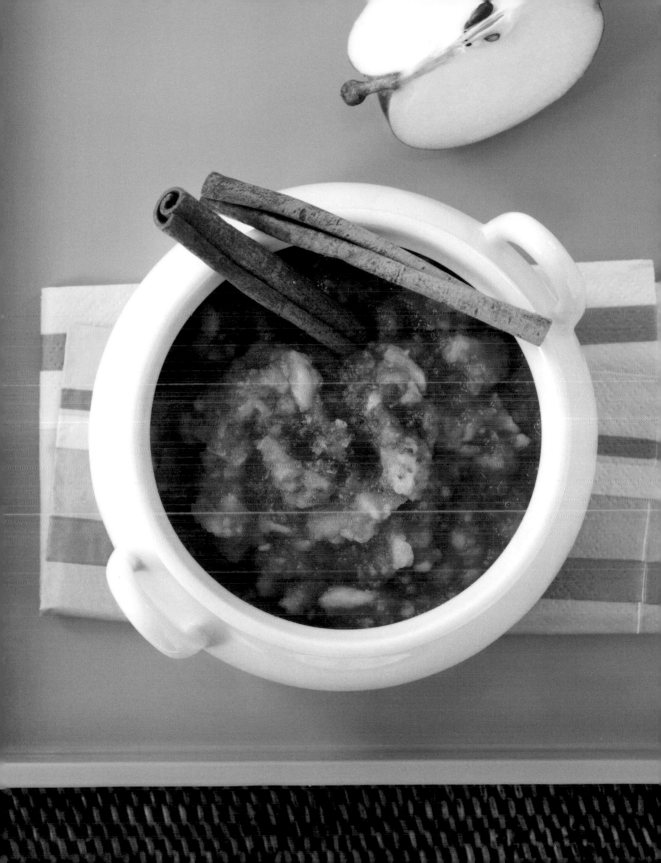

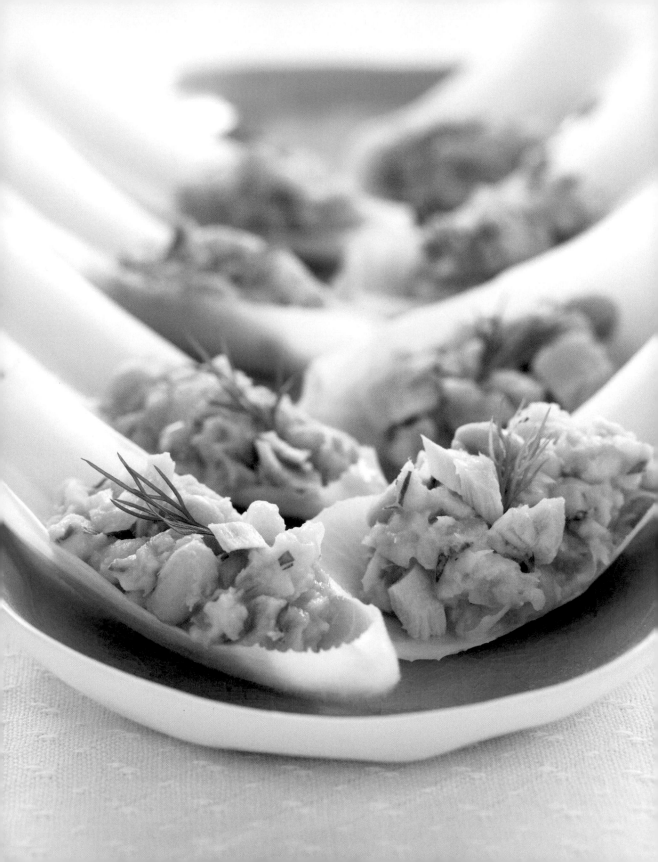

WHITE BEAN SPREAD WITH TUNA

This is an interesting way to get lean protein and complex carbs at the same time. This spread is versatile and delicious.

INGREDIENTS:

1 Tbsp / 15 ml best-quality olive oil

1 cup / 240 ml chopped Vidalia onion

3 cloves garlic passed through a garlic press

1 can white beans of your choice – white kidney beans, pinto, navy or other

2 Tbsp / 30 ml lemon or lime juice

2 Tbsp / 30 ml chopped fresh parsley or cilantro, trimmed

1 tsp / 15 ml fresh dill, chopped

8 oz / 224 g albacore tuna, water packed

Sea salt and fresh ground black pepper to taste

PREPARATION:

1 Heat oil in small frying pan and sauté onions until just translucent. Do not over-brown. Transfer pan contents to food processor. Add remaining ingredients. Pulse until just blended for a chunky version or longer for a smooth version.

2 Serve as shown, or on flat bread, in pita bread or wraps, or be creative!

TIP

I love this spread because it helps make the tuna less dry.

NUTRITIONAL VALUE PER SERVING:
Calories: 120 | Calories from Fat: 20 | Protein: 10g | Carbs: 10g
Dietary Fiber: 2g | Sugars: 1g | Fat: 2g | Sodium: 254mg

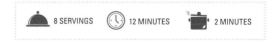

8 SERVINGS   12 MINUTES   2 MINUTES

HIGH-FIBER BEAN DIP

Why settle for boring, high-calorie butter or margarine when you can have a superior spread for your bread, made with good-for-you high-fiber beans?

INGREDIENTS:

1 x 15 oz / 425 g can red kidney beans, rinsed and well drained

1½ tsp / 8 ml) extra virgin olive oil

1 tsp / 5 ml chili powder

1 tsp / 5 ml dried oregano

½ small onion, minced fine

1 clove garlic, minced

Pinch sea salt and fresh black pepper to taste

PREPARATION:

1 Blend the red kidney beans and olive oil until the mixture resembles a paste. Add remaining ingredients and mix well. Transfer to a bowl and cover with plastic wrap. Refrigerate.

2 Enjoy this bean dip with bread, veggies, in wraps, or just about anywhere else. I like to put it on grilled chicken for a change of flavor.

TIP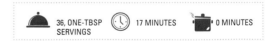

You can start from scratch with dry kidney beans, too, but using canned beans speeds up prep time.

NUTRITIONAL VALUE PER ONE-TBSP SERVING:

Calories: 15 | Calories from Fat: 2 | Protein: 0.7g | Carbs: 2g
Dietary Fiber: 0.7g | Sugars: 0.3g | Fat: 0.19g | Sodium: 25mg

36, ONE-TBSP SERVINGS   17 MINUTES   0 MINUTES

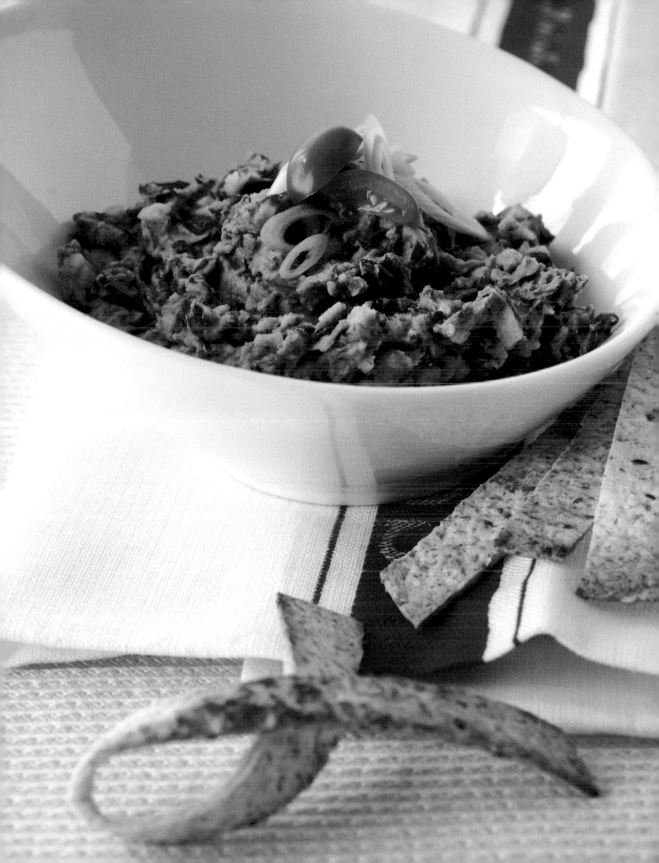

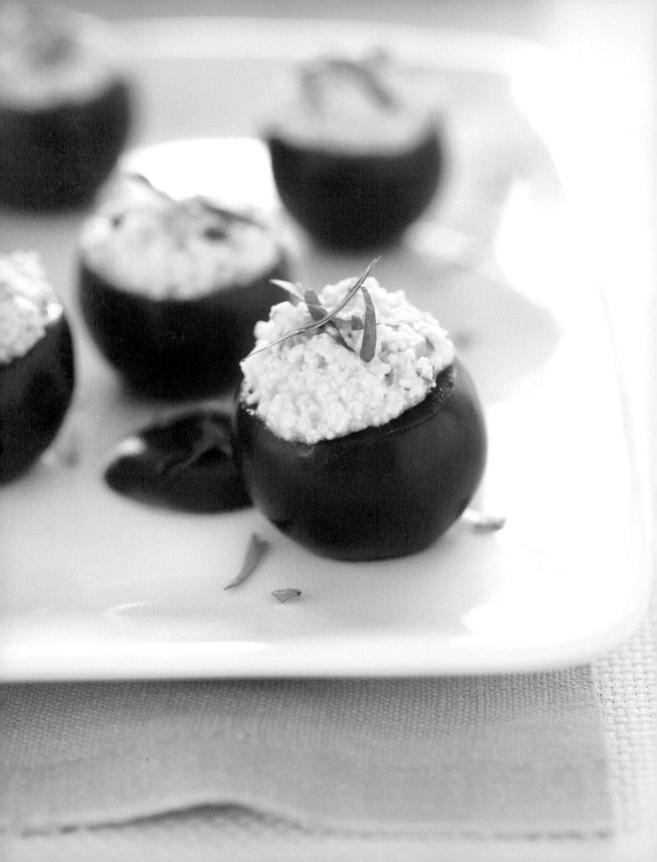

TOFU AND CURRY DIP

It is nice to have a variety of dips to choose from when offering crudités (raw vegetables). This version uses tofu as a base and keeps calories and fat down to a minimum.

INGREDIENTS:

6 oz / 168 g silken tofu

1½ Tbsp / 23 ml fresh lemon juice

2 Tbsp / 30 ml best-quality olive oil

¼ tsp / 1.25 ml sea salt

2 Tbsp / 30 ml chopped green onion

½ tsp / 2.5 ml curry powder

1 Tbsp / 15 ml parsley

2 cloves garlic, minced

PREPARATION:

1 Place all ingredients in a food processor and pulse until just combined. Do not over-process. Cover and refrigerate.

2 Serve with crudités as a healthy dip alternative, spread on wraps with grilled chicken, or anywhere else you would like a delicious shot of creamy flavor.

TIP

Don't you just love the look of tomatoes stuffed with this dip? Yummy too.

NUTRITIONAL VALUE PER ONE-TBSP SERVING:
Calories: 28 | Calories from Fat: 22 | Protein: 1g | Carbs: 0.5g
Dietary Fiber: 0g | Sugars: 0g | Fat: 2g | Sodium: 43mg

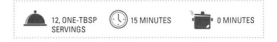 12, ONE-TBSP SERVINGS   15 MINUTES   0 MINUTES

ROASTED GARLIC – *The Wonder Spread*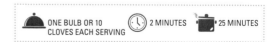

I first tasted this lovely roasted garlic spread at a restaurant in London, Ontario called Garlic's. The golden flesh is served with warmed bread. The flavor is superb, since roasting mellows the intensity of the garlic. Garlic is one of the most satisfying seasonings because of its rich, intense flavor, but it is also a nutritional powerhouse. Garlic is often used for its healing properties. Try it instead of fatty butter or margarine spreads.

INGREDIENTS:

As many full bulbs of garlic as you like.

Best-quality olive oil

PREPARATION:

1 Preheat oven to 400°F / 204°C. Using a sharp knife, cut off the pointed end of the garlic bulb, exposing the flesh. Remove the loose papery skins but not all the skin. Arrange the bulb(s) in a shallow baking dish. Drizzle olive oil over each bulb. Bake uncovered for 25 minutes or until the bulbs appear soft and golden in color.

2 Remove from the oven and turn cooked bulbs over, flesh side down. This allows the cooked garlic flesh to absorb the olive oil.

TO USE:

Squeeze the soft garlic out of the skins once the bulbs have cooled down. Place cooked flesh in a small colorful dish and serve with a hot meal.

This is an excellent alternative to butter and will impress guests at a dinner party.

When I make roasted soups, vegetables or meats I often place a bulb or two of garlic in the roasting pan. The roasting garlic imparts a wonderful flavor to the rest of the ingredients.

NUTRITIONAL VALUE PER ONE-BULB SERVING:

Calories: 57 | Calories from Fat: 50 | Protein: 0g | Carbs: 1g
Dietary Fiber: 0g | Sugars: 0g | Fat: 5g | Sodium: 1mg

ONE BULB OR 10 CLOVES EACH SERVING   2 MINUTES   25 MINUTES

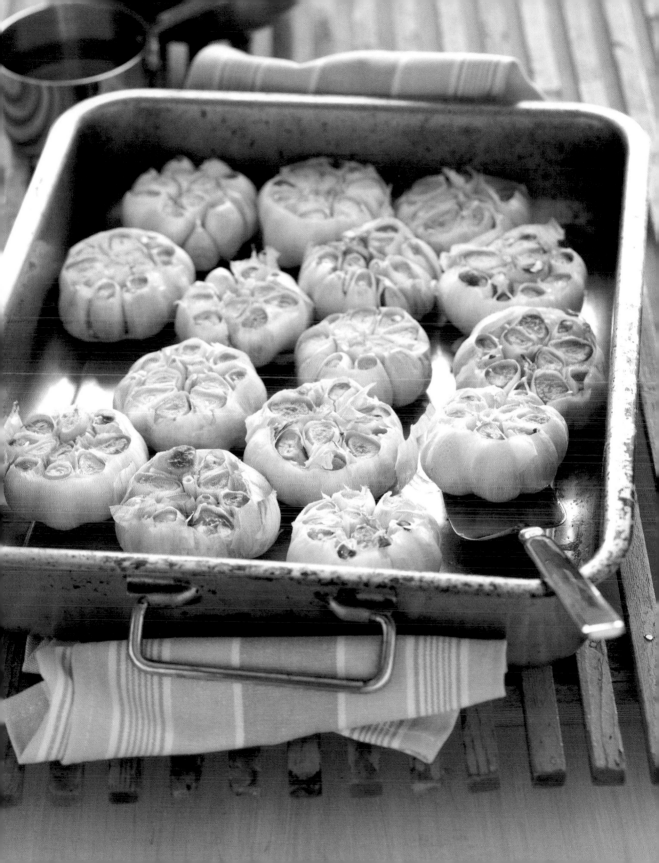

VARIATIONS: I have hidden all sorts of vegetables in this recipe. You can add parsnips to the soup, and red peppers make a wonderful sweet version of the same soup or sauce.

FOR SOUP

Simply add remaining 4 cups / 960 ml stock to sauce to create a delicious soup. Your kids won't even know they are eating sweet potatoes!

SOUP OR SAUCE

I know! I know! This sounds funny. Is it soup or is it sauce? This is a versatile recipe that can be used as a sauce in a thicker format or as a soup when thinned with broth. It is delicious and hides a variety of healthy vegetables in the tomato-based broth. This is one of our favorite family meals. I put a pot of this on when I know the day is going to be busy and I won't have time to cook a meal. The soup or sauce is ready and I can whip up a meal by adding pasta or bread, depending on whether my family wants soup or sauce.

INGREDIENTS:

4 pounds / 1.8 kg plum tomatoes, halved

2 purple or sweet Vidalia onions

2 sweet potatoes

4 thick carrots

2 full heads garlic

¼ cup plus 2 Tbsp / 90 ml best-quality olive oil

8 cups / 1.9 L non-fat, low-sodium chicken
    or vegetable stock, divided (gluten free)

3 organic chicken or vegetable bouillon cubes
    (gluten free if necessary)

2 Tbsp / 30 ml dried basil

1 Tbsp / 15 ml dried oregano

1 tsp / 5 ml sea salt

Black pepper

PREPARATION:

1 Preheat oven to 350°F / 177°C. Coat a large, flat roasting pan with ¼ cup / 60 ml of olive oil.

2 Wash the tomatoes and cut them in half lengthwise. Place them cut side down in the roasting pan. Peel the onions and cut into chunks. Toss overtop the tomatoes. Wash the sweet potatoes and cut into chunks. Peel carrots and cut into chunks. Toss both of these in the pan with the tomatoes. Remove loose papery skins from the garlic bulbs, keeping them as intact as possible. Remove the pointed top part of the garlic with a flat knife. Set the garlic amongst the vegetables in the roasting pan. Pour 2 tablespoons / 30 ml of olive oil over the heads of garlic (1 tablespoon / 15 ml per head). Place a sheet of parchment paper over the vegetables and place in the oven to roast for 45 minutes. Remove from oven and let cool.

NEXT STEP:

1 When vegetables have cooled, remove skins from tomatoes and sweet potatoes. Squeeze roasted garlic from each clove into pan. If any vegetables have blackened edges, remove them. Place contents of roasting pan in a large stock pot. Pour 4 cups / 960 ml chicken broth over contents and bring to a boil. Add the bouillon cubes, reduce heat and let simmer for 10 minutes. Purée contents with a hand blender right in the pan. The mixture can be a bit coarse. If sauce is too thick add a bit more stock. Add the basil, oregano, black pepper and salt.

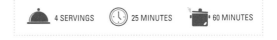

4 SERVINGS   25 MINUTES   60 MINUTES

NUTRITIONAL VALUE PER SERVING:

Calories: 512 | Calories from Fat: 193 | Protein: 19g | Carbs: 65g
Dietary Fiber: 11g | Sugars: 28g | Fat: 21g | Sodium: 1739mg

DIVINE TUSCAN BEAN SPREAD

This delicious bean spread evokes the flavor and exotic beauty of Tuscany. Prepare it on a warm summer day with delicious home-baked bread or lovely chicken breasts grilled on an open wood flame. Wonderful!

INGREDIENTS:

1 head garlic, remove only loose papery skins

1 x 15 ounce / 420 g can chick peas, rinsed and well drained

1 x 15 oz / 420 g can cannellini or navy beans, rinsed and well drained

½ cup / 125 ml freshly squeezed lemon juice

2 tsp / 30 ml ground Tuscan spices, toasted

Pinch cumin, ground and toasted

4 Tbsp / 60 ml extra virgin olive oil, divided

¼ cup / 60 ml finely chopped cilantro

¼ cup / 60 ml finely chopped basil

Sea salt

Fresh ground black pepper

PREPARATION:

1 Prepare garlic head for roasting: slice top points off so that the oil can soak in. Place garlic head on sheet of parchment paper or foil. Drizzle 1 tablespoon / 15 ml olive oil over garlic. Loosely wrap garlic in parchment or foil. Place in preheated 300°F / 150°C oven. Roast for 15 minutes or until golden brown. Remove from heat. Carefully open paper or foil and let cool.

2 In a food processor combine garlic and all remaining ingredients except herbs. Process until mixture resembles a thick paste. Add more or less olive oil to adjust to desired thickness. Add the fresh herbs and pulse lightly. Transfer to a serving bowl. Serve immediately or cover with plastic wrap and refrigerate. Keeps for four days.

NUTRITIONAL VALUE PER ONE-TBSP SERVING:
Calories: 47 | Calories from Fat: 17 | Protein: 1g | Carbs: 6g
Dietary Fiber: 1g | Sugars: 0g | Fat: 1g | Sodium: 99mg

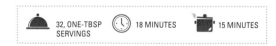

32, ONE-TBSP SERVINGS   18 MINUTES   15 MINUTES

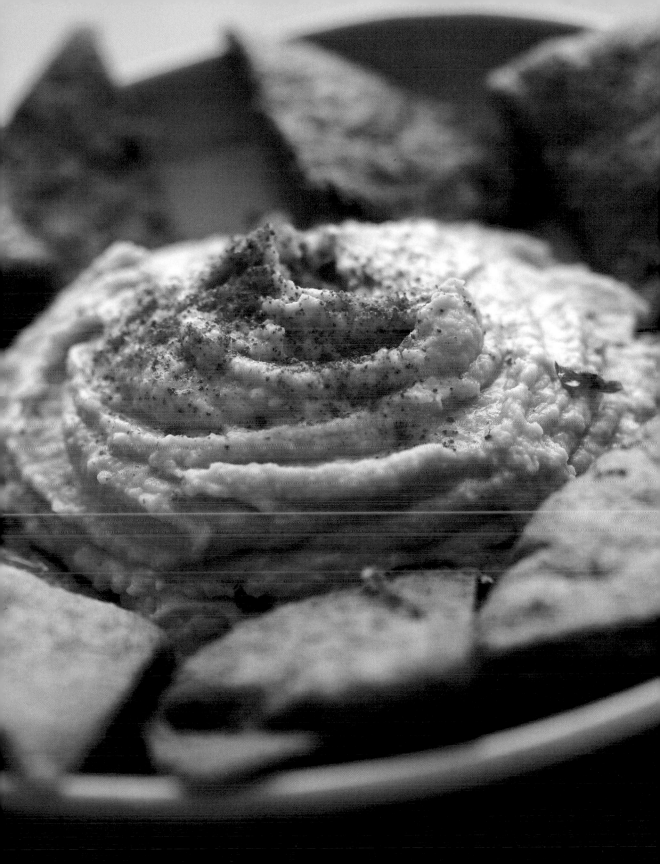

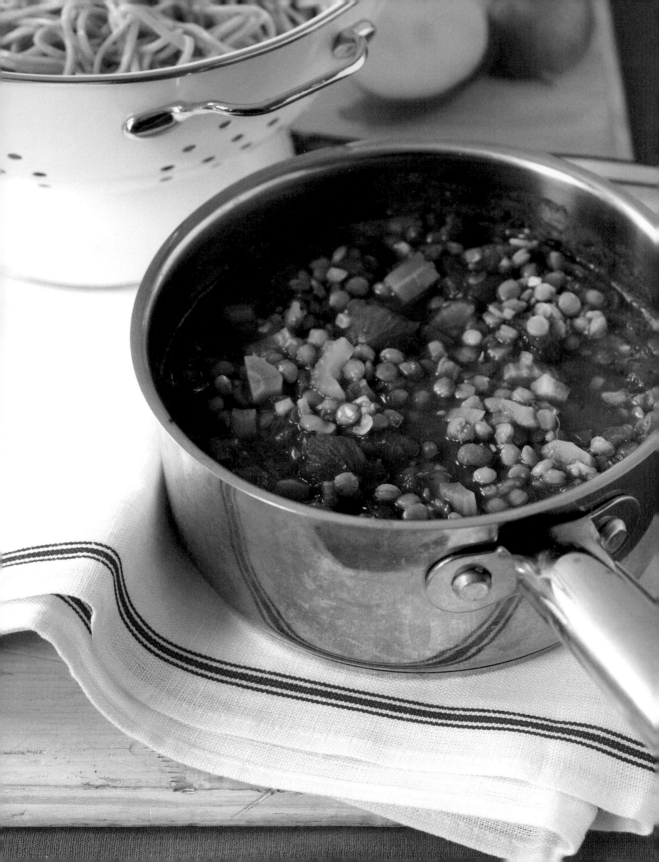

LENTIL TOMATO SAUCE

Lentils are an ideal source of plant-based protein, excellent for vegetarians as well as the rest of us. It was not so long ago that lentils were considered food for livestock. Recently, this tiny legume has achieved something of a cult status. This sauce is a delicious way to serve lentils to those who need some coaxing. The tomatoes and pasta make it seem like you're eating the traditional spaghetti version, but it contains much more nutritional value and Clean-Eating benefits.

INGREDIENTS:

4 Tbsp / 60 ml olive oil, rice bran oil or avocado oil

½ cup / 120 ml finely chopped carrots

1 large onion, peeled and finely chopped

6 cloves garlic, minced

2 ribs celery, washed and finely chopped

1½ cups / 360 ml lentils, well rinsed

½ tsp / 2.5 ml dried thyme

1 x 28 oz / 784 g can whole tomatoes

4 cups / 960 ml low-sodium, low-fat chicken or
    vegetable stock (gluten free if necessary)

Sea salt and fresh ground black pepper to taste

⅔ cup / 160 ml low-fat yogurt (optional)

1½ pounds / 680 g brown rice pasta, rice noodles,
    soba noodles, or buckwheat noodles

PREPARATION:

1 Heat oil in a large skillet over medium heat. Add carrots, onions, garlic and celery. Cook 5 minutes or until vegetables are soft. Add lentils and thyme. Continue cooking a few minutes more, stirring until lentils are coated. Add tomatoes to lentil mixture, breaking them up a bit. Add 4 cups / 960 ml chicken stock or water. Bring mixture to a boil. Reduce heat, cover and simmer, stirring occasionally. The lentils are done when they start to soften a little. Season with sea salt and ground black pepper. Add yogurt if using immediately.

2 Meanwhile have a large pot of water ready. Add sea salt, 2 Tbsp / 30 ml olive oil and bring to a boil. Add pasta and cook al dente. Toss with lentil sauce and serve.

TIP

Puy lentils are a lovely green lentil grown in France. They keep their shape during cooking.

NUTRITIONAL VALUE PER SERVING:
Calories: 641 | Calories from Fat: 87 | Protein: 23g | Carbs: 113g
Dietary Fiber: 13g | Sugars: 16g | Fat: 9g | Sodium: 447mg

8 SERVINGS   17 MINUTES   40 MINUTES

EAT-CLEAN HUMMUS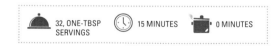

Hummus is my favorite way to jazz up food when I have run out of ideas and want a taste change. It is easy to make and store-bought varieties do not compare. Try to make this version yourself. It keeps in the fridge for several days.

INGREDIENTS:

4 cloves garlic

2 cups / 480 ml canned chickpeas, rinsed and well drained

1 tsp / 5 ml sea salt

⅓ cup / 80 ml tahini

Juice of 2 fresh lemons

1 Tbsp / 15 ml fresh olive oil

PREPARATION:

1 Place all ingredients in food processor. Pulse for a few minutes until well combined but still coarse. Adjust seasonings. Transfer to serving bowl and serve or cover with plastic wrap. Keeps well.

NUTRITIONAL VALUE PER ONE-TBSP SERVING:
Calories: 35 | Calories from Fat: 15 | Protein: 1g | Carbs: 4g
Dietary Fiber: 0.7g | Sugars: 0g | Fat: 1g | Sodium: 94mg

32, ONE-TBSP SERVINGS   15 MINUTES   0 MINUTES

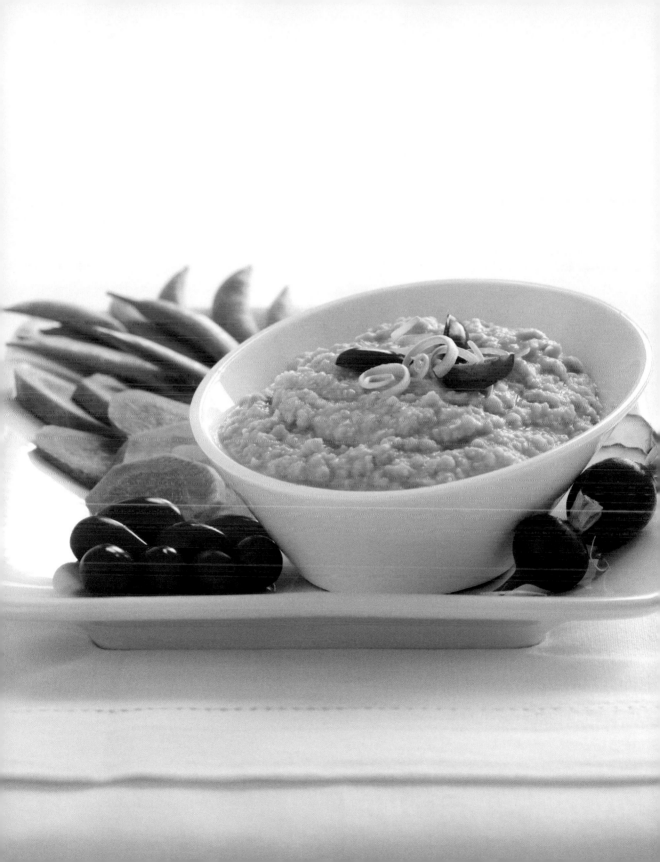

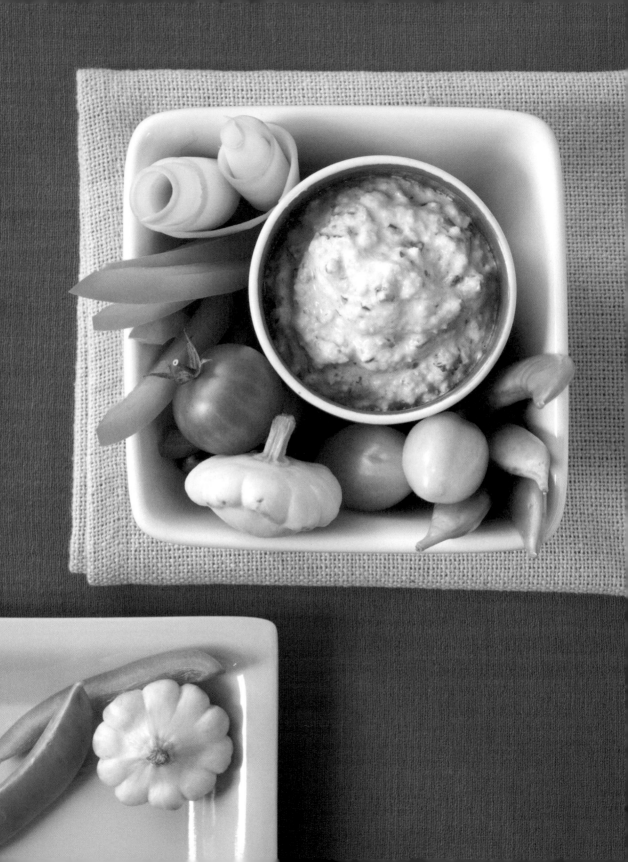

ZUCCHINI HUMMUS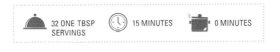

Here's a novel approach to hummus – add zucchini to it. When your garden is overflowing with summer zucchini this is just one more way to make good use of it.

INGREDIENTS:

2 cups / 480 ml chopped unpeeled young zucchini

⅔ cup / 160 ml tahini (sesame seed paste)

¼ cup / 60 ml water

¼ cup / 60 ml chopped fresh parsley

¼ cup / 00 ml chopped fresh basil

Juice of 2 fresh lemons

2 cloves garlic

½ tsp / 2.5 ml sea salt

PREPARATION:

1 Place all ingredients in food processor. Purée and serve with crudités or pita chips.

NUTRITIONAL VALUE PER ONE-TBSP SERVING:

Calories: 33 | Calories from fat: 24 | Protein: 1g | Carbs: 1g
Dietary Fiber: 0.3g | Sugars: 0g | Fat: 2g | Sodium: 27mg

32 ONE-TBSP SERVINGS   15 MINUTES   0 MINUTES

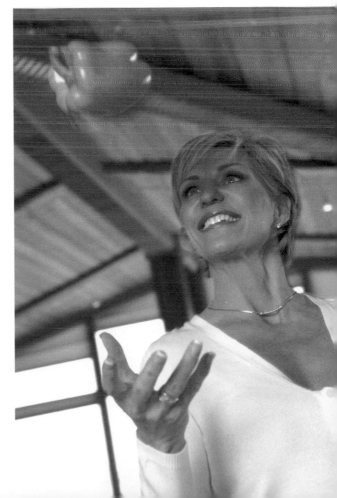

YOGURT CHEESE

No, this is not the high-fat, dense cheese you may be thinking about. This cheese is made with low-fat, plain yogurt. And boy does this cheese have legs! It can do a million things for your Clean-Eating cooking. Let's get started.

INGREDIENTS FOR THE YOGURT CHEESE:

2 quarts / 1.9 L low-fat plain yogurt, dairy or
   soy based

METHOD FOR YOGURT CHEESE:

1 Place 4 layers of damp cheesecloth in a fine mesh sieve or colander. Place the colander over a bowl.

2 Add yogurt and let it drain overnight in the refrigerator.

3 Discard the water from the bowl.

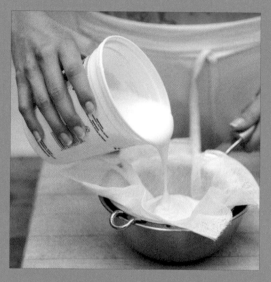

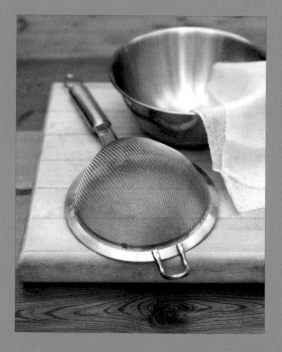

WHAT NEXT?

The result of the draining process will leave you with a soft, creamy cheese-like product. In fact, it is lower in calories than cream cheese but can be used in its place. It is also lower in lactose, higher in protein, and lower in sodium than cream cheese. The best part is that it is all natural.

You now have a wonderful base into which you can mix just about anything, since yogurt cheese readily takes on the flavors of whatever you choose to mix with it. It is sinfully rich and makes you think you are eating something very naughty – but you aren't.

HERE'S WHAT YOU CAN DO WITH
YOGURT CHEESE

HERBED SPINACH YOGURT CHEESE DIP

Into 1½ cups / 360 ml of yogurt cheese mix 2 cloves minced garlic, ½ cup / 125 ml minced fresh basil, 2 teaspoons / 10 ml avocado oil, pinch sea salt and 1 package frozen spinach, thawed and well drained. Mix well and chill. Serve with crudités and baked pita chips.

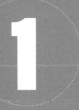

YOGURT CHEESE WHIPPED CREAM

Mix 1½ cups / 360 ml yogurt cheese with 1 teaspoon / 5 ml best-quality vanilla and 1 teaspoon / 5 ml ground cinnamon. Blend ingredients well and use as a topping in place of whipped cream.

CAKE FROSTING

On those occasions you need to whip up a birthday cake try this icing alternative. Into 2 cups / 480 ml yogurt cheese mix ½ cup / 120 ml sifted confectioner's sugar and ½ teaspoon / 2.5 ml best-quality vanilla. Mix well and frost cake. Refrigerate.

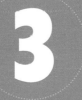

CHOCOLATE MOUSSE

Into 1 cup / 240 ml yogurt cheese mix 3 tablespoons / 45 ml melted dark chocolate that has been mixed with 1 teaspoon / 5 ml organic honey or agave nectar. Blend ingredients well and refrigerate.

GARLIC AND WHITE BEAN SPREAD

The many ways to jazz up bread, besides butter, are astounding. Beans make wonderful spreads, and this one is divine. Use whatever can of beans you have in the house. Spreads like these are super fast to prepare. Try it!

INGREDIENTS:

2 Tbsp / 30 ml extra virgin olive oil

2 cloves garlic, peeled

2 tsp / 10 ml minced fresh rosemary

1 x 16 ounce / 448 g can white beans, undrained

PREPARATION:

1 Place olive oil, garlic and rosemary in medium skillet. Heat until ingredients begin to sizzle. Add beans and liquid to pan. As the beans begin to cook, mash them with a potato masher. Cook until the mixture looks like a spread. It should be a little loose, but it will thicken as it cools.

2 Place in serving bowl and cover with plastic wrap. Refrigerate.

NUTRITIONAL VALUE PER ONE-TBSP SERVING:
Calories: 22 | Calories from fat: 7 | Protein: 1g | Carbs: 2g
Dietary Fiber: 1g | Sugars: 0g | Fat: 0.8g | Sodium: 1mg

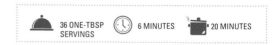

36 ONE-TBSP SERVINGS   6 MINUTES   20 MINUTES

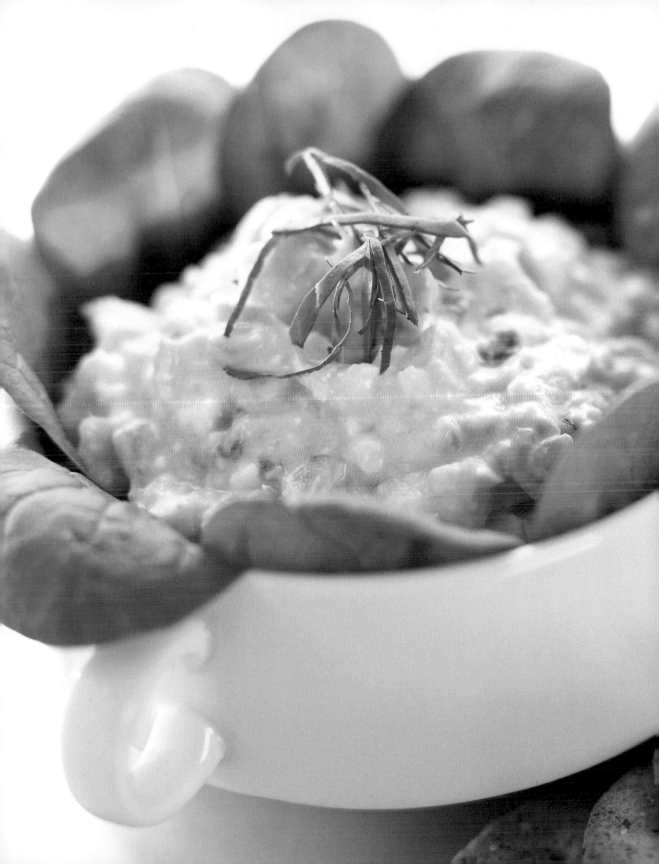

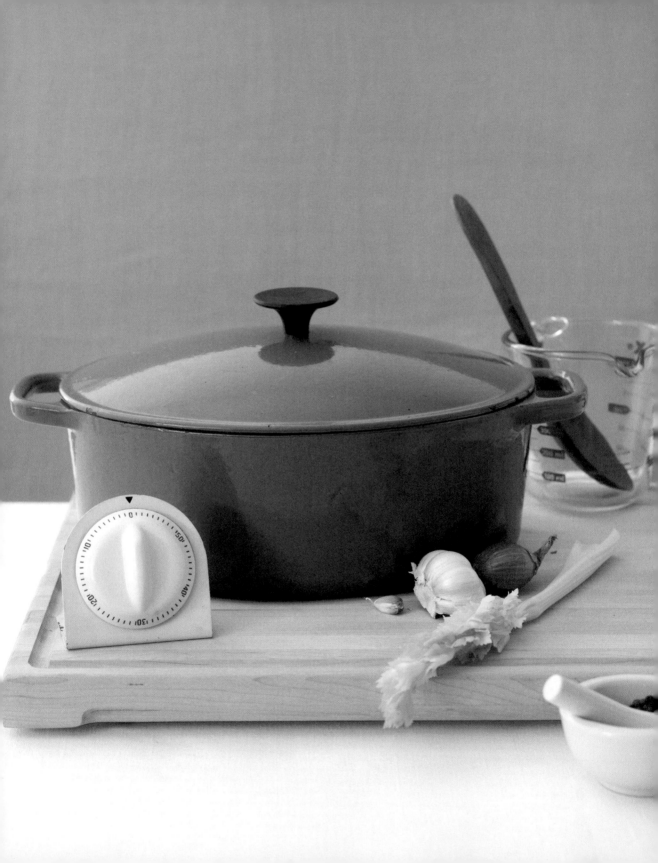

5

One-Dish
& Easy Meals

When life is getting the better of you and you face the possibility of missing a meal because of a hectic schedule, there is no better option than a one-dish meal. I often rely on these when I know I won't be able to whip anything else up in the kitchen. Throw a slew of gorgeous ingredients into a slow cooker and presto! Dinner is ready. I call them "sittable" dinners. They can sit around for hours, ever at the ready to feed a hungry crowd.

IN A CANADIAN STEW

This is my all-time-favorite stew recipe. It's excellent and simple to make. I always make planned leftovers. There are loads of vegetables in this stew and the flavors only get better as it sits in the fridge for a few days. On a night when I am planning a treat for myself, I open a good bottle of red wine and sip it while I chop vegetables. I usually do this on Friday nights!

INGREDIENTS:

1½ lbs / 700 g lean beef tenderloin or bison, cut
    into one-inch cubes

2 leeks, whites and light green only, cut into chunks
    and well rinsed

3 or 4 medium sized cooking onions, peeled and cut
    into chunks

3 carrots, peeled and cut into chunks

3 parsnips, peeled and cut into chunks

1 – 10 oz / 280 g can whole plum tomatoes

1 – 10 oz / 280 g can small potatoes (trust me,
    they have to be canned!)

Several cloves garlic

4 Tbsp / 60 ml best-quality olive oil

½ cup / 120 ml whole-wheat flour

Sea salt and black pepper

1 tsp / 5 ml dried oregano

1 tsp / 5 ml dried basil

1 cup / 240 ml low-sodium, low-fat chicken stock

1 cup / 240 ml light beer

TIP

Try this hearty and nutritious stew with dense whole-grain bread on a cold night. Enjoy a glass of wine alongside if it's a treat night.

PREPARATION:

1 Cut meat into one-inch cubes. Place whole-wheat flour, salt, ground black pepper, oregano and basil in a large plastic container with a tight-fitting lid. Shake the contents so they mix. Now place the cubed meat in the container and shake until coated. Meanwhile in a large Dutch oven heat the oil and sauté the garlic and onions until soft. Add remaining vegetables, except canned potatoes, and cook 5 minutes longer. Gently remove cubed and seasoned meat from container and add to the cooking vegetables. Cook until meat is browned. You will notice the mixture getting sticky. This is caused by the flour seasoning on the meat. When it gets too sticky add the chicken stock and light beer.

2 Bring to a boil and then reduce heat to a simmer. Stir the stew until the sauce becomes evenly smooth. Now add canned, drained potatoes. Don't be tempted to use regular potatoes as they become too mushy. Cook over low heat for another 30 minutes or until vegetables are tender.

NUTRITIONAL VALUE PER SERVING:

Calories: 315 | Calories from Fat: 95 | Protein: 20g | Carbs: 35g
Dietary Fiber: 6g | Sugars: 8g | Fat: 10g | Sodium: 314mg

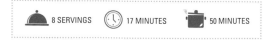

8 SERVINGS   17 MINUTES   50 MINUTES

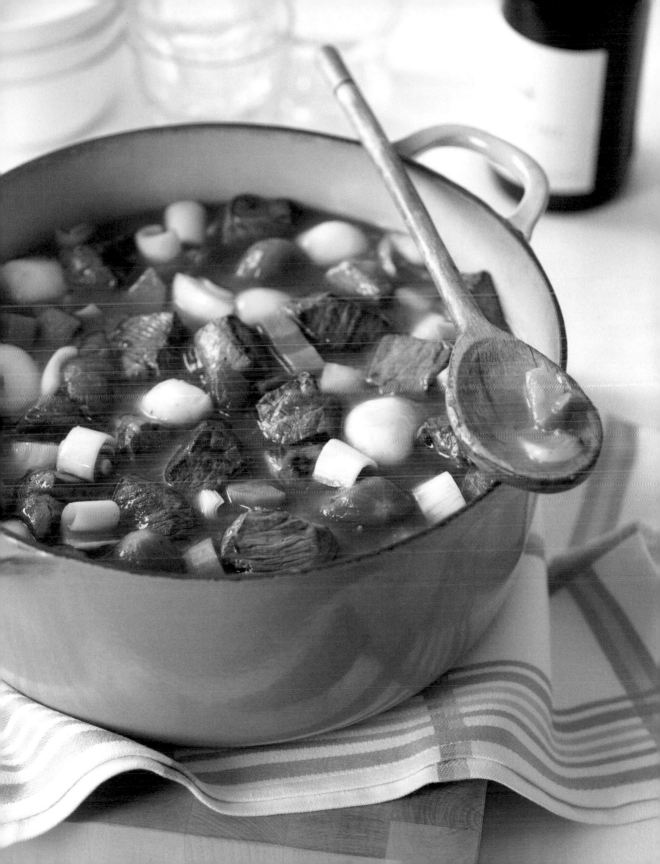

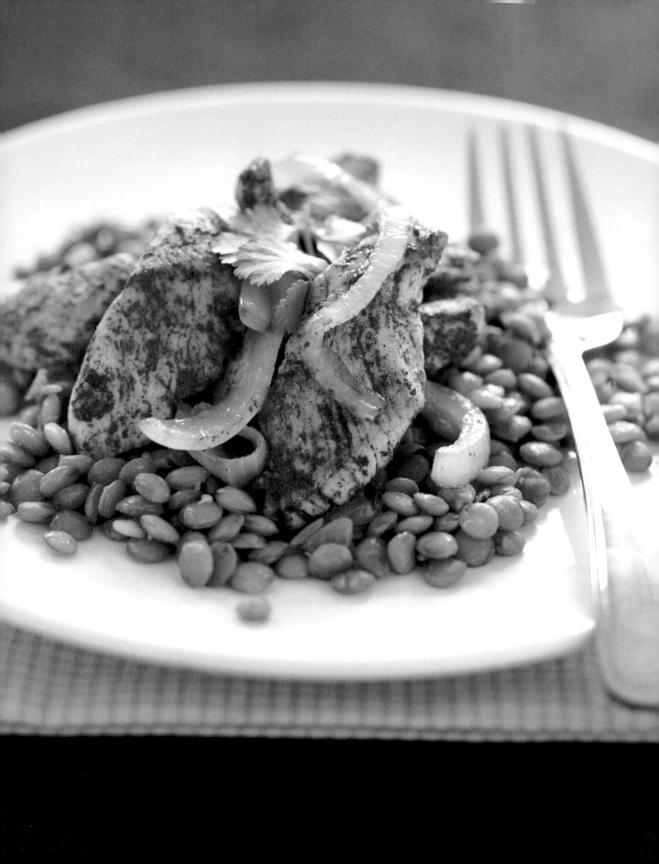

MOROCCAN CHICKEN AND LENTILS

Spices fire up your metabolism and this dish features several. The rich blend of ingredients in combination with the superb nutritional content of this one-dish meal makes it a must for your Clean-Eating table.

INGREDIENTS:

8 cups / 2 L water

3 tsp / 15 ml sea salt, divided

1 lb / 454 g dried lentils, rinsed, drained and picked over

1 cup plus 2 Tbsp / 270 ml best-quality olive oil

½ cup / 120 ml red wine vinegar

3 Tbsp / 45 ml ground cumin, divided

2 Tbsp plus 2 tsp / 40 ml chili powder

2 garlic cloves, peeled and minced

1 large onion, peeled and chopped

2 lbs / 908 g skinless, boneless chicken breast or turkey breast, thinly sliced

¼ tsp / 1.25 ml ground cinnamon

1 cup / 240 ml chopped fresh parsley or cilantro

PREPARATION:

1 Combine water and 1 tsp salt in stock pot over high heat. Add lentils. Bring to a boil. Cover and reduce heat to medium. Simmer until lentils are soft, about 20 to 25 minutes. Drain well. Rinse under cold water and drain well. Place in large bowl and set aside.

2 In small bowl, mix 1 cup olive oil, vinegar, 2 Tbsp cumin, 2 Tbsp chili powder, garlic and 1 tsp sea salt. Pour this dressing over lentils. Toss gently and let cool.

3 In large skillet heat 2 Tbsp olive oil. Add onion and sauté until well cooked, about 5 minutes. Onion should appear dark brown and soft. Add chicken or turkey and sauté 2 minutes more. Add 1 tsp / 5 ml sea salt, 1 Tbsp / 15 ml cumin, 2 tsp / 10 ml chili powder and cinnamon. Sauté until poultry is cooked through.

4 Arrange lentils on a large serving platter. Place sliced chicken on top of lentils. Use remaining dressing and pour over chicken. Sprinkle with chopped parsley. Serve at room temperature.

NUTRITIONAL VALUE PER SERVING:
Calories: 391 | Calories from Fat: 181 | Protein: 28g | Carbs: 25g
Dietary Fiber: 5g | Sugars: 3g | Fat: 20g | Sodium: 564mg

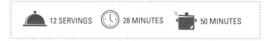

12 SERVINGS   28 MINUTES   50 MINUTES

STUFFED PUMPKINS

Pumpkins were valued by First Nations peoples for their nutritional value. The flesh from these beautifully colored orbs sustained many tribes in the earliest days of North America. Pumpkins can be prepared as sweet or savory and their interesting shapes make them perfect for use as a serving dish, too. Your family and dinner guests will be impressed with this dish served in their very own pumpkin!

INGREDIENTS:

1 x 4 to 5 lb / 2 kg sugar pumpkin or
    6 small sugar pumpkins

2 tsp / 10 ml sea salt

1 tsp / 5 ml dry mustard

1 Tbsp / 15 ml extra virgin olive oil

1½ lbs / 672 g lean ground venison or bison

7 green onions, trimmed and chopped

4 cloves garlic passed through a garlic press

1½ cups / 360 ml cooked wild rice

4 egg whites + 1 yolk, beaten

1 tsp / 5 ml dried sage, crumbled

½ tsp / 2.5 ml fresh ground black pepper

TIP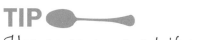

Use an acorn squash if you can't find a pumpkin. Just slice off the point so the squash can sit flat.

PREPARATION:

1 Preheat oven to 350°F / 177°C.

2 Cut the top from each pumpkin and remove seeds and strings. Prick the inside flesh with a fork. In a small bowl mix the sea salt and dry mustard. Rub the interior of the pumpkin with this mixture. Set pumpkins aside.

3 In a large skillet heat olive oil. Add ground meat, onion and garlic. Sauté over medium high until meat is browned. Remove from heat. Drain excess oil. Add cooked wild rice, eggs, sage and pepper. Mix well with clean hands. Stuff each pumpkin with the meat / rice mixture.

3 Place the pumpkin(s) in a shallow baking dish or lasagna pan. Add water until half of the baking dish is full.

4 Bake for 1 to 1½ hours or until pumpkin is tender. If using individual pumpkins, cooking time may be less. If using a large pumpkin cooking time may be more. When serving a large pumpkin, cut it into six wedges and serve. When serving individual pumpkins, place on individual serving plates.

NUTRITIONAL VALUE PER SERVING:
Calories: 345 | Calories from Fat: 99 | Protein: 32g | Carbs: 30g
Dietary Fiber: 2g | Sugars: 4g | Fat: 11g | Sodium: 665mg

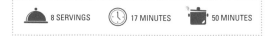
8 SERVINGS   17 MINUTES   50 MINUTES

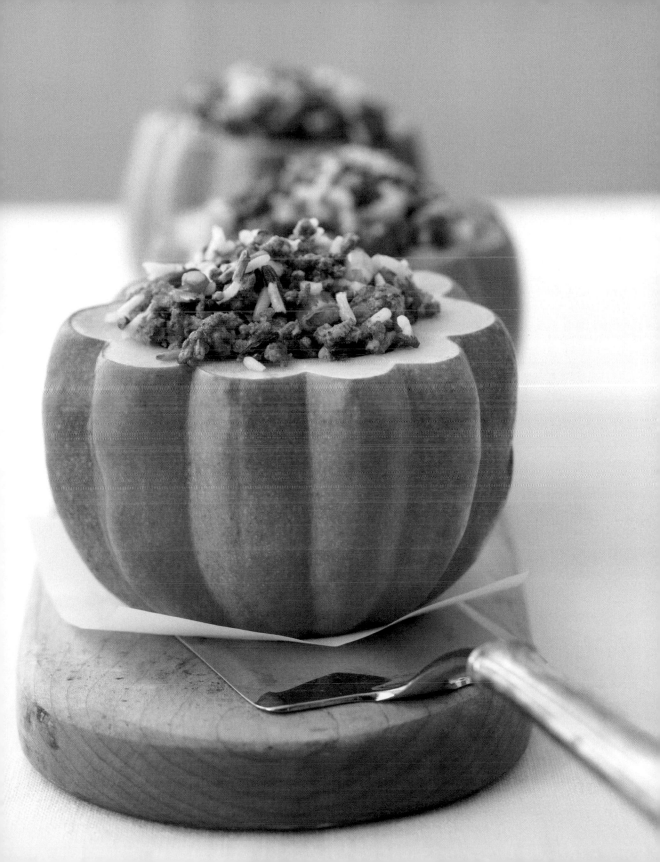

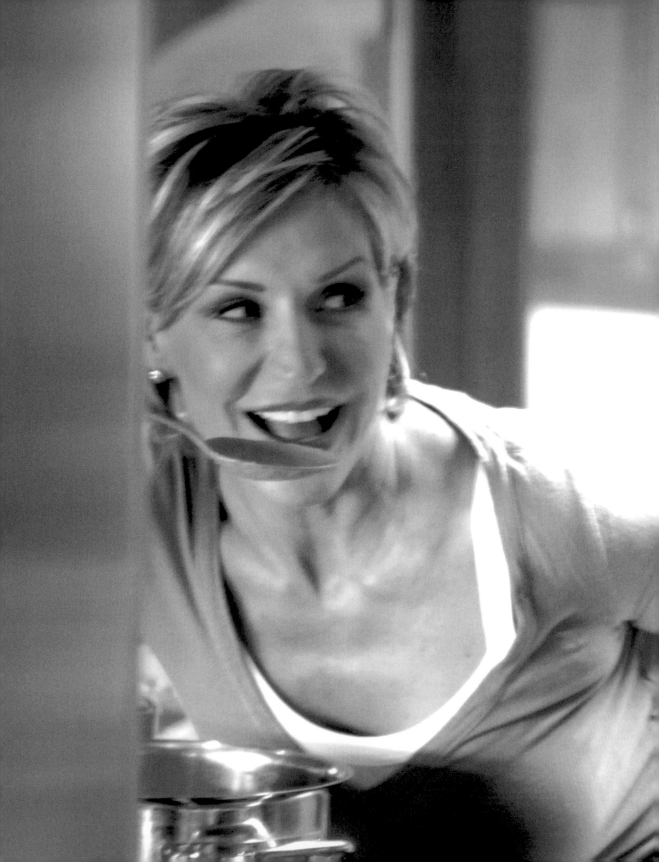

"I'll let you in on a little secret ... I don't spend hours in the kitchen! One-dish meals are my favorite way to save time and avoid doing dishes. They should be called one-dish wonders!"

VEGETARIAN CHILI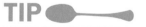

Beans are an ideal source of Clean-Eating protein and even those who aren't vegetarian love this "meaty" meatless chili recipe. It is still a satisfying version of chili without losing out on hearty flavor. Use leftovers in a wrap for lunch the next day.

INGREDIENTS:

2 Tbsp / 30 ml cumin seeds, toasted*

2 Tbsp / 30 ml extra virgin olive oil

1 medium yellow onion, peeled and chopped

1 large red bell pepper, chopped

1 large carrot, peeled and grated

1 head roasted garlic

    (see page 129 for Roasted Garlic)

3 Tbsp / 45 ml chili powder

¼ tsp / 1.25 ml red pepper flakes

Sea salt and fresh ground black pepper

1 cup / 240 ml canned white kidney beans, rinsed and drained

1 cup / 240 ml canned great Northern beans, rinsed and drained

1 cup / 240 ml canned red kidney beans, rinsed and drained

1 cup / 240 ml canned black beans, rinsed and drained

1 cup / 240 ml canned corn kernels, rinsed and drained

2½ cups / 600 ml water or low-sodium vegetable stock (gluten free if necessary)

2 tsp / 10 ml crumbled, dried oregano

2 tsp / 10 ml crumbled, dried basil

4 squares dark (75% or more cocoa) organic chocolate

28 oz / 784 g canned tomatoes

Juice of one fresh lime

Juice of one fresh lemon

PREPARATION:

1 In a Dutch oven, warm olive oil over medium heat. Add onion, pepper and grated carrot and sauté until onion becomes soft and translucent. Stir in chili powder, toasted cumin seeds, red pepper flakes, sea salt and black pepper. Cover and cook over low heat for 10 minutes, stirring occasionally.

2 Add all remaining ingredients. Blend well. Cover and let simmer for 20 minutes. Remove from heat and serve immediately. This recipe can be served over brown rice for a hearty variation. Leftovers are perfect in a wrap.

TIP

*To toast cumin seeds: place seeds in a skillet and warm over medium heat until you begin to smell the spices. Shake the pan vigorously so the seeds don't stick and burn. Remove from heat and set aside.

NUTRITIONAL VALUE PER SERVING:

Calories: 329 | Calories from Fat: 72 | Protein: 15g | Carbs: 56g
Dietary Fiber: 15g | Sugars: 9g | Fat: 8g | Sodium: 1190mg

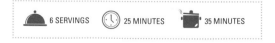

6 SERVINGS   25 MINUTES   35 MINUTES

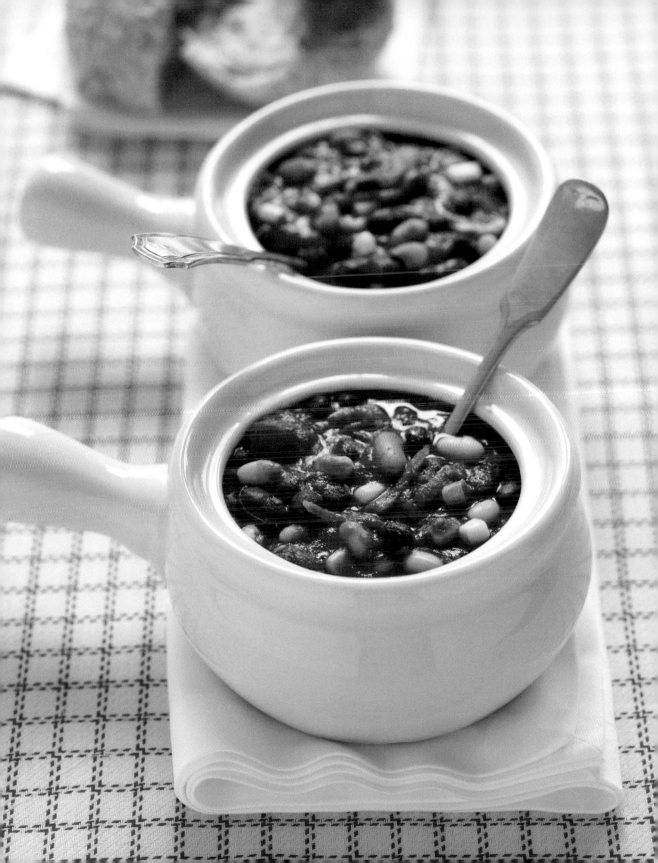

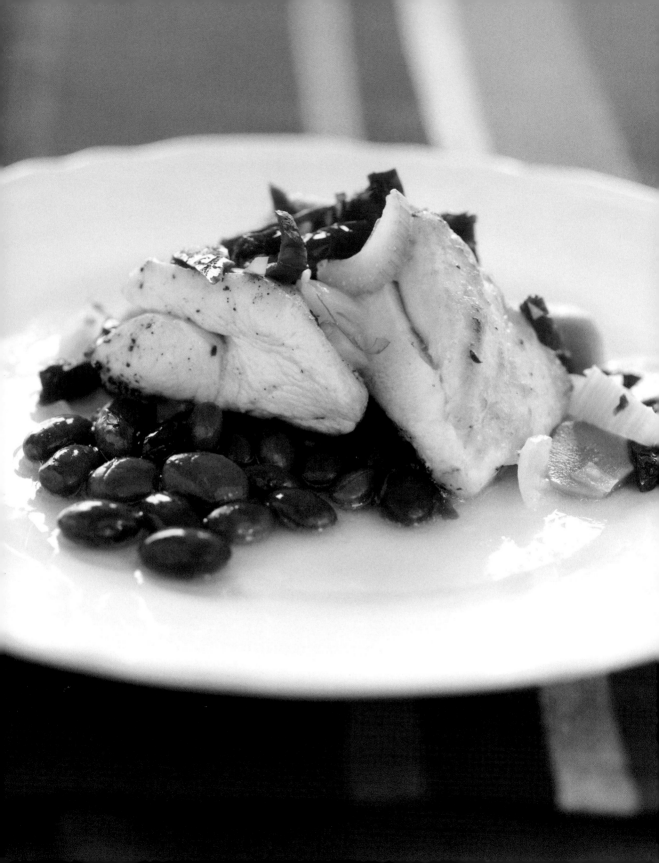

SLOW-COOKER CHICKEN CASSOULET

Cassoulet is a traditional French dish that is more like a stew. The basic ingredients include beans and meat, and it requires a long, slow cooking time. This is the perfect recipe for a slow cooker.

INGREDIENTS:

1 x 15 oz can / 420 g navy beans, pinto beans or
    black-eyed peas, rinsed and well drained

4 boneless, skinless chicken breasts or
    1 small skinless boneless turkey breast cut into
    4 large pieces

Sea salt and fresh ground black pepper

2 Tbsp / 30 ml extra virgin olive oil

1²/₃ cups / 400 ml low-sodium chicken stock (gluten
    free if necessary)

1 medium onion, peeled and chopped

4 celery stalks, trimmed and chopped

4 garlic cloves passed through a garlic press

¼ cup / 60 ml sundried tomatoes
    (not those packed in oil)

3 large carrots, peeled and cut into chunks

¼ cup / 60 ml fresh basil, chopped fine

1 tsp / 5 ml thyme

2 Tbsp / 30 ml fresh minced parsley

PREPARATION:

1 Spread half of the beans in the bottom of your slow-cooker pot.

2 Season poultry with pepper and sea salt. Heat olive oil over medium heat in a skillet. Brown the poultry on both sides in the skillet for about 5 minutes each side. Place the browned chicken on top of the beans in the slow cooker. Top with remaining beans and the chicken stock. Use water if you don't have chicken stock.

3 Sauté the onions, celery, garlic, sundried tomatoes, carrots and herbs using the same skillet. Spread this mixture over the ingredients in the crock pot. Cover and put on slow heat for several hours.

TIP

Serve with Ezekiel bread and one of the spreads from the previous chapter.

NUTRITIONAL VALUE PER SERVING:

Calories: 261 | Calories from Fat: 57 | Protein: 24g | Carbs: 24g
Dietary Fiber: 6g | Sugars: 3g | Fat: 6g | Sodium: 553mg

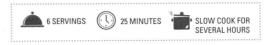

6 SERVINGS   25 MINUTES   SLOW COOK FOR SEVERAL HOURS

LENTIL STEW

Okay, so I have persuaded you to try lentils. Here is another recipe that will extend your lentil cooking powers and nourish your body and soul. This is a complete meal in a dish since it contains loads of complex carbohydrates as well as muscle-building protein.

INGREDIENTS:

1 cup / 240 ml Puy lentils

1 large onion, diced

4 cloves garlic, passed through garlic press

1 Tbsp / 15ml avocado or extra virgin olive oil

2 large carrots, coarsely chopped

2 ribs celery, diced

2 medium sweet potatoes, sliced

4 bay leaves

½ cup / 125 ml wheat berries or wild rice

1 Tbsp / 15 ml brown rice miso

½ tsp / 2.5 ml dried thyme

1 - 1 ½ cups low-sodium chicken stock or
    vegetable stock
    – if needed (gluten free if necessary)

Sea salt and pepper

PREPARATION:

1 Prepare lentils according to package instructions. Lentils should be chewy, not soft.

2 In a large skillet, sauté onion and garlic together for about 2 minutes in oil. Add remaining vegetables and bay leaves and continue to cook 5 minutes more. Add wild rice or wheat berries and continue to cook 35 minutes. If stew is too thick, dilute with water or stock.

3 Mix one tablespoon of water with the miso and add to stew. Add cooked lentils. Cover and simmer another 15 minutes. Season with salt and pepper and thyme. Remove from heat and serve.

TIP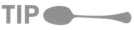

Gabriella Caruso, the wonderful art director here at Robert Kennedy Publishing, tells me that in her home country of Italy it is said that if you eat lentils you will grow rich — I don't know if that's true, but you will certainly be rich in health. Eat up!

NUTRITIONAL VALUE PER SERVING:

Calories: 240 | Calories from Fat: 28 | Protein: 11g | Carbs: 42g
Dietary Fiber: 13g | Sugars: 4g | Fat: 3g | Sodium: 164mg

6 SERVINGS   10 MINUTES   1 HOUR

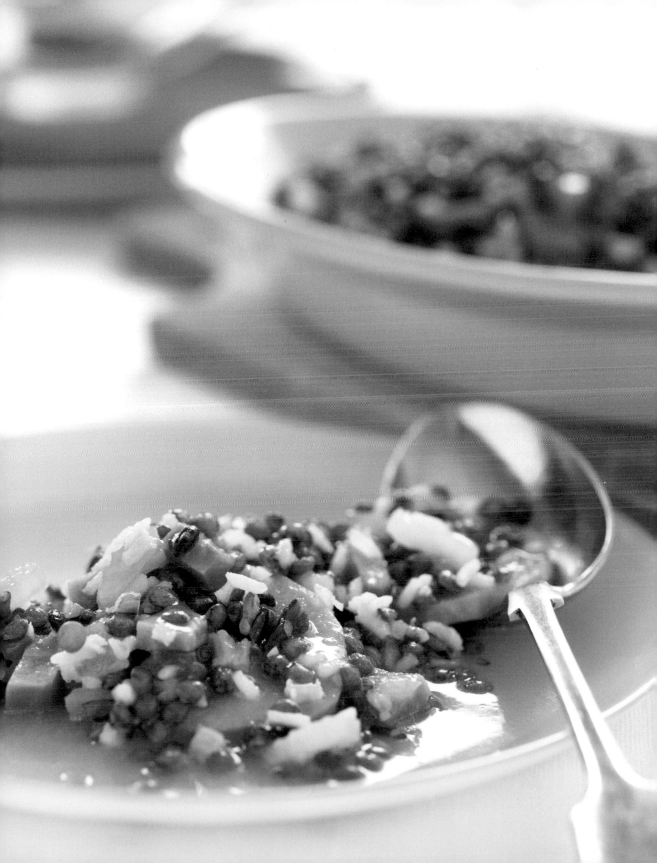

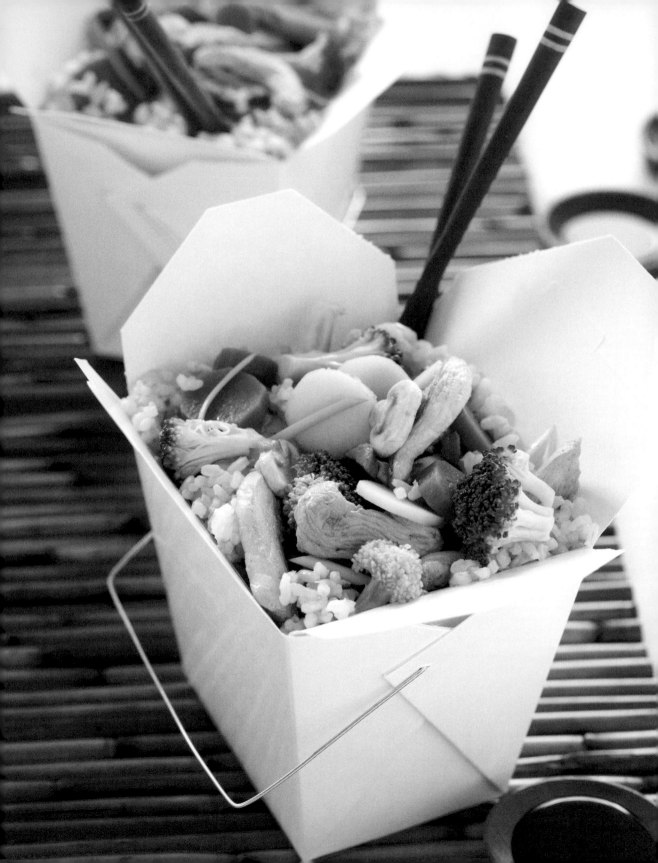

CHINESE CHICKEN AND RICE

Will there ever be enough ways to prepare chicken? It is the most versatile protein source available. This is a quick but healthy version of a popular favorite. Add your favorite vegetables to this dish to tailor it to your own palate or to that of your family. Brown rice makes it even healthier.

INGREDIENTS:

1 pound boneless, skinless chicken breasts, cut into julienne strips. If vegetarian, use tofu, cut into cubes

2 cups / 480 ml water

1 cup / 240 ml brown rice

½ tsp / 2.5 ml sea salt

2 Tbsp olive oil

2 cloves garlic, minced

1½ cups / 360 ml broccoli florets

1 cup / 240 ml sliced mushrooms

½ cup / 120 ml sliced water chestnuts

1 cup / 240 ml penny-sliced carrots

1 cup / 240 ml green onions, sliced

MARINADE:

2 Tbsp / 30 ml extra virgin olive oil

1 Tbsp / 15 ml minced ginger root

2 tsp /10 ml low-sodium soy sauce or gluten-free tamari

1 clove garlic, minced

Dash hot pepper sauce

PREPARATION:

1 Combine all marinade ingredients. Place chicken in marinade and let stand for 1 hour in refrigerator. Meanwhile, preheat oven to 350°F / 177°C. Prepare a six-quart covered casserole dish with cooking spray. Add rice, water and salt and bake for 40 minutes or until all the liquid is absorbed.

2 Meanwhile, heat olive oil in a large skillet and gently sauté garlic until just fragrant. Add sliced chicken and sauté until no longer pink. Add chopped vegetables and cook until just soft. Remove from heat. Add the cooked vegetable mixture to the rice when it is finished baking. Serve piping hot for a delicious Clean-Eating meal.

NUTRITIONAL VALUE PER SERVING:

Calories: 269 | Calories from Fat: 60 | Protein: 21g | Carbs: 30g
Dietary Fiber: 3g | Sugars: 12g | Fat: 6g | Sodium: 380mg

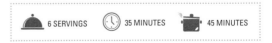 6 SERVINGS · 35 MINUTES · 45 MINUTES

STIR-FRY 101

Here's the scoop on how to create your own fabulous stir-fry any day of the week. Let your kids get in on the creative process. There is no right or wrong ingredient list. Whatever happens to be in your refrigerator often works. Well, maybe not those leftover pizzas … Be sure to have a steaming hot dish of brown rice ready to serve with your stir-fry creation.

CLEAN-EATING INGREDIENT LIST:

If serving 4 people use 1 lb / 454 g of lean protein

Lean protein choices: beef tenderloin; boneless, skinless chicken or turkey breast; firm tofu; large shrimp

2 tsp / 10 ml **low-sodium soy sauce or tamari**

2 tsp / 10 ml **lemon juice**

4 cloves **garlic,** passed through a garlic press

1 Tbsp / 15 ml **fresh grated ginger root**

4 **scallions,** trimmed and chopped

2 Tbsp + 1 tsp / 35 ml **extra virgin olive, canola** or **avocado oil**

1 tsp / 5 ml **toasted sesame oil**

2 lbs / 908g of **fresh vegetables** cut into-bite sized pieces for the stir-fry *(see chart to the right)*

Please note: To avoid gluten, make sure to use gluten-free tamari rather than soy sauce, and make sure any stock is gluten free.

INSTRUCTIONS:

1 Marinate the protein choice – beef, poultry, tofu or shrimp – in soy sauce or tamari and lemon juice, in a small glass bowl.

2 In another small bowl, mix garlic, ginger, scallions, 2 Tbsp / 30 ml oil and sesame oil.

3 In a large skillet heat 1 tsp / 5 ml oil over high heat. Add protein choice and brown. Transfer to a bowl and cover with a plate.

4 Stir-fry the vegetables in batches, adding more oil as you go if needed. Transfer each cooked batch to the bowl containing the cooked protein and cover.

5 Put ginger and garlic mixture in the skillet and heat through. Place all cooked ingredients back in the skillet and toss while reheating the mixture. You can add a stir-fry sauce at this point *(recipe for stir-fry sauce follows).*

NUTRITIONAL VALUE PER SERVING:

Calories: 182 | Calories from Fat: 57| Protein: 25g | Carbs: 9g
Dietary Fiber: 2g | Sugars: 3g | Fat: 6g | Sodium: 351mg

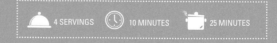
4 SERVINGS   10 MINUTES   25 MINUTES

GARLICKY STIR-FRY SAUCE

INGREDIENTS:

½ cup / 120 ml **low-sodium chicken stock,**
    vegetable stock or **water**

4 Tbsp / 60 ml **fresh-squeezed lemon juice**

4 Tbsp / 60 ml **fresh-squeezed orange juice**

2 Tbsp / 30 ml **hoisin sauce**

2 Tbsp / 30 ml **low-sodium soy sauce or tamari**

2 Tbsp / 10 ml **corn starch**

4 cloves **garlic,** passed through a garlic press

1 tsp / 5 ml **toasted sesame oil**

Pinch sea salt

INSTRUCTIONS:

1 Whisk all ingredients together in a small bowl.

2 Add the sauce to the stir-fry mixture near the end of the cooking process. Heat through until mixture is bubbly.

NUTRITIONAL VALUE PER SERVING:

Calories: 42 | Calories from Fat: 10 | Protein: 1g |
Carbs: 6g | Dietary Fiber: 0.25g | Sugars: 3g | Fat: 1g |
Sodium: 662.5mg

4 SERVINGS   8 MINUTES   0 MINUTES

STIR-FRY VEGGIES

Some vegetables take longer to cook in the stir-fry process so it is important to know which are fast cooking and which are slow. Here's your handy reference:

STIR-FRY VEGGIES' COOKING TIMES

1 - 5 MINUTES	Onions
	Sweet peppers
	Mushrooms
	Asparagus
	Bok choy
	Carrots
	Celery
	Garlic
	Edamame

FAST COOKING	Spinach
	Green onions
	Nappa cabbage
	Snow peas
	Leafy greens
	Zucchini
	Corn
	Water chestnuts

LONG COOKING MORE THAN 5 MINUTES	Hard squash
	Green or yellow beans
	Broccoli
	Broccoli rabe
	Cauliflower
	Hard cabbage varieties – green or purple

EAT-CLEAN CHICKEN AND RICE

While the name may suggest a boring recipe, it is quite deceiving. This Clean-Eating meal is loaded with flavor from delicious seasonings and a wide variety of vegetables. A one-dish meal that will satisfy both your tummy and your taste buds; what more could you ask for?

INGREDIENTS:

6 boneless, skinless chicken breasts, cooked
1 Tbsp olive oil
1 medium onion, peeled and chopped
4 cloves garlic, passed through a garlic press
1 tsp / 5 ml chopped fresh thyme
1 tsp / 5 ml fresh rosemary
Sea salt (+ more for seasoning) along with ground black pepper
3 cups / 720 ml low-sodium chicken broth (gluten free if necessary)
1½ cups / 360 ml brown rice
¾ lbs / 336 g fresh broccoli florets
1 cup / 240 ml carrots, peeled and cut into penny slices, then parboiled
½ cup / 120 ml edamame, frozen

PREPARATION:

1 In a large skillet, heat olive oil over medium temperature. Add onion, garlic, thyme, rosemary and sea salt. Cover and cook over low heat until the onion has softened — about 10 minutes. Add chicken broth. Stir in the brown rice and cook uncovered over high heat for 5 minutes. Cover and reduce heat to low. Cook for 20 minutes.

2 Place the chicken breasts over the rice in the skillet. Cook for another 15 minutes, making sure the chicken is heated through. Once the chicken is done remove it from the pan and put it on a clean platter. Cover it with tin foil or another plate.

3 Add the broccoli, edamame and parboiled carrots to the rice mixture. Heat through 10 minutes. Season with sea salt and pepper. Remove from heat. Serve rice immediately, along with one chicken breast.

NUTRITIONAL VALUE PER SERVING:
Calories: 356 | Calories from Fat: 71 | Protein: 35g | Carbs: 44g
Dietary Fiber: 4g | Sugars: 2g | Fat: 7g | Sodium: 616mg

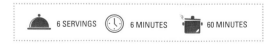

6 SERVINGS   6 MINUTES   60 MINUTES

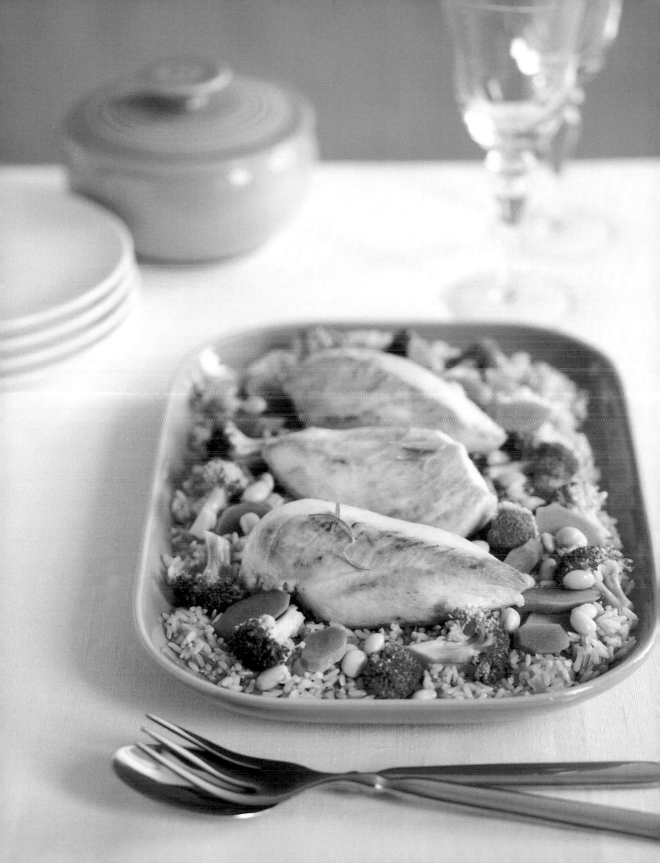

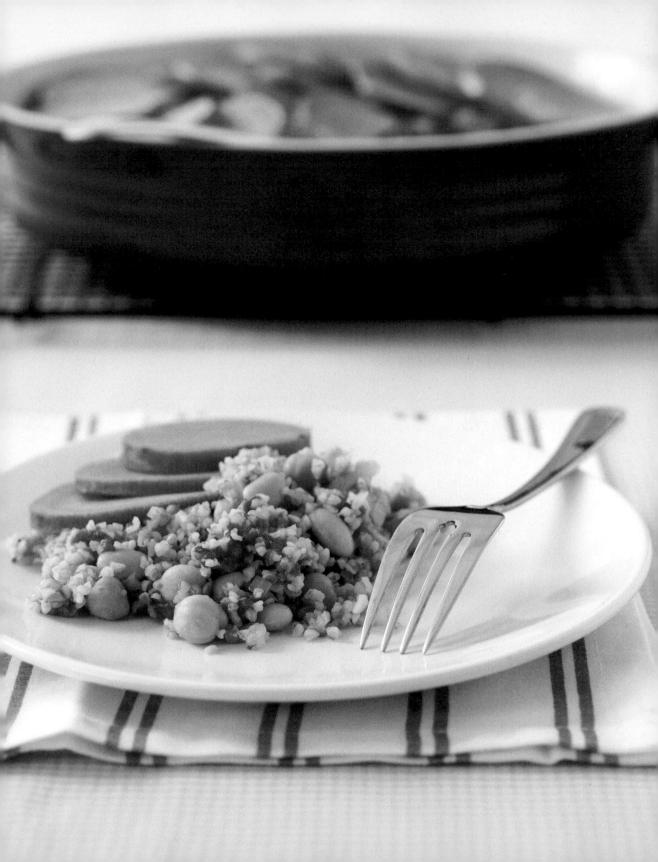

SHEPHERD'S PIE WITHOUT THE SHEEP

Shepherd's pie is a food I recall from my childhood as the ultimate comfort food. I adore its simplicity and mouthwatering taste and texture. My mom made a wonderful shepherd's pie, which I have borrowed and changed a little to suit Clean-Eating menus. Hope you don't mind, Mom.

INGREDIENTS:

1 tsp / 5 ml extra virgin olive oil

1 medium onion, peeled and chopped

2 ribs celery, trimmed and chopped

4 cloves fresh garlic, passed through a garlic press

¾ cup / 180 ml bulgur or wheat berries (if you can't eat wheat use buckwheat or brown rice instead)

1 tsp / 5 ml crumbled, dried oregano

1 tsp / 5 ml crumbled, dried basil

1 tsp / 5 ml crumbled, dried parsley

Pinch red pepper flakes

1½ cups / 360 ml low-sodium vegetable stock (gluten free if necessary) or water

1 cup / 240 ml canned stewed tomatoes

2 sweet potatoes

1 cup / 240 ml chickpeas, drained and rinsed

1 cup / 240 ml frozen edamame

Sea salt and fresh ground black pepper

PREPARATION:

1 Preheat oven to 400°F / 204°C. In a large skillet heat olive oil. Add onion, celery, garlic, grain choice, oregano, basil, parsley and red pepper flakes. Cook until onion and celery become soft – about 5 minutes. Add stock or water and tomatoes. Allow mixture to come to a boil. Reduce heat and cover. Cook until the bulgur or grain you are using is tender.

2 Scrub sweet potatoes and cook. You can do this in the microwave (depending on size about 4 minutes) or bake them in the oven (about 45 minutes at 450°F / 232°C). Let cool when done.

3 Add chickpeas, edamame, and salt and pepper to the tomato and grain mixture. Stir well. Place all these ingredients in a prepared 6-quart casserole dish. Slice the cooked potato on top. Season with salt and pepper.

4 Bake in oven for about 15 minutes.

NUTRITIONAL VALUE PER SERVING:
Calories: 381 | Calories from Fat: 61 | Protein: 16g | Carbs: 63g
Dietary Fiber: 13g | Sugars: 8g | Fat: 6g | Sodium: 217mg

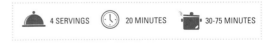

4 SERVINGS   20 MINUTES   30-75 MINUTES

WHITE CHICKEN CHILI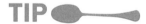

Anyone preferring a lean, mean white chili with a kick to it will enjoy the depth of flavor in this recipe. Not only does this white chili load up on lean protein but it is chock full of fiber, complex carbohydrates and tummy-satisfying nourishment. The fiery chiles will certainly heat up your metabolism, too.

INGREDIENTS:

3 medium Poblano chiles, stemmed, seeded and chopped

2 medium Jalapeno chili peppers, seeded and deveined, chopped

2 Vidalia onions, peeled and chopped

2 ribs celery, trimmed and chopped

1 large leek, white only, well rinsed and chopped

6 cloves garlic, passed through a garlic press

2 Tbsp / 30 ml ground cumin

2 Tbsp / 30 ml crumbled, dried oregano

2 Tbsp / 30 ml crumbled, dried basil

1 tsp / 5 ml fresh rosemary

1 Tbsp / 15 ml extra virgin olive oil

Sea salt and freshly ground black pepper

8 cups / 1.9 L water or low-sodium chicken stock (gluten free if necessary)

2 x 15 oz / 420 g cans navy beans, cannellini beans or other small white bean or combination, drained and rinsed

3 lbs / 1.4 kg boneless, skinless chicken breasts (about 3 double breasts), cooked and cubed

Juice from 2 fresh limes

Juice from 2 fresh lemons

½ cup / 120 ml chopped fresh cilantro leaves

4 green onions, trimmed and chopped for garnish

NUTRITIONAL VALUE PER SERVING:

Calories: 249 | Calories from Fat: 34 | Protein: 32g | Carbs: 24g
Dietary Fiber: 4g | Sugars: 5g | Fat: 0.3g | Sodium: 592mg

PREPARATION:

1 In a large saucepan or Dutch oven, place all chiles, onions, celery, leeks, garlic cloves, cumin, oregano, basil, rosemary, olive oil, sea salt and black pepper. Cook over medium heat until onions become translucent – about 10 minutes.

2 Add 8 cups / 1.9 L cooking liquid, beans and cubed chicken and bring mixture to a boil. Reduce heat and let mixture simmer for 40 minutes. Add lime and lemon juices, cilantro and green onions. Remove from heat and serve immediately.

TIP

I like to serve chili over brown rice. This gives me another serving of whole grains and it makes a perfect Clean-Eating meal.

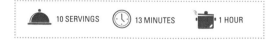

10 SERVINGS   13 MINUTES   1 HOUR

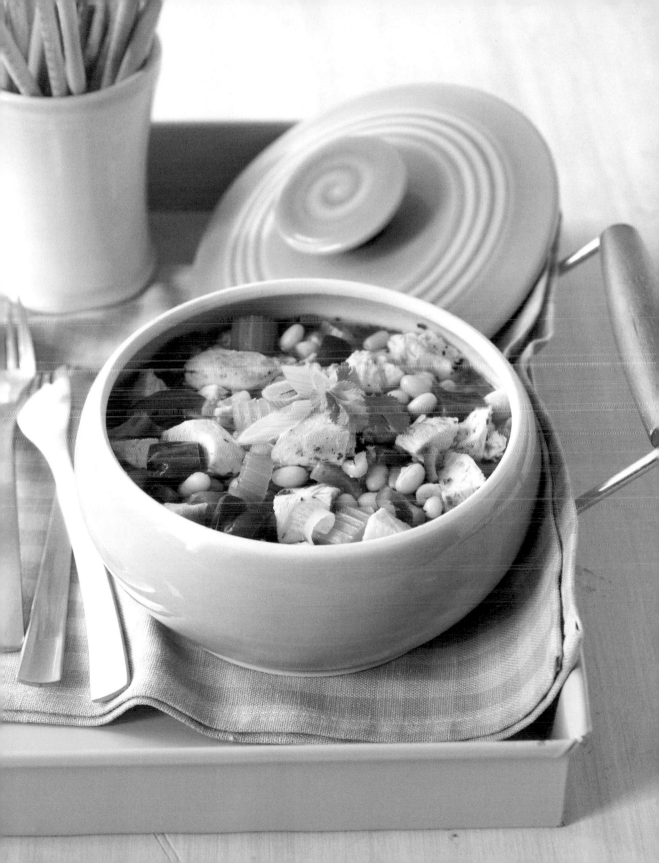

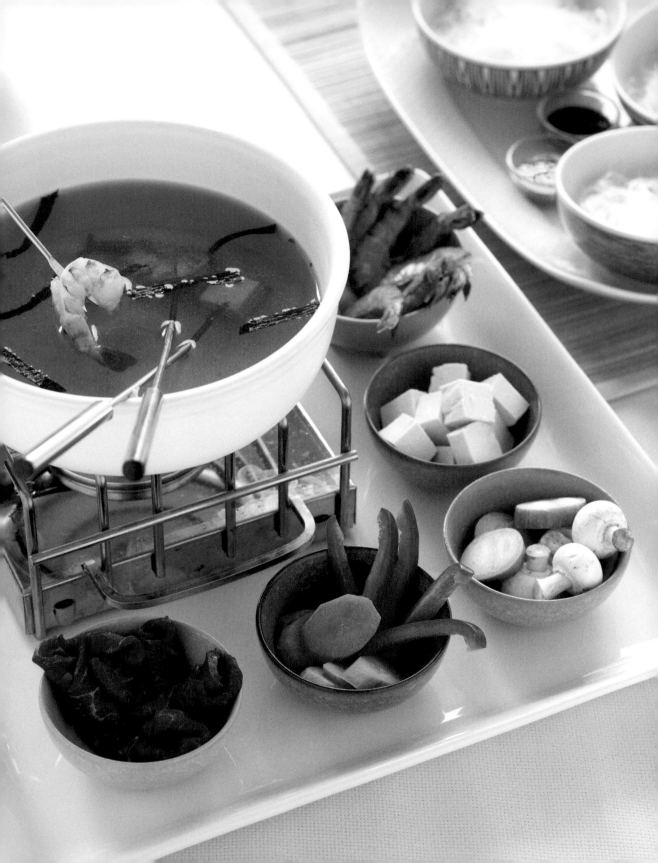

SHABU SHABU

Shabu shabu is a traditional Japanese fondue recipe and gets its name from the swishing sound that is made as the food is swished in the broth. Our family loves this as it is an intimate dinner experience. We all dip our chopsticks into the simmering pot and rub elbows with each other. A roar of laughter occurs every time someone drops food into the broth, which is often. We always make shabu shabu on Christmas Eve, but you can enjoy it any time!

INGREDIENTS:

½ lb / 227 g rice noodles or vermicelli

2 pieces of seaweed or kombu

1 lb / 454 g thinly sliced, lean beef or bison tenderloin

OR 1 lb / 454 g thinly sliced turkey breast or chicken breast

OR for vegetarians, 1 lb / 454 g firm tofu cut into 1" cubes

OR for fish lovers, 1½ lbs / 681 g large tiger shrimp, peeled and deveined

½ cup / 240 ml shallots, cut into 1-inch pieces

2 large carrots, peeled and thinly sliced – penny slice style

1 lb / 454 g button mushrooms, cleaned

1 large red sweet pepper, cut into strips

6 cups / 1.5 L low-sodium chicken or vegetable broth or plain water or combination (gluten free if necessary)

TIP

I always serve steaming bowls of brown rice with shabu shabu. This makes for a fun and truly delicious Clean- Eating meal.

PREPARATION:

1 Cook the rice noodles in a large pot of boiling water according to package instructions. Drain the noodles well and set aside.

2 Rinse the seaweed.

3 Bring low-sodium chicken broth to a boil. Add the seaweed and boil for another minute. Have a fondue pot ready. Strain the boiled broth and seaweed mixture into the fondue pot.

4 Have all the vegetables and meat in separate bowls on the table. Place the fondue pot in the middle where everyone can reach it. Keep the chicken broth hot. Offer both conventional cutlery and chopsticks with which to eat. Cook the food in the fondue pot.

ACCOMPANIMENTS: Provide several small bowls of favorite dipping sauces including ponzu, soy, tamarind, black bean garlic, chili garlic or plum.

NUTRITIONAL VALUE PER SERVING:

Calories: 391 | Calories from Fat: 21 | Protein: 34g | Carbs: 61g
Dietary Fiber: 3g | Sugar: 4g | Fat: 2g | Sodium: 1188mg

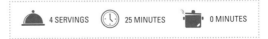

4 SERVINGS   25 MINUTES   0 MINUTES

SLOW-COOKER CHESTNUT STEW

I have to admit I have never really known what to do with chestnuts. All that roasting and shelling put me off. Chestnuts were a rarity on our plates, but there is good news. Fully cooked and cleaned chestnuts are available today. They should not be overlooked since they are a valuable source of important nutrients including protein, complex carbohydrates, vitamins and minerals. This recipe is wonderful on a blustery night when nothing but a heaping bowl of thick stew will satisfy the soul. This may be the meal you choose to drink a glass of red wine with to complete the experience.

INGREDIENTS:

3 lbs / 1.4 kg lean, boneless bison or beef, cut into 1
    inch chunks

⅓ cup / 80 ml amaranth flour or flour of your choice

½ tsp / 2.5 ml sea salt

½ tsp / 2.5 ml ground black pepper

1 Tbsp / 15 ml crumbled dried oregano

1 Tbsp / 15 ml crumbled dried basil

3 Tbsp / 45 ml extra virgin olive oil

1 large sweet onion, peeled and chopped fine

4 cloves garlic, passed through a garlic press

2 thick carrots, peeled and chopped

2 thick parsnips, peeled and chopped

4 ribs celery, trimmed and chopped

2 sweet potatoes, peeled and cut into one inch
    chunks

1 cup / 240 ml steamed chestnuts, chopped

1 Tbsp / 15 ml tomato paste

3 cups / 725 ml water or beef or vegetable stock,
    low sodium (gluten free if necessary)

PREPARATION:

1 In a container with a lid place the flour, sea salt, pepper, oregano and basil. Put the lid on the container and shake. Now add the cubed bison or beef to the flour and shake again to coat each piece with flour and seasonings. Set aside.

2 In a large skillet, place 1½ Tbsp / 23 ml olive oil and set over medium-high heat. Remove the meat cubes from the flour mixture one at a time. This ensures no excess of flour, and the coating on each cube will not be disturbed. Place the meat in the skillet. You may have to brown it in batches. Once the meat is nicely browned, remove from the skillet. Place the meat in the bowl of a slow cooker. Add all remaining ingredients to the slow cooker, mix gently and set to high. Cook covered for 6 hours. Serve hot!

NUTRITIONAL VALUE PER SERVING:

Calories: 454 | Calories from Fat: 203 | Protein: 42g | Carbs: 16g
Dietary Fiber: 5g | Sugar: 3g | Fat: 22g | Sodium: 151mg

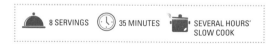

8 SERVINGS   35 MINUTES   SEVERAL HOURS' SLOW COOK

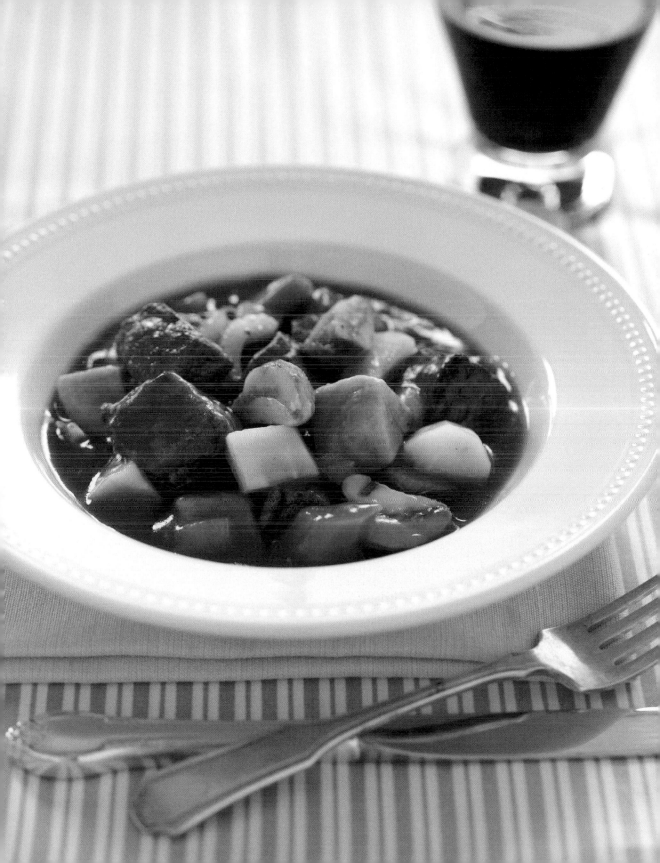

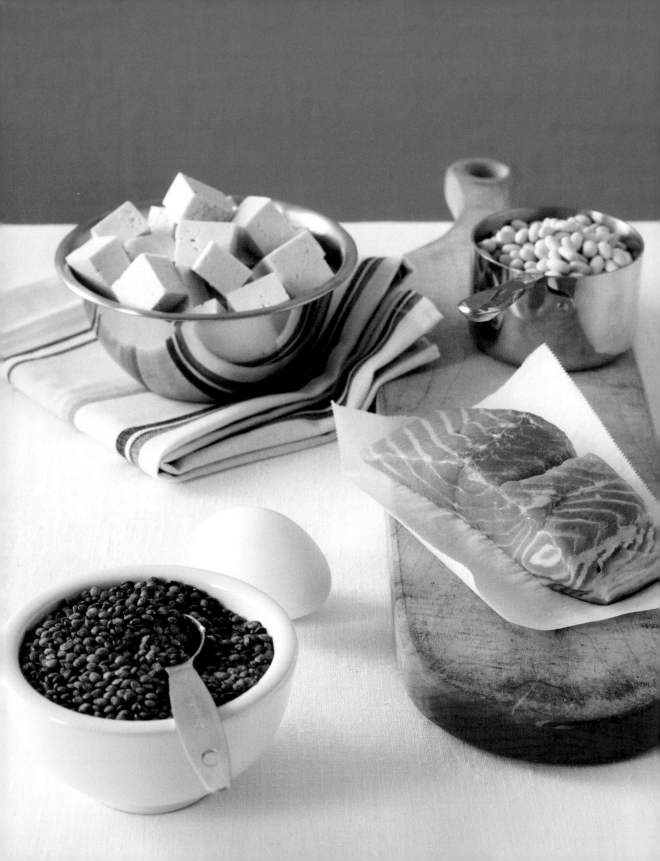

6

Proteins

It's easy to think Clean Eating might fall into the category of a high-protein diet. In fact Eating Clean advocates pairing lean protein with complex carbohydrates at every meal. There is never an abnormally high or low consumption of this essential building material. Besides, what is a "high-protein diet?" High relative to what? The body can assimilate 25 grams of protein at each meal. Clean Eating supports that number. It would be better to say Clean Eating is a diet well balanced in carbohydrate and protein consumption.

LOW-FAT TURKEY BURGERS

I love a great-tasting burger just like anyone else, but the fat content of a regular one is way too high for my Clean-Eating purposes. I played around with a few turkey-based burger recipes and this one always comes up as the family favorite. I think you'll agree it is just as delicious as a regular burger but is much lower in fat and calories.

INGREDIENTS:

1 cup / 240 ml high-protein cereal flakes

½ cup /120 ml skim milk

3 tsp / 15 ml instant low-sodium chicken bouillon

3 Tbsp / 45 ml minced onion

2 egg whites

1 lb / 454 g lean ground turkey

PREPARATION:

1 Combine first five ingredients in a large bowl. Let the milk soak into the cereal flakes for 5 minutes. Add lean ground turkey. Mix well with clean bare hands. Shape into patties and grill.

2 Serve hot with lightly toasted Ezekiel buns or whole-grain buns. Avoid high-fat condiments such as mayonnaise. But definitely add mustard, low-sodium, low-sugar ketchup, lettuce and slices of fresh tomato. Enjoy!

NUTRITIONAL VALUE PER SERVING:
Calories: 209 | Calories from Fat: 51 | Protein: 29g | Carbs: 9g
Dietary Fiber: 1g | Sugars: 1g | Fat: 5g | Sodium: 810mg

6 SERVINGS   20 MINUTES   15 MINUTES

EGGS – THE PERFECT EAT-CLEAN PROTEIN

Have you ever asked yourself whether a white egg or a brown egg is better? Most of us have but the truth is there is no nutritional difference. Both colors deliver equally lean, perfect protein. In fact egg whites are the standard against which all other proteins are measured. Egg whites contain all essential amino acids and are a rich source of complete protein. Eggs are also rich in B vitamins, iron and minerals.

When you are in a pinch trying to decide what to eat always consider egg whites since they are an ideal Clean-Eating food. Each whole egg contains an average of 71 calories but the egg white contains only

about 16 calories. There is so much easily digestible protein in an egg white you will want to eat plenty of them. Just throw out the yolks or eat one yolk for every five or six egg whites.

The body can assimilate only about 25 grams of protein at a time. If one egg white contains about 4 grams of protein you'll need to eat about 5 to 7 egg whites to get the ideal amount. I'm giving a range because eggs vary in size and people vary in size. Egg whites are considered to be the "perfect food." They are portable, coming in their own handy carrying case, and they are mighty nutritious.

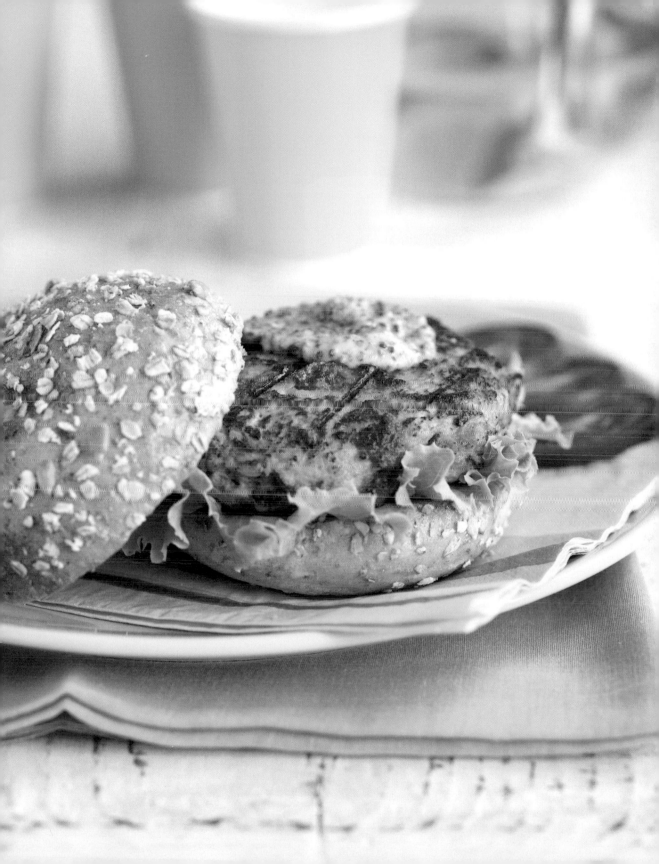

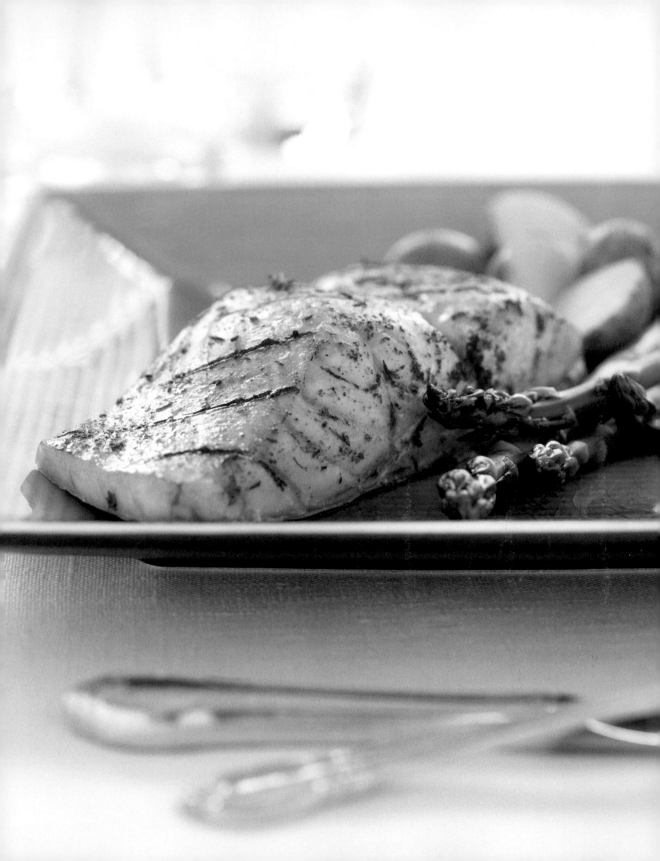

SALMON IN BRINE

Brine is a salt and seasoning solution used to saturate meat or other foodstuffs with flavor and moisture. Brining is often done with turkey and other poultry since it has a tendency to be dry. Salmon benefits from the process too, since there is a fine line between perfectly grilled salmon and the shoe leather that often comes off the grill.

POTLATCH SEASONING FOR SALMON:

2 tsp / 10 ml sea salt

¾ tsp / 4 ml ground cumin

½ tsp / 2.5 ml crumbled, dried oregano leaf

¼ tsp / 1.25 ml garlic powder

¼ tsp / 1.25 ml chili powder

½ tsp / 2.5 ml freshly ground black pepper

Mix all ingredients well.

BRINED POULTRY

This is a wonderful way to prepare a small turkey or chicken. Make the same brine and allow to cool. Place the uncooked bird in the brine solution and let marinate. Whole birds usually require more marinating time. I put mine in the fridge overnight. The trick here is to find a container deep enough to cover the meat completely. I like to add the usual poultry seasonings – parsley, sage, rosemary and thyme – to the chilled brining solution. Use whole seasonings if possible. Once the poultry has been sufficiently brined, rinse and dry. Then roast in the usual way.

A WORD OF ADVICE:

If you are on a low-sodium diet for medical reasons, use smaller portions of this dish.

HOW TO BRINE:

1 Heat 6 to 8 cups (about 1.7 L) of water in a large saucepan. Add 2 cups / 480 ml kosher salt and 1 cup / 240 ml organic sugar to the water. Add ¼ cup / 60 ml dried juniper berries and 4 tablespoons / 60 ml potlatch seasoning – see recipe at left. Bring brine to an optimal heat to allow the salt and sugar to dissolve. No rolling boil! Remove from heat and allow to cool. The brine then needs to be refrigerated. Place about 4 pounds / 1.8 kg of salmon in the brine. The fish should be completely covered with brine solution. Let the fish soak for about 2 hours. Remove the fish from the brine with a slotted spoon and rinse. Let the fish sit on a plate that has been covered in a few layers of paper towel.

2 Preheat your grill to high.

3 Brush salmon fillets with a coating of extra virgin olive oil – this will prevent the fish from sticking to the grill. Grill the first side for 5 minutes. Turn over and grill the other side for 4 minutes. The idea is to have the meat feel firm but not solid after cooking. If you are using a meat thermometer, let it register 130°F / 54°C. Remove the fish from the grill and place on a heated platter. Cover with another dish or tin foil until ready to serve.

TURKEY BREAST
with Leek and Oatmeal Stuffing

Oatmeal turns up not only for breakfast, but for dinner as well. Try this novel idea for stuffing, using wholesome leeks and oatmeal in place of breadcrumbs.

INGREDIENTS:

1 Tbsp / 15 ml olive oil

½ yellow onion, peeled and chopped

1 small leek, well rinsed and chopped

¼ cup / 60 ml rolled oats

½ tsp / 2.5 ml dried sage

½ cup / 120 ml dried rosemary

½ cup / 120 ml dried thyme

Sea salt and black pepper

1 boneless, skinless turkey breast, approximately
   3 pounds

PREPARATION:

1 In medium skillet coated with olive oil, sauté onion and leek until soft. Be careful not to burn. Add oatmeal, herbs, spices, salt and pepper, and stir. Let stuffing mixture cool slightly.

2 Butterfly the turkey breast to create a pocket in which to place the stuffing. Fill the pocket with the stuffing mixture. Use kitchen twine to tie the breast if necessary.

3 Place in shallow roasting pan and cover with parchment paper. Bake at 350°F / 177°C for about 60 minutes, depending on size of breast. Serve immediately.

NOTE: Remember if you cannot tolerate gluten, purchase oats guaranteed uncontaminated by other grains.

NUTRITIONAL VALUE PER SERVING:
Calories: 202 | Calories from Fat: 30 | Protein: 31g | Carbs: 11g
Dietary Fiber: 4.5g | Sugars: 0.56g | Fat: 3g | Sodium: 122mg

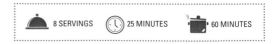

8 SERVINGS   25 MINUTES   60 MINUTES

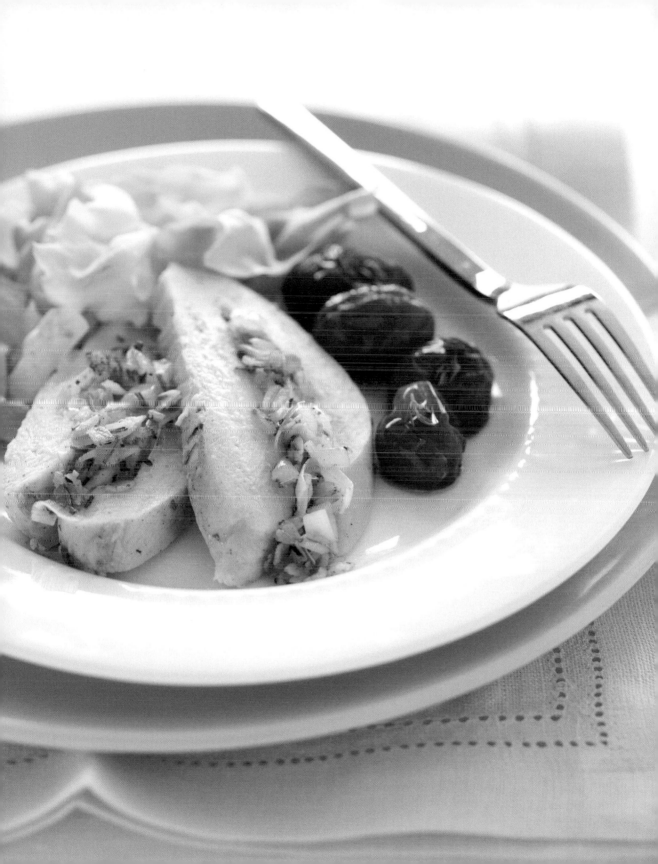

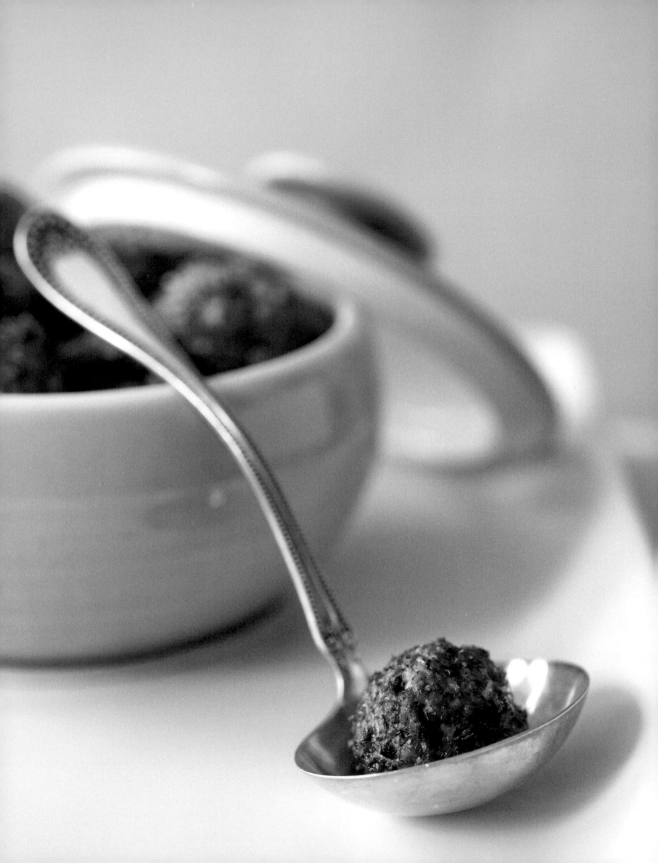

EVERY DAY IS A MEATBALL DAY!

When you feel like something fun for dinner, make meatballs. The kids love them and cold meatballs sliced onto your lunchtime pita are delicious. Much better than processed meat! Enjoy these with spaghetti too.

INGREDIENTS:

1½ lbs / 672 g lean ground turkey or chicken or if vegetarian, use textured vegetable protein

½ cup / 120 ml finely chopped onion

1 egg, lightly beaten

1 cup / 240 ml oat bran or breadcrumbs

2 Tbsp / 30 ml fresh parsley, finely chopped

2 Tbsp / 30 ml fresh basil, finely chopped

2 Tbsp / 30 ml fresh oregano, finely chopped

2 cloves garlic, passed through a garlic press

1 tsp / 5 ml sea salt

1 tsp / 5 ml freshly ground black pepper

PREPARATION:

1 Preheat oven to 400°F / 204°C.

2 In a large bowl place egg and breadcrumbs or oat bran. Add spices and mix well. Add remaining ingredients and mix well. Using an ice cream scoop make meatballs and place on prepared cookie sheet. Place in hot oven and bake for 20 minutes or until golden.

TIP

Make it gluten free by making your own breadcrumbs. Simply use day-old gluten-free bread and place it in a food processor. Pulse until crumbs are of the correct texture.

NUTRITIONAL VALUE PER SERVING:

Calories: 170 | Calories from Fat: 24 | Protein: 30g | Carbs: 11g
Dietary Fiber: 2g | Sugars: 0.8g | Fat: 2g | Sodium: 327mg

 6 SERVINGS | 30 MINUTES | 20 MINUTES

TOFU CABBAGE ROLLS 🍃 🐂 🌾

Many of you have requested more ideas for vegetarian eating. I consider tofu to be a wonder food. It takes on the flavor of whatever you are cooking it with, so it is never boring. Quite the opposite of what you might think when you open up a block of commercially prepared tofu – it does look boring, and a little scary! Think of it as a blank page upon which you can write anything. Don't tell the kids what it is until after they eat it!

INGREDIENTS:

½ purple onion, chopped fine

3 cloves garlic, put through garlic press

1 cup / 240 ml grated carrot

1 rib celery, chopped fine

1 Tbsp / 15 ml extra virgin olive oil

1 block tofu – about one pound medium firm

¼ cup / 60 ml fresh basil, chopped

¼ cup / 60 ml fresh parsley, chopped

3 Tbsp / 45 ml low-sodium soy sauce or gluten-free tamari

4 quarts / 3.8 L water

6 large green or savoy cabbage leaves

(have a few extra leaves handy in case one gets damaged while cooking)

PREPARATION:

1 In large nonstick skillet, sauté onion, garlic, carrot and celery in olive oil. Crumble tofu into skillet. Add herbs. Cook a few minutes more until heated through. Add soy sauce or tamari and mix well. Remove from heat and set aside.

2 In medium saucepan bring 4 quarts water to a boil. Place cabbage leaves in boiling water. Reduce heat and let cabbage cook briefly until it just changes color. Remove from water immediately and run under cold water. Set on paper towel to drain.

3 Divide tofu mixture among the six cabbage leaves. Roll cabbage carefully so tofu mixture doesn't fall out and leaves don't split. Place cabbage rolls in steamer basket and steam for 10 minutes. If you don't have a steamer you can use a grill pan to grill the rolls with a little cooking spray. Serve hot!

NUTRITIONAL VALUE PER SERVING:
Calories: 158 | Calories from Fat: 82 | Protein: 13g | Carbs: 9g
Dietary Fiber: 3g | Sugars: 2g | Fat: 9g | Sodium: 488mg

6 SERVINGS   25 MINUTES   35 MINUTES

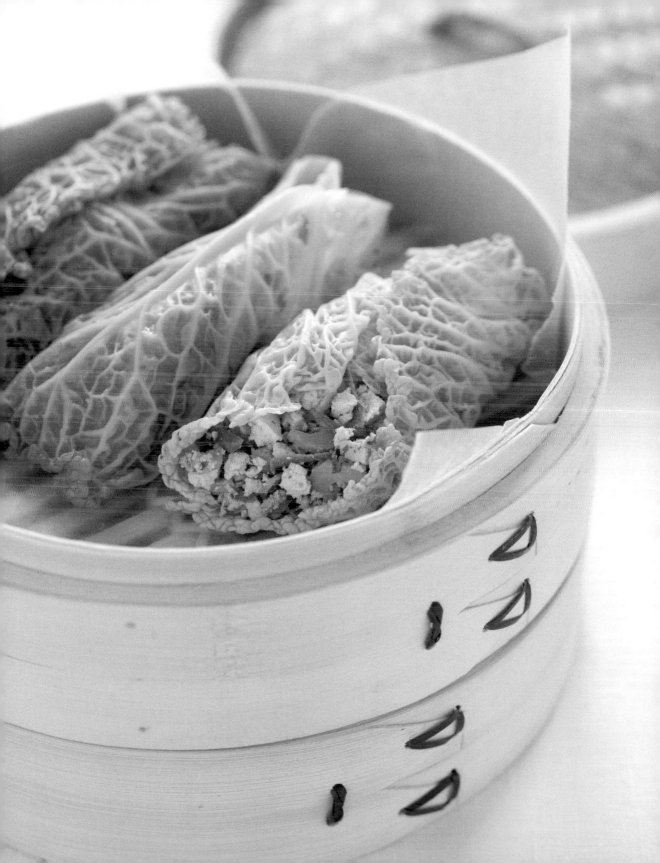

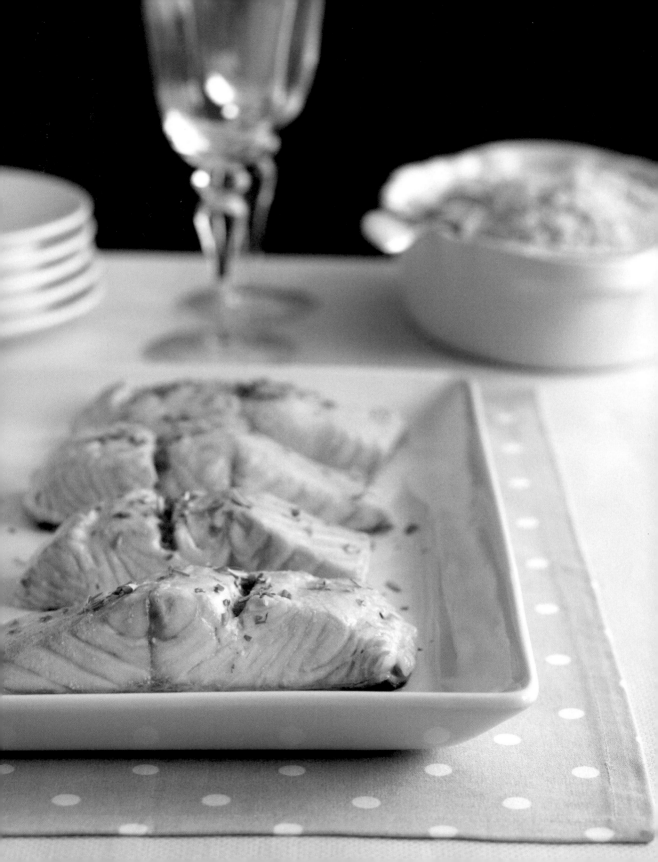

SUMMER ROASTED SALMON

I like to incorporate fish into my weekly menus. It is easy to prepare (easier than you might think) and is a fantastic source of readily digestible lean protein. Combine it with complex carbs from brown rice and fresh vegetables and you have an ideal Clean-Eating meal. This is something I often serve to guests.

INGREDIENTS:

4 x 6-oz salmon fillets, fresh from a reliable source
    if possible

2 tsp / 30 ml best-quality olive oil

Sea salt and fresh black pepper

Juice of one lemon

1 bunch fresh green onions, trimmed

¼ cup / 60 ml combined fresh chopped parsley,
    rosemary, thyme, chives

PREPARATION:

1 Preheat oven to 450°F / 232°C.

2 Prepare a baking dish with a light coating of cooking spray or olive oil. Place salmon fillets in the baking dish skin side down. Brush a coating of olive oil onto the salmon. Sprinkle each fillet with some sea salt and black pepper. Squeeze the juice of the lemon over the salmon. Lay the green onions on top.

3 Roast the fillets in the oven for about 10 minutes. Remove from heat. Remove the wilted green onions. Dust each fillet with a generous helping of the chopped herbs. Serve hot.

NUTRITIONAL VALUE PER SERVING:

Calories: 200 | Calories from Fat: 59 | Protein: 78g | Carbs: 1g
Dietary Fiber: 0.5g | Sugars: 0.5g | Fat: 6g | Sodium: 109mg

4 SERVINGS   10 MINUTES   10 MINUTES

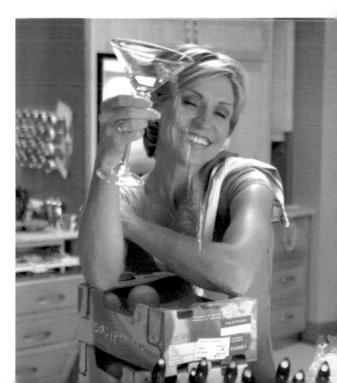

TURKEY WALDORF SALAD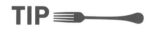

When it is just too hot to cook and you still want your lean protein try this beautiful salad. It tastes great all year round but is perfect in the heat of the summer.

INGREDIENTS:

½ turkey breast, roasted and cooled, skin removed, cut into ½" cubes – approx. 1½ lbs

4 ribs celery, trimmed and chopped

1 cup / 240 ml cored and chopped red apple

1 bunch green onions, trimmed and chopped

½ cup / 120 ml walnuts

½ cup / 120 ml fresh cilantro, chopped

1 cup / 240 ml yogurt cheese *(you may need more depending on how big your turkey breast is)*

(for Yogurt Cheese recipe see page 141)

Juice of one fresh lemon

Sea salt and freshly ground black pepper

PREPARATION:

1 Place turkey, celery, apple, green onion, walnuts and cilantro in large salad bowl. Set aside.

2 In small mixing bowl, whisk yogurt cheese with lemon juice, sea salt and pepper. Pour dressing over salad ingredients. Mix until dressing coats other ingredients. Chill.

TIP

Use firm nectarines in place of apples when making this recipe in the summer. It's crazy, but good.

NUTRITIONAL VALUE PER SERVING:

Calories: 240 | Calories from Fat: 28 | Protein: 11g | Carbs: 42g
Dietary Fiber: 13g | Sugars: 4g | Fat: 3g | Sodium: 164mg

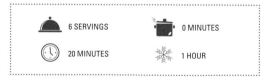

6 SERVINGS   0 MINUTES

20 MINUTES   1 HOUR

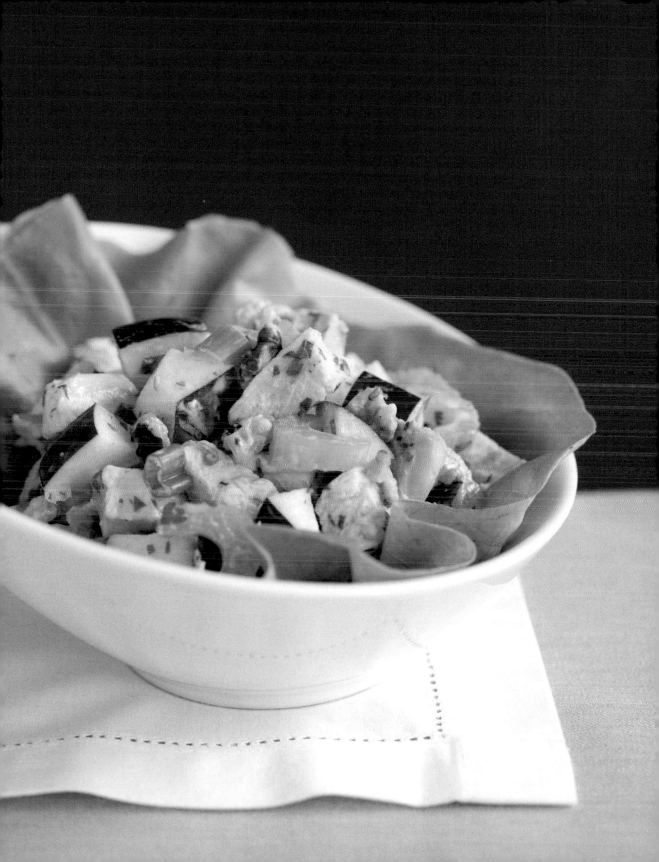

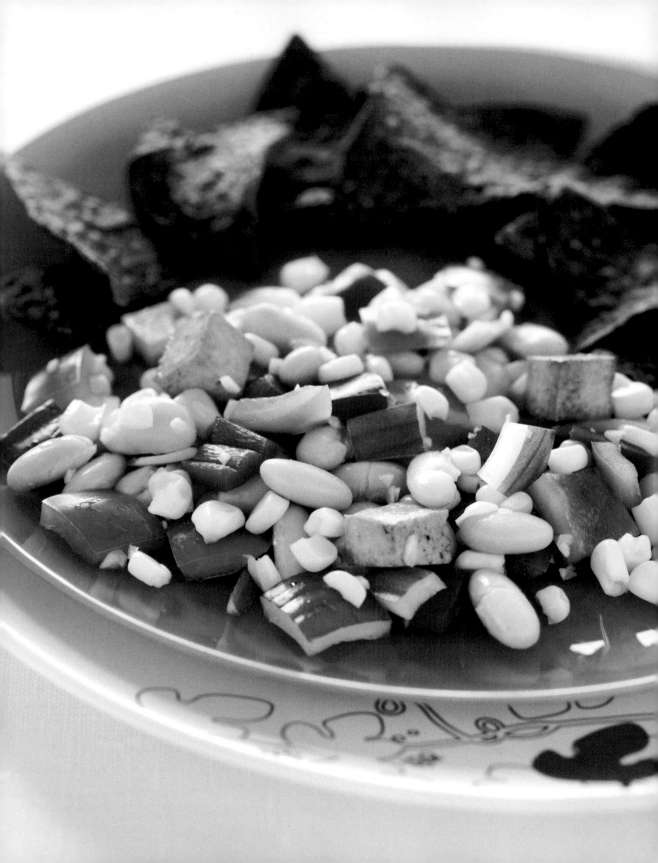

ARRIBA TOFU SALAD

This delicious and zesty salad will satisfy any of you who love the picante flavors of Latin America. Kidney beans provide fiber and protein while tofu kicks the protein up a notch. Corn and peppers round out the nutritional value of this dish. Serve it as an appetizer or main dish.

INGREDIENTS:

1 cup / 240 ml firm tofu

1 cup / 240 ml white kidney beans, drained and rinsed

1 cup / 240 ml fresh corn kernels

1 red bell pepper, seeded and deveined, chopped

1 green bell pepper, seeded and deveined, chopped

1 purple onion, peeled, chopped

2 cloves garlic, put through a garlic press

DRESSING:

⅛ cup / 30 ml pumpkin oil

⅛ cup / 30 ml avocado oil

2 Tbsp / 30 ml tamari (gluten-free)

1 Tbsp / 15 ml fresh lime juice

Sea salt and black ground pepper to taste

NUTRITIONAL VALUE PER SERVING:

Calories: 211 | Calories from Fat: 69 | Protein: 15g | Carbs: 22g | Dietary Fiber: 7g | Sugars: 7g | Fat: 7g | Sodium: 866mg

4 SERVINGS   13 MINUTES   0 MINUTES

PREPARATION:

1 Cut tofu into one-inch cubes. In medium bowl add beans, corn, peppers, onion and garlic.

2 In a separate medium bowl mix dressing ingredients. Combine with tofu. Mix until tofu is thoroughly coated. Add to vegetables and mix well. Add salt and pepper to taste.

TIP

A Clean-Eating Super Bowl snack: Serve the salad with blue corn chips and guacamole.

I DON'T EAT MEAT!

Many of you are vegetarian and I admit I don't want to eat chicken every day all day long either. Fortunately, there are many protein alternatives to fit with the Clean-Eating lifestyle. The list is long and plentiful, but here are a few ideas:

- Soy beans and other soy products
- Legumes
- Nuts and seeds
- Sea vegetables and seaweed
- Grains, especially amaranth, quinoa, oatmeal
- Spirulina
- Bee pollen and royal jelly
- Goat's milk
- Hemp and hemp products

PROTEIN
THE MAGIC INGREDIENT

While Eating Clean you will notice that you consume protein at every meal. Eating protein every two or three hours is one of the Clean-Eating principles. Protein is required to build lean muscle mass. It is also required to repair and maintain muscle and tissue.

HOW DO YOU KNOW HOW MUCH PROTEIN TO EAT?

Many other diets will have you perform fancy calculations to determine the correct amount of protein to eat. They don't take into consideration that the average body cannot absorb any more than 25 grams of protein at a given meal. When you consume extra protein the extra calories are stored as fat the same as if you had consumed extra calories from other food macronutrients.

The real skill is learning how to identify what 25 grams of protein looks like. Don't forget that protein is not well absorbed unless it is consumed with complex carbohydrates from fresh fruit and vegetables and from whole grains.

WHAT DOES
25 GRAMS
OF PROTEIN LOOK LIKE?

FOOD ITEM	AMOUNT TO MAKE 25 GRAMS OF PROTEIN	NUMBER OF CALORIES
Egg whites	5 – 7 whites	115
Low-fat yogurt	2 cups / 480 ml	220
Low-fat cottage cheese	1 cup / 240 ml	115
Whey protein powder	⅓ cup / 80 ml	165
Soy protein powder	1 ounce / 28 g	112
Tofu	1 cup / 240 ml	360
Skinless turkey breast	5 ounces / 140 g	225
Skinless chicken breast	5 ounces / 140 g	232
Salmon	5 ounces / 140 g	166
Tuna	5 ounces / 140 g	155
Bison	5 ounces / 140 g	123
Lean beef tenderloin	4 ounces / 112 g	183
Quinoa	2 cups cooked / 480 ml	234
Almonds or pine nuts	¾ cup / 180 ml	621
Ezekiel 4:9 cereal	1½ cups / 360 ml	600
Soybeans/edamame	1 cup / 240 ml	254
Natural peanut butter	6 Tbsp / 90 ml	600
Almond butter	6 Tbsp / 90 ml	570
Lentils	1½ cups / 360 ml	265

LESLEY'S CHICKEN STACKS

esley is one of my best friends. She has successfully battled breast cancer and at the age of 60-something looks totally amazing! She trains hard and Eats Clean to keep herself healthy and looking great. We enjoyed this entrée at a friendly gathering recently.

INGREDIENTS:

1 medium Sicilian eggplant

2 medium yellow zucchini

2 fresh Roma tomatoes

4 x 5 oz / 140 g boneless, skinless chicken breasts,
    slightly flattened

Sea salt and black pepper to taste

Fresh basil leaves

PREPARATION:

1 Line a baking sheet with parchment paper. Cut the eggplant into ¾"- thick slices. Slice zucchini into lengths. Slice tomatoes thickly. Pat chicken breasts dry and season with sea salt and pepper. Place four pieces of eggplant on the baking sheet. Now add slices of tomato and zucchini. Add basil as well. Top with a chicken breast.

2 Place in preheated 350°F / 177°C oven. Bake for 20 to 25 minutes or until chicken is done. Remove from oven. Place on serving platter or plate and sprinkle plate with parsley. Place the bundle in the middle and serve immediately.

TIP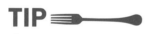

As an alternative to chicken you can top the cooked veggie stacks with shrimp. Use the largest shrimp available
– precooked and deveined. Butterfly the shrimp and
place on the top of each cooked stack.

NUTRITIONAL VALUE PER SERVING:

Calories: 164 | Calories from Fat: 15 | Protein: 28g | Carbs: 7g
Dietary Fiber: 4g | Sugars: 3g | Fat: 0.1g | Sodium: 80mg

4 SERVINGS   20 MINUTES   25 MINUTES

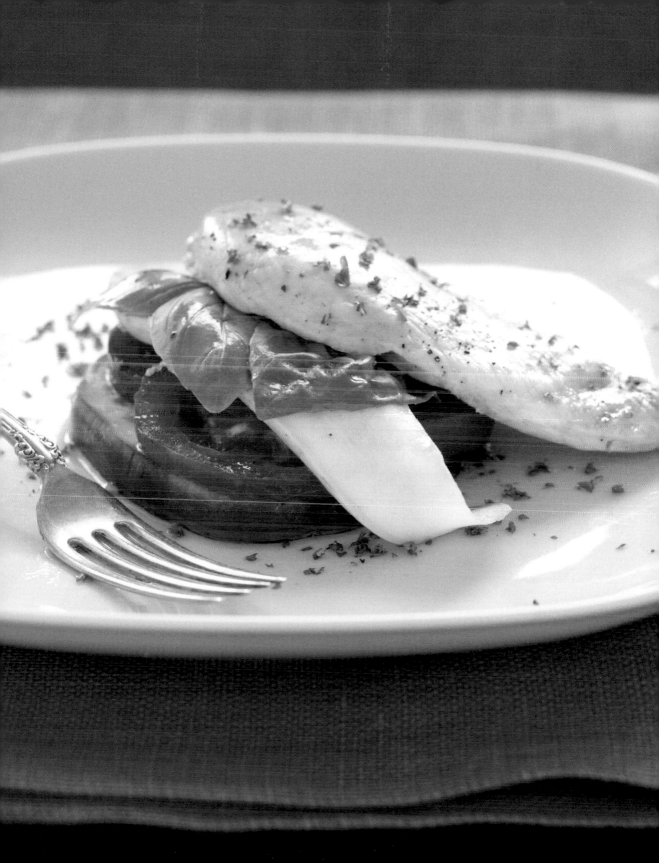

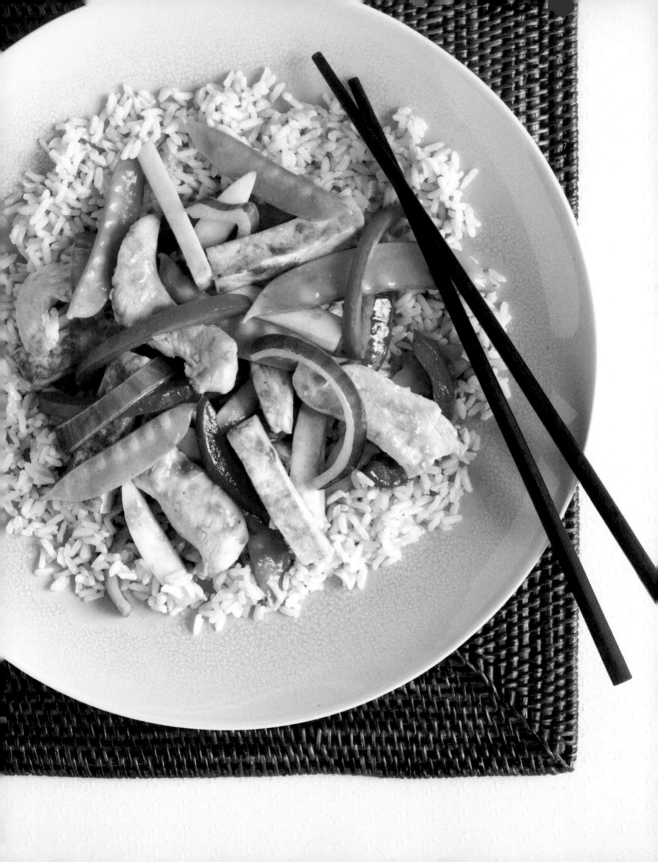

CHICKEN STRIPS AND TOFU SZECHUANESE

Hello! Join me and whip up a creative, easy and Clean-Eating supper with chicken and/or tofu. You decide! Get smart and make planned leftovers. You will want to have them for a Clean-Eating lunch the next day.

INGREDIENTS:

Safflower or olive oil

1 lb / 454 g lean, skinless chicken breast, cut into strips

OR 1 lb / 454 g well drained firm tofu, cut into strips

OR combination of both to equal one pound

Sea salt and freshly ground black pepper

½ cup / 120 ml red pepper, cut into strips

½ cup / 120 ml firm green or yellow zucchini, cut into strips

⅓ cup / 80 ml purple onion, cut into strips

⅓ cup / 80 ml snow peas, trimmed

2 cloves garlic, passed through garlic press

1 tsp / 5 ml freshly grated ginger

SAUCE INGREDIENTS:

Sea salt

Freshly ground black pepper

2 tsp potato flour or quinoa flour

3 tsp low-sodium soy sauce or gluten-free tamari

3 tsp rice vinegar

1 tsp organic honey

1 cup low-sodium vegetable broth or water (gluten free if necessary)

NUTRITIONAL VALUE PER SERVING WITH CHICKEN:

Calories: 234 | Calories from Fat: 93 | Protein: 24g | Carbs: 12g | Dietary Fiber: 4g | Sugar: 6g | Fat: 10g | Sat Fat: 0.05g | Sodium: 548mg

PREPARATION:

1 Place some of the oil in a nonstick skillet or wok. Brown chicken or tofu strips in batches over medium-high heat. Season with sea salt and black pepper. Remove from skillet or wok and transfer to a serving bowl.

2 In same skillet with a little more oil, stir-fry vegetables and garlic and ginger until just done, but still bright in color. Add sauce mixture (see preparation details below) to skillet. Bring to a boil and stir constantly. Add chicken or tofu or both if using. Heat through. Serve over brown rice.

SAUCE PREPARATION:

1 Mix all dry ingredients in small bowl.

2 Add liquid ingredients and mix well. Ensure there are no lumps.

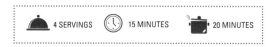
4 SERVINGS   15 MINUTES   20 MINUTES

PUY LENTILS

I encourage everyone to give lentils a try. Not only is this tiny green legume loaded with protein, but also with fiber and minerals. If you buy the beautiful Lentils Verte du Puy you will taste lentils as they ought to taste. These little gems are not at all floury and keep their shape even after long cooking times. The lentils you may be used to seeing are not the same as Puy lentils – I suggest you give these a try!

INGREDIENTS:

1 medium purple onion, peeled and chopped

1 large stalk celery, chopped

1 large carrot, peeled and chopped

1 medium bunch chard, stems and leaves, well
   rinsed and chopped

1 tsp / 5 ml sea salt

2 tsp / 10 ml extra virgin olive oil

1¾ cup / 420 ml low-sodium chicken or vegetable
   broth or water (gluten free if necessary)

1 cup / 240 ml Puy lentils, rinsed and drained

1 tsp / 5 ml fresh thyme, chopped

1 tsp / 5 ml fresh oregano, chopped

2 tsp / 10 ml fresh lemon juice

2 tsp /10 ml avocado oil

Sea salt and black pepper for seasoning

PREPARATION:

1 In large stock pot place onion, celery, carrot, chard stems, 2 teaspoons / 10 ml olive oil and ½ teaspoon/ 2.5 ml sea salt. Cover and cook over medium-low heat, stirring often, until vegetables become soft.

2 Add broth, lentils and herbs. Bring to a full boil. Reduce heat and cover. Stir occasionally and make sure the lentils are just getting soft. This takes about 30 minutes.

3 Add chard leaves and cook until the leaves soften – not more than 10 minutes. Add lemon juice and avocado oil. Season with salt and pepper.

NUTRITIONAL VALUE PER SERVING:

Calories: 151 | Calories from Fat: 14 | Protein: 10g | Carbs: 25g
Dietary Fiber: 5g | Sugars: 4g | Fat: 1g | Sodium: 453mg

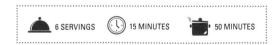

6 SERVINGS   15 MINUTES   50 MINUTES

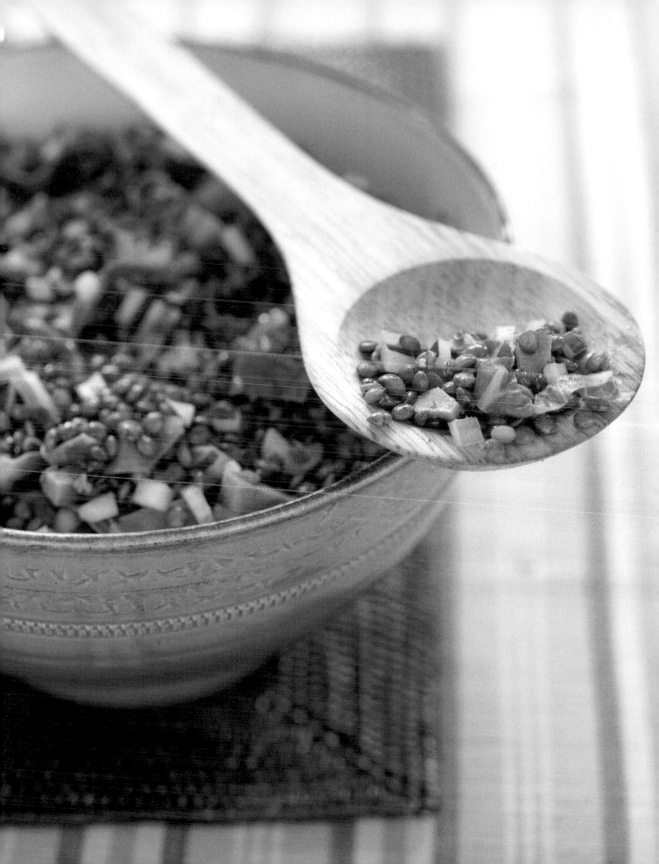

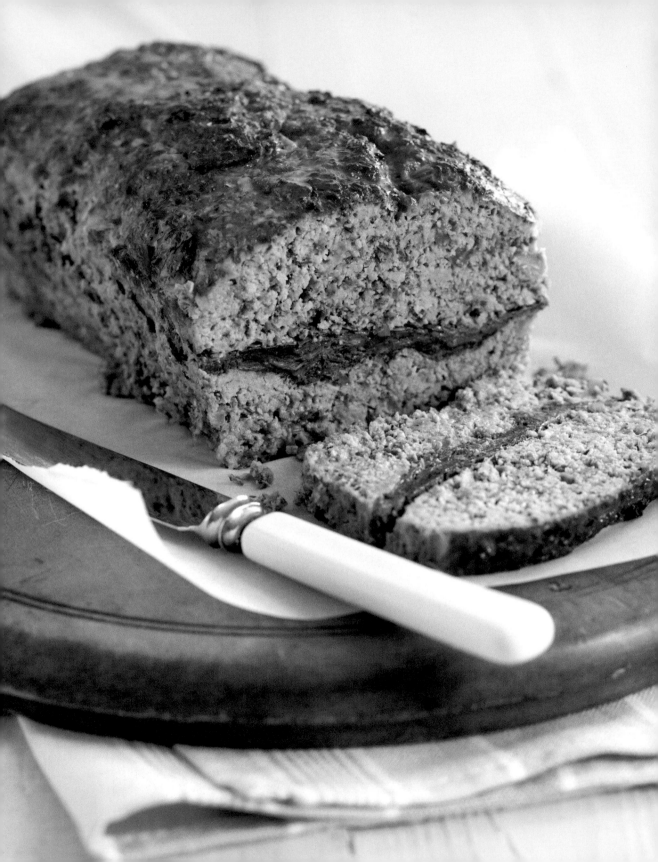

TURKEY LOAF TO LIVE BY

Who wants to eat turkey loaf, meatloaf or any other loaf? You do! This recipe makes the most of lean ground turkey and delicious fresh herbs. Serve it hot one night for supper and cold in your wrap the next day for lunch. Let's eat!

INGREDIENTS:

2 Tbsp / 30 ml best-quality olive oil

2 purple onions or Vidalia onions, finely chopped

½ cup / 120 ml finely chopped celery

Sea salt and fresh ground black pepper

6 cups / 1.4 L baby spinach leaves, washed

6 cups / 1.4 L baby arugula leaves

1 tsp / 5 ml water

1 cup / 240 ml basil leaves

¼ cup / 60 ml minced cilantro

4 egg whites + one yolk

1 Tbsp / 15 ml tomato paste mixed with one tablespoon water

¾ cup / 180 ml low-sodium chicken or vegetable
stock (gluten free if necessary)

2½ lb / 600 ml ground turkey breast, no skin or fat
included, or textured vegetable protein

¾ cup / 180 ml oat bran (if you don't have oat bran
use oatmeal that has been ground in the
blender) – uncontaminated for gluten free

¼ cup / 60 ml ground flax seeds

Cooking spray

NUTRITIONAL VALUE PER ONE-INCH SLICE:

Calories: 222 | Calories from Fat: 49 | Protein: 33g | Carbs: 11g
Dietary Fiber: 3g | Sugars: 2g | Fat: 5g | Sodium: 139mg

10 SERVINGS   20 MINUTES   1 HOUR 30 MINUTES

PREPARATION:

1 Preheat oven to 375°F / 190°C. Make sure there is a rack in the center of the oven. Heat olive oil in a nonstick pan and cook onions and celery until they are translucent but not brown. Season with salt and pepper and transfer to a small bowl to cool.

2 Add baby spinach and arugula leaves to the pan with one teaspoon of water. Cook until the greens are wilted. Remove from heat and let cool. Add basil and cilantro to the wilted greens and mix well.

3 In a large bowl add egg whites, yolk, tomato paste mixture and stock. Mix well. Add ground turkey or TVP, oat bran and flax seeds along with cooked onions and celery. Spray clean hands with cooking spray and mix the turkey concoction well.

4 In a 10" loaf pan coated with cooking spray, place half of the turkey mixture. Spread evenly. Using clean hands, transfer wilted greens and herbs to loaf pan. Distribute evenly on top of the turkey mixture already in the pan. Now place remaining ground turkey mixture on top of the wilted greens. Make the top smooth with your hands.

5 Bake the turkey loaf for 1½ hours or until a meat thermometer registers 160°F / 71°C. Remove loaf from the oven and let cool for 15 minutes so everything sets properly. Once cool, remove loaf from pan and cut into one-inch-thick slices using a very sharp knife. Arrange on a serving platter and serve immediately. Refrigerate leftovers and use for lunch.

APRICOT AND CHICKEN CURRY À LA RENÉ

The first time I tasted this delectable chicken was at a dinner my then-bachelor brother prepared for me. He was incredibly proud of his efforts and with good reason. It really is a delicious meal, especially with the addition of brown rice. I had to try the recipe for myself when I got home and had a difficult time finding garam masala. Don't worry, it's easy to find once you know what it is. It's a blend of dry roasted spices often used in Pakistani/Indian cuisine. It literally means "hot mixture." Thanks René!

INGREDIENTS:

3½ lbs / 1.5 kg chicken breasts, skinless and boneless

½ tsp / 2.5 ml chili powder

1 Tbsp / 15 ml garam masala

1, one-inch piece fresh ginger root, grated

2 cloves garlic, crushed

½ cup / 120 ml fresh orange juice

¼ cup / 60 ml fresh lemon or lime juice

1 cup / 240 ml dried apricots

⅔ cup / 160 ml low-sodium, low-fat chicken stock (gluten free if necessary)

2 Tbsp / 30 ml best-quality olive oil or rice bran oil

2 sweet onions, finely sliced

2 Tbsp / 30 ml white wine vinegar

1 x 14 oz / 392 g can chopped tomatoes, Mexican salsa style

Sea salt and fresh ground pepper to taste

NUTRITIONAL VALUE PER SERVING:

Calories: 401 | Calories from Fat: 89 | Protein: 57g | Carbs: 27g
Dietary Fiber: 3g | Sugars: 15g | Fat: 9g | Sodium: 762mg

6 SERVINGS   40 MINUTES   1 HOUR 30 MINUTES

PREPARATION:

1 Pat chicken breasts dry with paper towel. Flatten each piece with a wooden mallet or the flat side of a cleaving knife.

2 Prepare a marinade of chili powder, garam masala, ginger root, garlic, orange juice and lemon or lime juice. Place chicken breasts in marinade and let stand for 2 – 3 hours in the refrigerator.

3 In a separate bowl, cover dried apricots with water. Soak for 2 – 3 hours. Drain.

4 Preheat oven to 350°F / 177°C. Remove chicken breasts from marinade and stuff with drained apricots cut into thirds. Tie each breast with kitchen string or use toothpicks to keep the meat rolled tightly. Reserve the marinade. Coat a shallow covered casserole dish with olive oil. Put a layer of onions on the bottom. Place stuffed chicken breasts in the casserole. Pour reserved marinade and chicken stock over top of the chicken breasts. Cover with Mexican salsa tomatoes. Drizzle with white wine vinegar. Season with sea salt and pepper. Cover and bake for 1½ hours. Serve with baked brown rice.

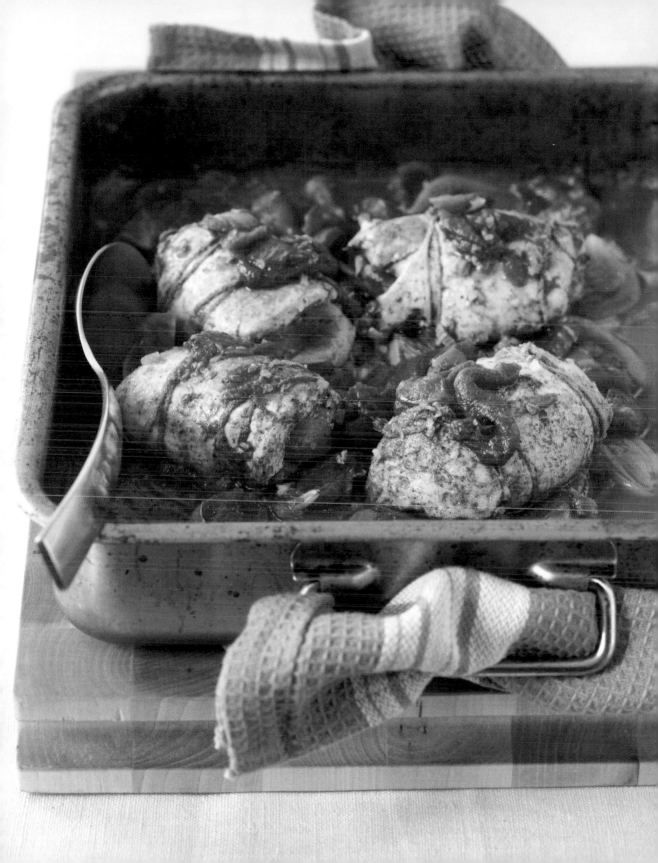

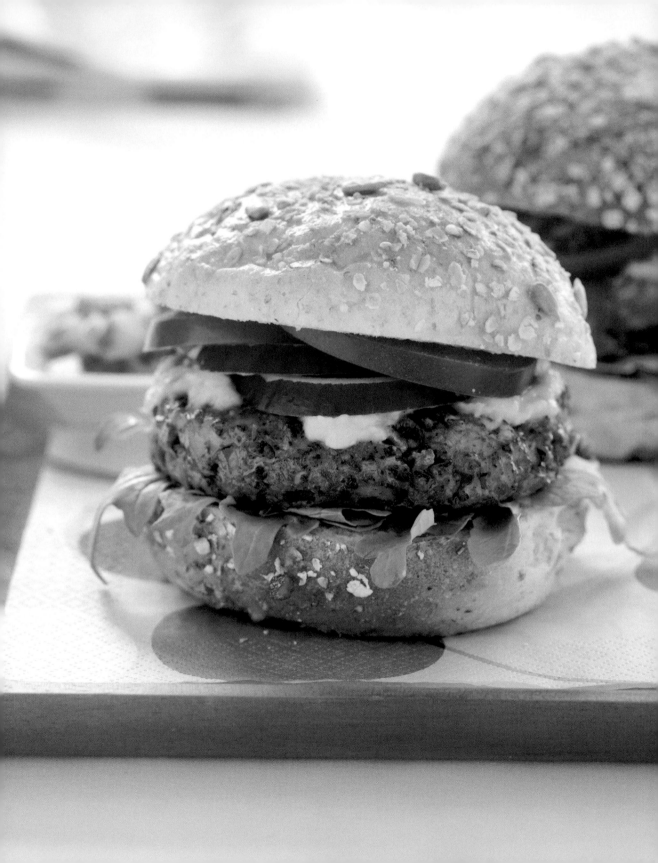

EAT-CLEAN TUNA BURGERS 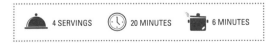 (without bun)

Is there anything better than a juicy burger? I think this version is superb! It provides the fun of eating a burger but not the guilt of eating unwanted fat. Adding zippy purple onions to the mix along with peppers and a surprising dash of molasses not only sharpens the flavor but increases the nutritional profile of this main course. Make it a meal by adding a Farmstand Tomato Salad. (See recipe on page 213)

INGREDIENTS:

2 lbs / 908 g fresh tuna steak – the flesh should be
     deeply colored and mild smelling

4 cloves garlic, passed through a garlic press

2 Tbsp / 30 ml low-sodium soy sauce or gluten-free
    tamari

2 Tbsp / 30 ml unsulfured molasses

3 green onions, finely chopped

½ sweet red pepper, finely chopped

½ sweet purple or Vidalia onion, finely chopped

2 tsp / 10 ml sesame oil

1 Tbsp / 15 ml mixed herbal seasoning of your
    choice

Olive-oil-based cooking spray

4 Ezekiel grain buns or other hearty buns

Sea salt and black pepper

CONDIMENTS:

• Leaf lettuce or arugula leaves

• Sliced tomato

• Sliced purple onion

• Hummus

• Mango salsa*or commercial salsa of your choice

PREPARATION:

1 Place tuna in food processor and pulse until meat resembles texture of ground turkey or beef. In large mixing bowl combine garlic, soy sauce, molasses, green onions, red pepper, Vidalia onions, sesame oil, herbal seasoning, and salt and pepper to taste. Add tuna. With clean bare hands, mix all ingredients until uniformly distributed. Divide into four parts and shape into flat patties.

2 Coat grill pan with olive oil spray. Place over medium heat. Place patties in grill pan, cook for 2 minutes and flip. Cook for another 2 minutes. This will make a rare burger. If you want your burger medium to well done, cook for another 2 minutes on both sides.

3 Meanwhile, cut buns in half (if they aren't already separated) and toast lightly. Spread bottom half with hummus. Place lettuce greens of your choice on top and set the burger on top of that. Add condiments of your choice and serve immediately.

NUTRITIONAL VALUE PER SERVING:
Calories: 391 | Calories from Fat: 41 | Protein: 28g | Carbs: 61g
Dietary Fiber: 3g | Sugars: 6g | Fat: 0.4g | Sodium: 768mg

4 SERVINGS   20 MINUTES   6 MINUTES

* See page 116 for the Super Easy Mango Salsa recipe

ROAST STUFFED PORK TENDERLOIN

Pork tenderloin is a delicious and lean source of protein. Preparing it according to this recipe makes it a perfect special Sunday entrée. Add steamed veggies and baked sweet potatoes and you've got a meal. Don't like pork? Use boneless turkey breast instead.

INGREDIENTS:

½ cup / 120 ml cooked broccoli

¼ cup / 60 ml finely chopped parsley

½ cup / 120 ml breadcrumbs (use gluten-free bread if desired)

¼ cup / 60 ml fine oat bran (uncontaminated)

⅓ cup / 80 ml chopped walnuts

⅓ cup / 80 ml finely chopped apricots

2 Tbsp / 30 ml water or low-sodium chicken stock (gluten free if necessary)

2 pork tenderloins (or one large turkey breast)

1 Tbsp / 15 ml black peppercorns, coarsely chopped

1 tsp / 5 ml dried sage

1 tsp / 5 ml dried rosemary

1 tsp / 5 ml dried thyme

Sea salt

PREPARATION:

1 In a medium bowl combine broccoli, bread crumbs, oat bran, walnuts, parsley, chopped apricots and 2 tablespoons / 30 ml water or low-sodium chicken stock. Mix well and set aside.

2 Place pork tenderloins (or turkey breast) on cutting board and butterfly them – cut them in half lengthwise almost all the way through but not quite. Using the blade of a large wide knife, such as a cleaver, flatten the pork tenderloins. Spoon the stuffing into each of the tenderloins or turkey if using.

3 Fold one side over the other and tie with kitchen twine, starting at the end of the tenderloin or turkey breast and moving to the other end. Sprinkle with dried herbs, black peppercorns and sea salt. Place in shallow casserole dish. Bake in preheated 350°F / 177°C oven for 25 to 40 minutes, or until a meat thermometer reads 160°F / 71°C. Remove meat from oven and cover with foil. Let stand for 5 minutes.

4 Serve pork or turkey with unsweetened apple-sauce. It is delicious!

NUTRITIONAL VALUE PER SERVING:

Calories: 229 | Calories from Fat: 63 | Protein: 26g | Carbs: 14g
Dietary Fiber: 1g | Sugars: 1g | Fat: 7g | Sodium: 87mg

8 SERVINGS   30 MINUTES   25 - 40 MINUTES

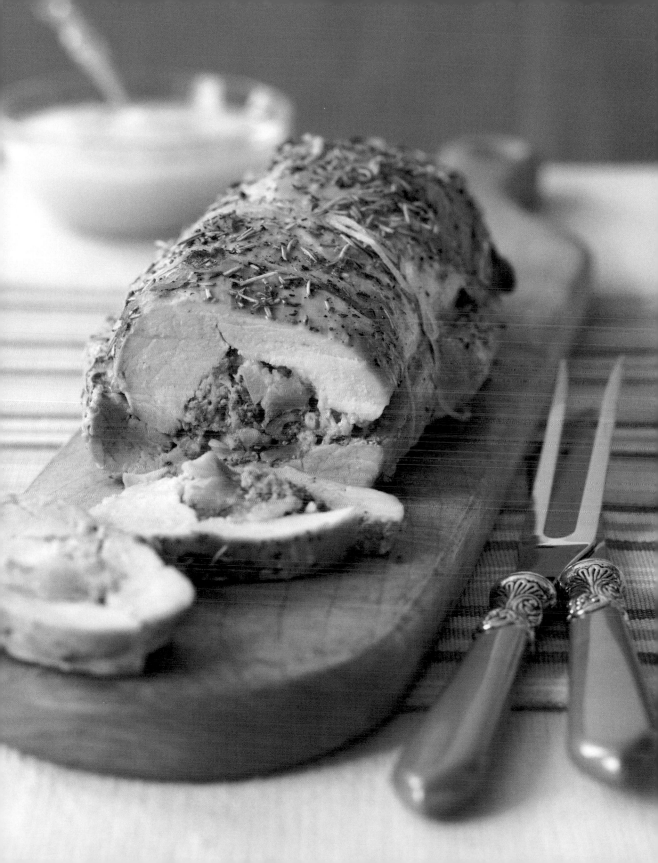

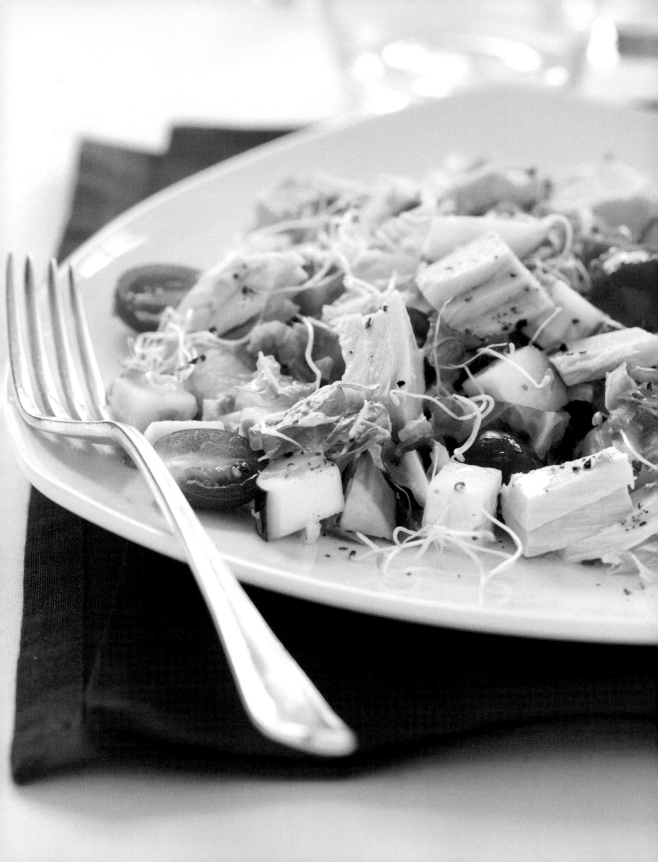

MORE THAN A TUNA SALAD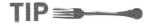

Tuna is one of those ingredients you should always have in your cupboard. Somehow it can always be turned into a quick Clean-Eating meal. This version of tuna salad packs loads of nutrients and a hefty dose of flavor.

INGREDIENTS:

2 x 3 oz / 84 g cans water-packed albacore tuna, broken into chunks

1 medium English cucumber, diced

½ cup / 120 ml sprouts – use alfalfa, broccoli or any combination of your favorite sprouts

½ cup / 120 ml fresh radishes, trimmed and sliced

2 small, firm zucchini, chopped

½ cup / 120 ml grated carrot

1½ cups / 360 ml nappa cabbage, chopped fine

½ cup / 120 ml grape tomatoes, halved

Sea salt and black pepper

DRESSING:

¼ cup / 60 ml pumpkin, olive or avocado oil or oil of your choice (try hazelnut or walnut oil)

Juice of one fresh lemon or lime

PREPARATION:

1 In medium mixing bowl combine all salad ingredients.

2 Pour dressing over ingredients and season with sea salt and pepper. Serve immediately or cover and chill.

TIP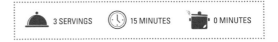

This tuna salad makes a perfect filling for pitas and wraps.

NUTRITIONAL VALUE PER SERVING:

Calories: 276 | Calories from Fat: 176 | Protein: 17g | Carbs: 11g
Dietary Fiber: 3g | Sugars: 5g | Fat: 19g | Sodium: 234mg

3 SERVINGS   15 MINUTES   0 MINUTES

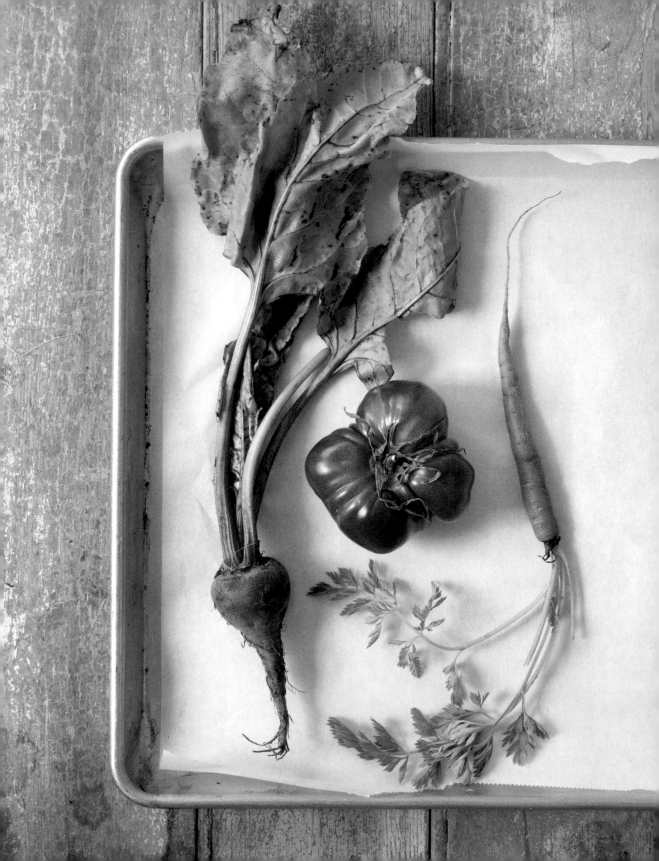

Vegetables

_7_

I have fond childhood memories of picking blushing red tomatoes from my father's brimming garden. The still-warm fruit we call a vegetable tasted like a perfect summer day. Baby cucumbers and green beans would fall prey to my hands as I stood under the leafy foliage, sampling the harvest.

Vegetables are a nutritional MUST. You may not have a garden, but with today's global economy your harvest is as near as the grocery store or farmer's market. Slice, dice, simmer and stew veggies solo or in mixed company to benefit from their nutritional storehouse. Try the Stuffed Peppers on page 220.

FARMSTAND TOMATO SALAD

Summer-ripe tomatoes are a rare and delicious treat. When your garden overflows with tomatoes make this salad and eat it for breakfast, lunch and dinner. I like it best at room temperature.

INGREDIENTS:

2 lbs / 908 g fresh tomatoes – try heirloom varieties for a welcome change

1 large clove garlic, passed through a garlic press

½ purple onion, peeled and sliced into very thin rings

Handful fresh basil leaves, shredded

3 Tbsp / 45 ml extra virgin olive oil or avocado oil

2 Tbsp / 30 ml white balsamic vinegar

Sea salt

Freshly ground black pepper

PREPARATION:

1 Wash the tomatoes. Remove green crowns. Cut the tomatoes into one-inch chunks and place in a decorative glass serving bowl.

2 Add garlic, onion and shredded basil leaves. In a small glass jar with a lid, place the olive oil or oil of your choice, vinegar, salt and pepper. Shake vigorously. Pour over tomatoes and toss gently.

TIP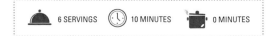

Add chopped cucumber and feta for a quick variation of Greek salad.

NUTRITIONAL VALUE PER SERVING:
Calories: 95 | Calories from Fat: 65 | Protein: 1g | Carbs: 5g
Dietary Fiber: 2g | Sugars: 5g | Fat: 7g | Sodium: 9mg

6 SERVINGS   10 MINUTES   0 MINUTES

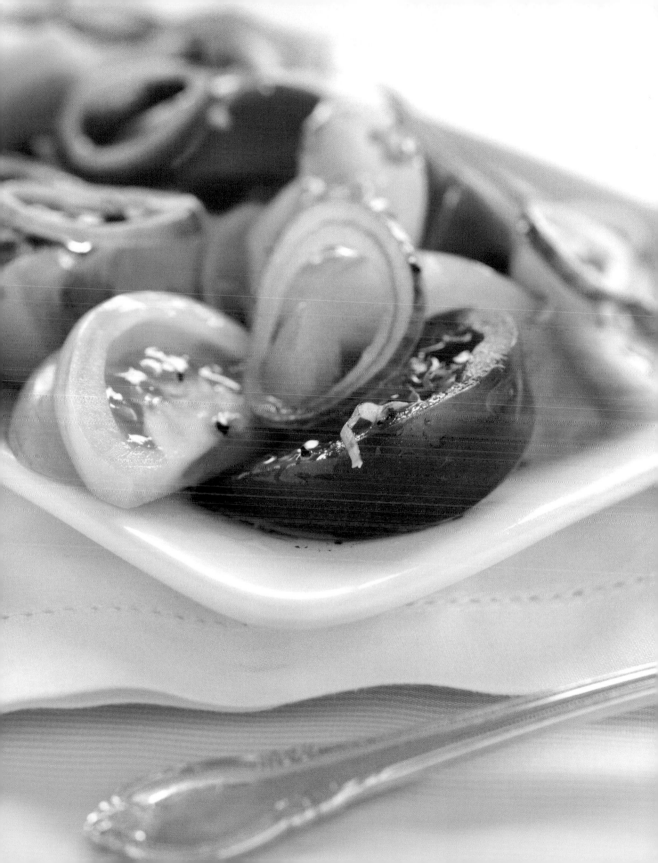

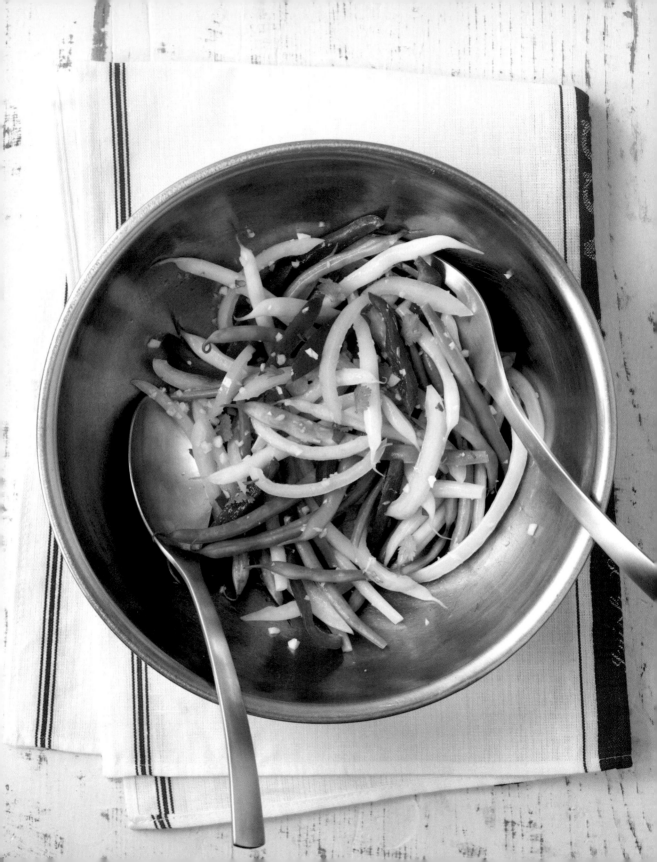

COLORFUL STRING BEANS

When string beans are plentiful there is nothing like eating them right off the vine. I remember eating beautifully colored green and yellow beans in my dad's garden in the heat of the summer. My dad grew loads of beans in his little garden and I still recall seeing the teepee-like structures he built for the beans to grow on. I would creep under the leaves and pinch a few of the prettiest beans. I love the crispy texture and juiciness of fresh beans. I still eat them raw. This recipe makes the most of fresh string beans in any color.

INGREDIENTS:

2 quarts / 1.9 L water

Sea salt

1 lb / 454 g fresh green or yellow beans or mix of
   both, trimmed (Sometimes you can find the
   unusual purple string bean, too. I encourage you
   to try these! Delicious!)

1 Tbsp / 15 ml extra virgin olive oil

3 cloves garlic, passed through a garlic press

½ red bell pepper, seeded and deveined, cut into
   strips similar in size to the string beans

½ yellow bell pepper, seeded and deveined, cut into
   strips similar in size to the string beans

⅓ cup / 80 ml chopped fresh cilantro

Fresh ground black pepper

PREPARATION:

1 Fill a big bowl with cold water and a few handfuls of ice cubes.

2 Meanwhile, in a large saucepan, bring 2 quarts / 1.9 L salted water to a rolling boil. Add fresh beans and cook until they just turn color – about 4 minutes. Drain the beans and place them in the cold water bath. Drain again and place on a layer of paper towel.

3 In a large skillet, heat olive oil over medium heat. Add garlic and bell peppers. Sauté briefly and add the drained beans. Cook until all vegetables are heated through. Season with cilantro, sea salt and black pepper. Serve immediately or chill in the refrigerator.

NUTRITIONAL VALUE PER SERVING:
Calories: 79 | Calories from Fat: 34 | Protein: 2g | Carbs: 11g
Dietary Fiber: 4g | Sugars: 3g | Fat: 3g | Sodium: 8mg

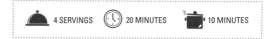
4 SERVINGS   20 MINUTES   10 MINUTES

SAUTÉED WILD MUSHROOMS

Wild mushrooms have a flavor all their own and if you have them growing nearby consider yourself lucky. They are high in nutritional content and flavor. If you can't find them wild, purchase a variety of commercially available mushrooms and prepare this dish to enjoy with lean protein.

INGREDIENTS:

2 Tbsp / 30 ml best-quality olive oil

¾ lb / 340 g wild or commercially available mushrooms: morels, oyster mushrooms, chanterelles, enokitake, shiitake, honey, button, portobello mushrooms

¼ cup / 60 ml sliced green onions

Sea salt and fresh ground black pepper

PREPARATION:

1 Clean mushrooms with a damp cloth, mushroom brush or paper towel. It is best not to immerse mushrooms in water as they absorb water and quickly become mushy. If your mushrooms are large, slice them so all mushroom pieces are roughly uniform.

2 Place olive oil in a large skillet and heat over medium high heat. Add mushrooms and green onions and sauté for a few minutes until just tender. Toss with sea salt and pepper and serve immediately.

WARNING!

Many wild mushrooms are extremely poisonous. Do not ever eat wild mushrooms unless you are well educated in all types of mushrooms and are very sure that those you pick are edible.

NUTRITIONAL VALUE PER SERVING:
Calories: 81 | Calories from Fat: 65 | Protein: 2g | Carbs: 3g
Dietary Fiber: 0.75g | Sugars: 1g | Fat: 7g | Sodium: 4mg

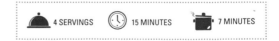
4 SERVINGS   15 MINUTES   7 MINUTES

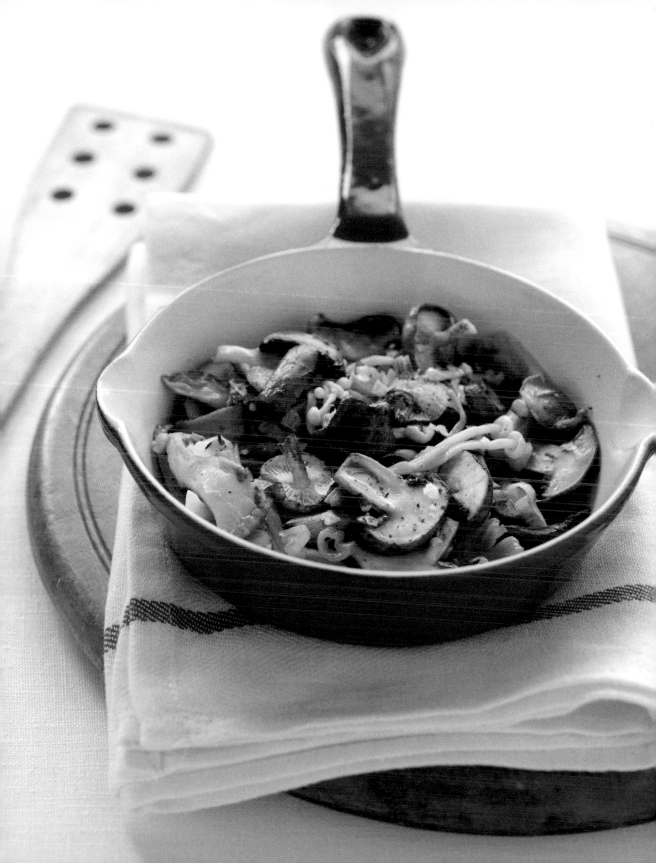

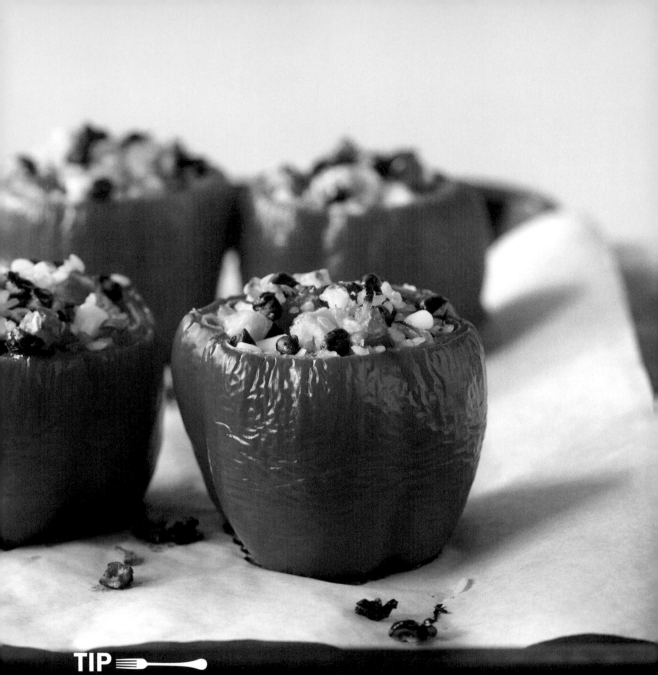

TIP

You can add cooked, lean ground chicken or turkey to the cooked rice mixture to make it a complete Clean-Eating meal. Simply brown one pound / 454 grams of ground chicken or turkey and add to the stuffing mixture. Then stuff and bake as usual.

STUFFED PEPPERS

In late summer and fall the harvest is sublime. Fresh fruits and vegetables in every color tantalize you into sampling each and every sun-kissed one. We often chop up colorful bell peppers and toss them into a dish. But they are a perfect vessel to hold their own little meal. Try this stuffed-pepper recipe, which makes the most of the late-summer bounty for a unique twist on peppers.

INGREDIENTS:

Water

Sea salt

4 large red bell peppers (you can really use any color) – make sure the peppers can sit upright nicely. Remove top, ribs and seeds.

2 cups / 480 ml cooked brown rice

1 tsp / 5 ml extra virgin olive oil

1 yellow onion, peeled and chopped

1 large carrot, peeled and grated

1 cup / 240 ml butternut squash, peeled and diced

3 cloves garlic, passed through a garlic press

2 cups / 480 ml fresh Roma tomatoes, diced and set over a fine-mesh sieve to drain

1 x 15 oz / 420 g can black beans, rinsed and drained

1 cup / 240 ml fresh corn kernels

½ cup / 120 ml fresh chopped cilantro

Juice of one fresh lime

Freshly ground black pepper

Cooking spray

NUTRITIONAL VALUE PER SERVING:

Calories: 302 | Calories from Fat: 30 | Protein: 11g | Carbs: 59g
Dietary Fiber: 12g | Sugars: 12g | Fat: 3g | Sodium: 518mg

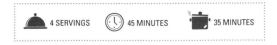

4 SERVINGS   45 MINUTES   35 MINUTES

PREPARATION:

1 Preheat oven to 350°F / 177°C. Place cooked brown rice in a bowl and let cool. Set aside.

2 Make sure there is a rack in the middle of the oven. Bring a large pot of salted water to a boil. Place the peppers in the boiling water and cook briefly. The peppers need to be just a little soft. Remove the peppers from the water and put them on a plate lined with paper towels, upside down so the water can drain out.

3 In a large skillet, heat olive oil and sauté onion, carrot and butternut squash. Cook for 10 minutes, covered. Add garlic and cook a few minutes more. Now add tomatoes, beans and corn. Cook for 5 minutes. Remove from heat.

4 Add vegetable mixture to cooled, cooked brown rice. Season with cilantro, lime juice, sea salt and black pepper. Mix with clean, bare hands until all ingredients are evenly distributed. Set aside.

5 Prepare a small baking pan with a light coating of nonstick spray. Place each of the peppers right side up in the pan. Stuff each pepper with brown rice filling. Don't pack the rice mixture too tightly. Bake for 20 minutes. Remove from heat and serve immediately.

OVEN-ROASTED VEGETABLES

Oven roasting brings out the flavor of vegetables like no other cooking method. The best part of oven roasting is its ease. Clean-Eating easy! I urge you to try it today. Gather up some of your favorites and have a good supply of extra virgin olive oil on hand. Any combination works well, but this is one I have tried often. I think you'll like it the way our family does.

INGREDIENTS:

2 large Spanish onions or sweet onions, cut in
    chunks
    OR 8 whole small onions
4 large sweet carrots, cut in chunks
2 peeled turnips, cut in chunks
½ lb / 227 g Brussels sprouts
6 small beets, peeled
8 – 10 small potatoes (not Idaho or russet bakers)
4 Tbsp / 60 ml extra virgin olive oil
1 tsp / 5 ml crushed dried rosemary
4 minced cloves garlic
1 Tbsp / 15 ml minced fresh marjoram
Sea salt and ground black pepper to taste
Cooking spray

PREPARATION:

1   Preheat oven to 375°F / 190°C. Peel all vegetables. Quarter the potatoes. Toss all vegetables in oil, rosemary, minced garlic and marjoram. Arrange the vegetables in a large roasting pan coated with cooking spray. Cover tightly with aluminum foil. Bake for 35 minutes.

2   Uncover and turn the vegetables with a large spoon. Add salt and pepper and roast at 425°F / 218°C for another 20 – 30 minutes or until the carrots and potatoes are thoroughly cooked and the edges are not burned.

NUTRITIONAL VALUE PER SERVING:
Calories: 371 | Calories from Fat: 90 | Protein: 9g | Carbs: 63g
Dietary Fiber: 10g | Sugars: 13g | Fat: 10g | Sodium: 155mg

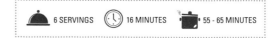

6 SERVINGS   16 MINUTES   55 - 65 MINUTES

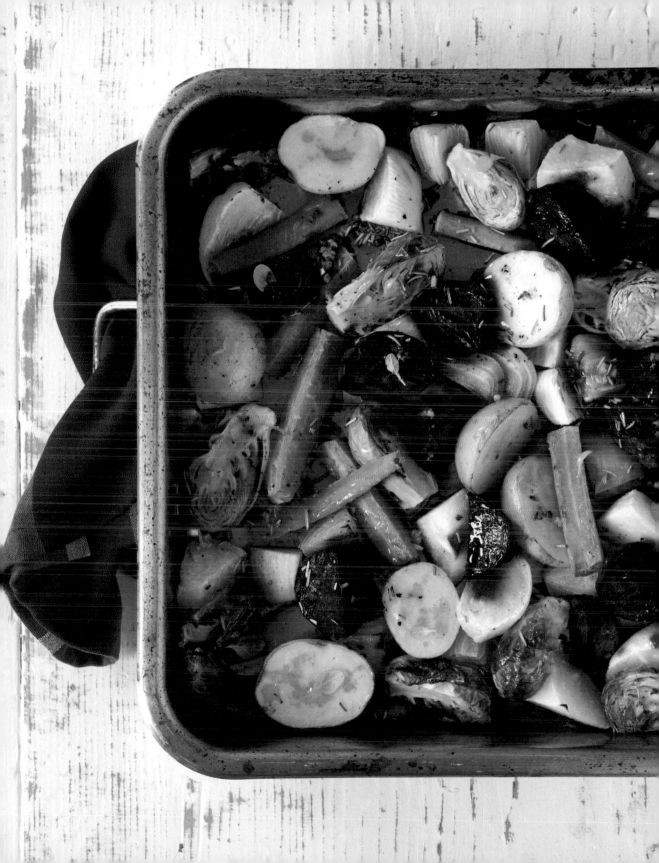

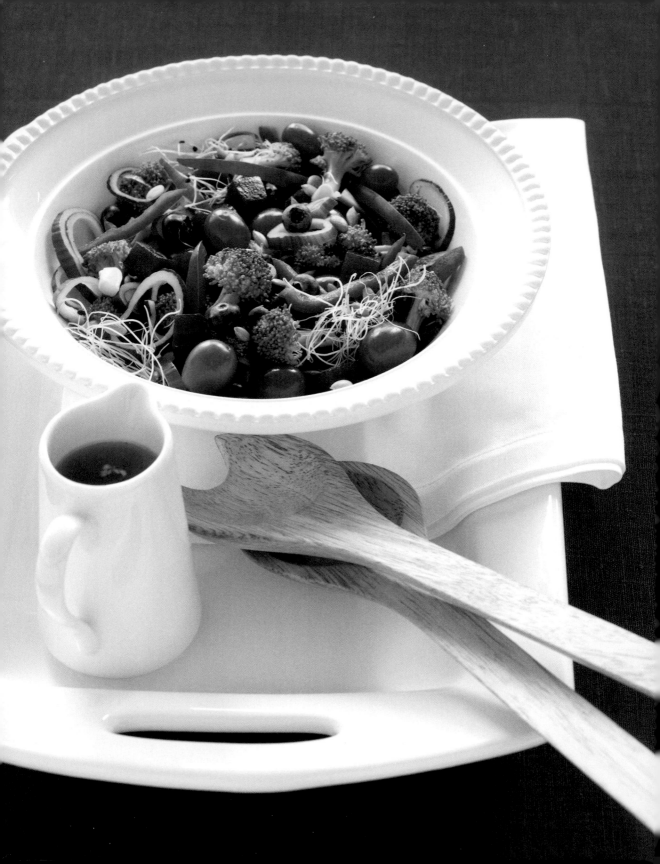

FIVE-B SALAD

A salad can be so many things, but it does not have to be Boring! Put a stop to dull iceberg lettuce salads topped with sad-looking tomatoes and doused with sickening dressings. Include this Clean-Eating salad in your new repertoire. It contains Broccoli, Bean sprouts, Bell pepper, Beets and Blueberries for a creative and health-charged meal.

INGREDIENTS:

2 cups / 480 ml bean sprouts – use alfalfa, broccoli onion, or any combination of sprouts

1 sweet red bell pepper, seeded, deveined and sliced into ribbons

3 cups / 720 ml broccoli florets, blanched and well drained

½ cup / 120 ml blueberries, fresh

½ cup / 120 ml cooked, diced purple beets, well drained

1 purple onion, peeled and sliced into thin rings

1 cup / 240 ml grape tomatoes

½ cup / 120 ml pumpkin seeds

DRESSING:

½ cup / 120 ml extra virgin olive oil, avocado oil, flaxseed oil, pumpkin oil or combination of any of these

2 Tbsp / 30 ml rice vinegar

3 cloves garlic, passed through a garlic press

6 Tbsp / 90 ml gluten-free tamari

PREPARATION:

1   In large decorative salad bowl combine the entire first list of ingredients. Cover and refrigerate or serve right away.

2   In small mixing bowl, whisk all dressing ingredients until well blended. Serve dressing on the side.

TIP

Complete your salad by serving it with albacore tuna and a pita wrap, a perfect Clean-Eating combination.

NUTRITIONAL VALUE PER SERVING:
Calories: 176 | Calories from Fat: 129 | Protein: 6g | Carbs: 8g
Dietary Fiber: 2g | Sugars: 3g | Fat: 14g | Sodium: 784mg

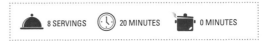
8 SERVINGS   20 MINUTES   0 MINUTES

GREEN BEAN, CORN AND TOMATO SALAD

At the end of the summer so many vegetables are coming into harvest it's hard to choose just one. A salad like this one is full of end-of-summer vegetables that taste delicious and are ideal for your Clean-Eating menu. This is a good salad to make if you've cooked too much corn the day before and have too many tomatoes ripening on the vines in your garden.

INGREDIENTS:

3 ears corn, husks and silks removed

1½ lb / 681 g green beans, topped and tailed

3 cloves garlic, peeled and smashed

4 Tbsp / 60 ml extra virgin olive oil or avocado oil

3 Tbsp / 45 ml red wine vinegar

½ sweet purple onion (about ½ cup), peeled and thinly sliced

1 medium tomato, red or yellow, sliced ½ inch thick

2 cups / 480 ml small tomatoes; try a combination of grape, cherry and sweet, halved

PREPARATION:

1 Place corn in a large pot of salted water. Bring water to a boil and cook for 5 minutes from that point. Remove from water and set aside on a cutting board to cool. Using a fine-mesh sieve, remove any corn silk remaining in the pot.

2 Add green beans to the pot and return to a boil, cooking until tender. The color should be bright green when done. Remove corn kernels from the cobs by standing each ear of corn on the flat end and running a knife down the side.

3 Remove green beans from boiling water and drain well. Put beans and corn in large bowl. Add garlic and 2 tablespoons / 30 ml oil. Toss and let stand for 30 minutes. Before serving, remove garlic pieces and add remaining tablespoon of oil, vinegar, onion and tomatoes. Toss gently. Season to taste with sea salt and freshly ground black pepper.

NUTRITIONAL VALUE PER SERVING:

Calories: 271 | Calories from Fat: 126 | Protein: 5g | Carbs: 40g
Dietary Fiber: 4g | Sugars: 4g | Fat: 10g | Sodium: 61mg

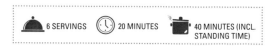

6 SERVINGS | 20 MINUTES | 40 MINUTES (INCL. STANDING TIME)

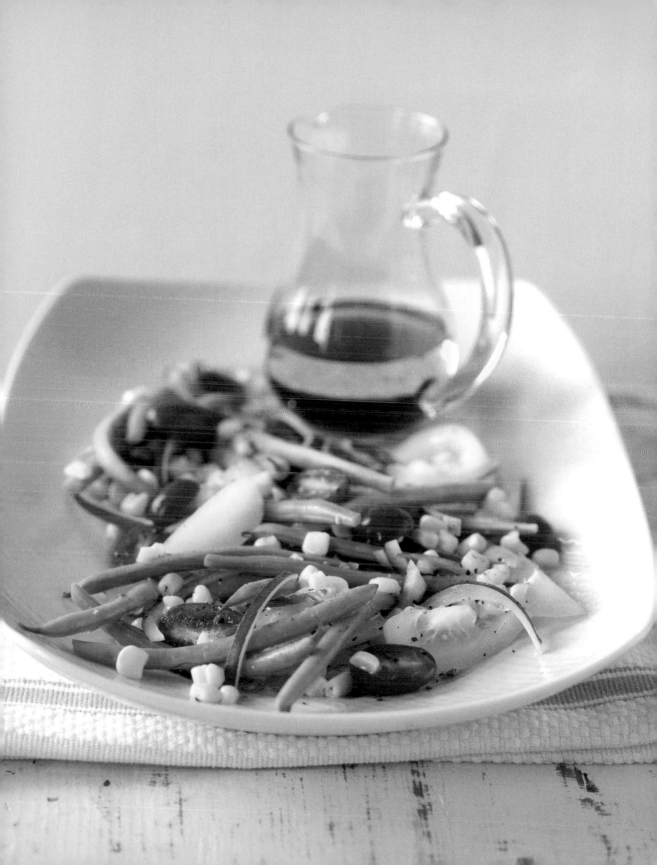

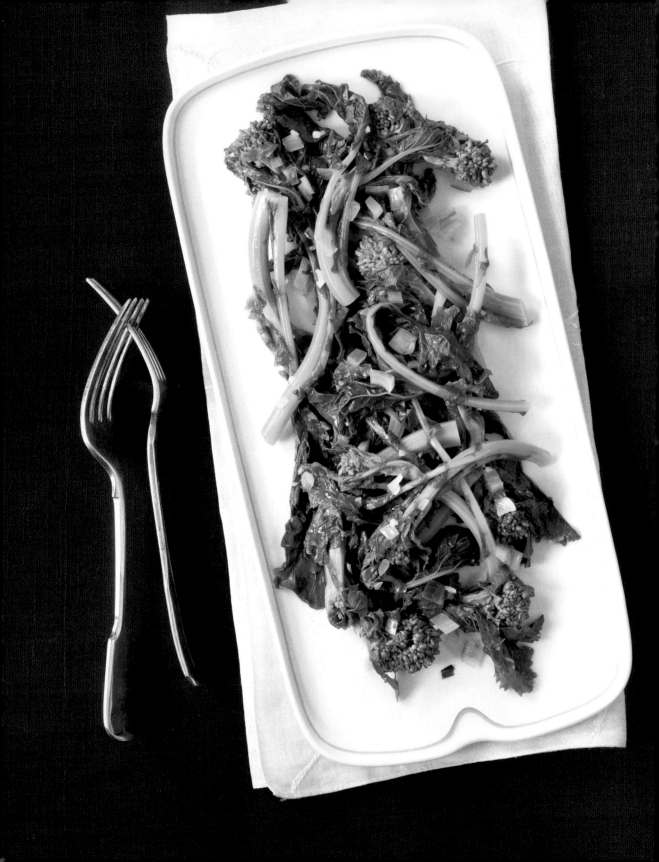

BROCCOLI RABE SAUTÉ

Sunday seems to be the day when I have a little more time to prepare an array of Clean-Eating surprises. The day I brought home broccoli rabe and served it sautéed was a memorable one. I had not seen much of this vegetable in the grocery stores, but I had visited one in the Little Italy area near where we live and noticed an abundance of it there. Lots of other shoppers were picking it up for their Sunday dinner, too. Try the slightly milder vegetable called "asparation." It is a hybrid cross of broccoli and Chinese kale. It will be a family favorite. This dish is so simple to make your even kids can do it.

INGREDIENTS:

1 lb / 454 g broccoli rabe or asparation, trimmed
1 medium purple onion, peeled and finely chopped
3 Tbsp / 45 ml best-quality olive or avocado oil
3 cloves garlic, passed through a garlic press
Coarse salt or sea salt
Black pepper

PREPARATION:

1   Fill a bowl with cold water and a few handfuls of ice cubes.

2   Meanwhile, in a large saucepan bring 2 quarts / 1.9 L water to a rolling boil. Add vegetables and a pinch of sea salt and cook until vegetables turn color. Once the broccoli or asparation has just turned color, remove from boiling water and place in ice water. Drain well and place on paper towels.

3   In a medium skillet heat olive or avocado oil until just hot. Add garlic and onion and cook until onions are soft, about 4 minutes. Add broccoli or asparation and cook over medium-high heat until al dente – tender but still crisp. Season with fresh ground black pepper and sea salt. Serve hot.

NUTRITIONAL VALUE PER SERVING:

Calories: 142 | Calories from Fat: 100 | Protein: 4g | Carbs: 7g
Dietary Fiber: 3g | Sugars: 1g | Fat: 11g | Sodium: 64mg

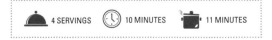
4 SERVINGS   10 MINUTES   11 MINUTES

SPECIALTY OILS

In our mother's kitchens anything that needed frying was done in butter, margarine or lard. But these fats are high in saturated and trans fats and are detrimental to health. Today we know that frying or sautéing should be done in oils much lower in saturated and trans fats. Gone are the days of reserving the bacon drippings in an old tin can.

A variety of healthy "nouveau" oils are now available to choose from, each with its own purpose and star qualities. Don't relegate yourself to using just corn or olive oil. Try any of these in your Clean-Eating cooking and get ready for a pleasant taste surprise.

STORAGE TIP

Please don't store any oils carelessly. These delicious oils are fragile and go rancid if stored incorrectly. Once the bottle has been opened, store it in a cool dark place far from the stove or even appliances that produce their own heat. If you store oil in the refrigerator, it may solidify. Don't worry, just set it on the counter for an hour before using and it will return to its liquid state.

PUMPKINSEED OIL

Styrian pumpkin seeds have no shell, which makes them perfect for pressing into this intensely colored oil. The resulting liquid is dark green tinged with red, thick and fragrant. Most pumpkinseed oil comes from the Austrian Styrian pumpkin. The oil is lovely in warm potato salad or drizzled over vegetables. Check the label before buying to make sure you are purchasing only pumpkinseed oil and not a product that has been blended with cheaper oils like sunflower or others.

Pumpkinseed oil cannot withstand high temperatures so do not use it as a replacement for olive oil when frying or sautéing. It will burn and destroy valuable nutrients.

HAZELNUT OIL

Hazelnut oil is highly fragrant with a sweet, nutty taste. It is pressed, of course, from hazelnuts. The light colored oil works well in dressings, marinades and baked goods. It has a relatively high smoke point so it can be used for general cooking. It keeps well in the refrigerator or in a cool dark place at less than 65°F. Like most oils hazelnut oil can go rancid quickly, so keep it cool.

WALNUT OIL

Walnut oil is cold pressed from dried walnuts. The flavor of walnut oil is fantastic and not to be missed in your Clean-Eating kitchen, although its use is not as extensive as that of other cooking oils. The reason for this is it is very much a specialty oil and therefore quite expensive. It is light in color, flavor and scent. Do not use walnut oil for pan frying because it has a low smoke point and goes rancid over heat. You will know it is rancid if you taste a bitter flavor after cooking. Use it mainly in cold dishes and dressings.

AVOCADO OIL

The best avocado oil is cold pressed from the flesh of the avocado and most often comes from Australia and New Zealand. But the Mexican people have long recognized the culinary value of the avocado not only as a fruit/vegetable but for its oil. The bright green oil is slightly thick and sticky with a smooth avocado flavor. It works well with lemon, chilis, salsas and strong herbs. If you are already cooking with olive oil then think of avocado oil in the same way. The oil has a high smoke point – it will not burn or smoke even at 500°F, which is higher than olive oil. The verdant green oil is loaded with potent antioxidants including vitamins D and E and a phytochemical called beta-sitosterol. This plant compound helps reduce levels of LDL "bad" cholesterol and balances levels of HDL "good" cholesterol. Give it a try next time you plan to sauté something.

RICE BRAN OIL

Rice bran oil is the new kid on the block when it comes to oils. The relatively "new" oil is pressed from the bran coating on rice kernels. This clear, almost colorless liquid possesses unique properties including an appealing nut-like flavor, many health benefits and a high smoke point, making it useful for frying. It contains loads of gamma-oryzanol and tocotrienols. Gamma-oryzanol is a potent antioxidant and it helps strengthen muscles. Best of all it converts fat to lean body mass! Tocotrienols are a unique form of vitamin E, a formidable antioxidant that helps protect against cellular damage and preserves youth. There are loads of reasons to include rice bran oil in your kitchen.

OIL SMOKE POINTS

OILS	FAHRENHEIT	CELCIUS
Flaxseed Oil	225	107
Pumpkinseed Oil	225	107
Hemp Seed Oil	330	166
Butterfat	350	177
Coconut Oil	350	177
Sesame Oil	350	177
Lard	370	182
Canola Oil	400	204
Walnut Oil	400	204
Extra Virgin Olive Oil	420	160
Cottonseed Oil	420	216
Almond Oil	425	218
Hazelnut Oil	430	221
Sunflower Oil	440	227
Olive Oil	440	227
Peanut Oil	440	227
Corn Oil	450	232
Palm Oil	450	232
Safflower Oil	450	232
Rice Bran Oil	490	254
Soybean Oil	495	257
Avocado Oil	520	271

CUCUMBER SALAD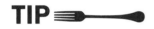

I remember this salad as a regular accompaniment to summer meals when growing up, especially when my dad's cucumbers were at their peak in his garden. It wouldn't matter if my mom put two, three or six cucumbers in the salad as it always disappeared. This simple recipe belies the delightful flavor. Yummy!

INGREDIENTS:

1 English cucumber (or two), washed, unpeeled and
   thinly sliced
½ cup / 120 ml ice cubes
¼ cup / 60 ml white vinegar
½ tsp / 2.5 ml sea salt

PREPARATION:

1   Into a decorative ceramic or glass serving bowl, measure the vinegar and sea salt. Stir well. Add sliced cucumber and toss so the vinegar mixture coats the cucumber.

2   Place the ice cubes on top of the cucumber and let sit until ready to serve. Otherwise, place in the refrigerator, covered, until ready to serve.

TIP

My Grandma, who lived to be 96, enjoyed this salad with thinly sliced green onions.

NUTRITIONAL VALUE PER SERVING:
Calories: 7 | Calories from Fat: 0 | Protein: 0g | Carbs: 0g
Dietary Fiber: 0g | Sugars: 0g | Fat: 0g | Sodium: 66mg

6 SERVINGS   5 MINUTES   0 MINUTES

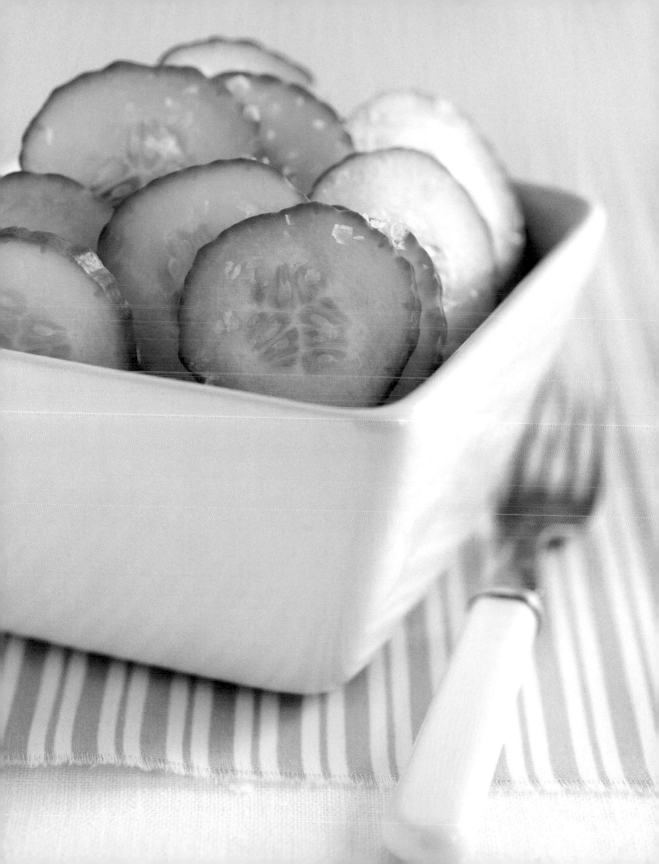

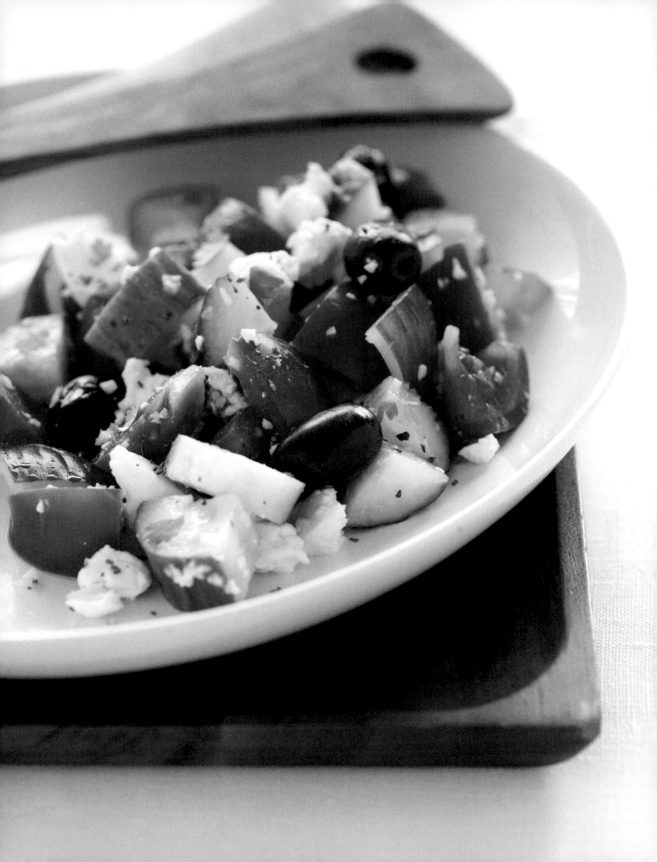

GREEK SALAD

One of my absolute favorite summer salads is this version of Greek salad. There is nothing better than fresh-off-the-vine tomatoes combined with crisp cucumbers. Fresh oregano and zesty lemon juice give the salad character. Add a grilled chicken breast and you have a meal. Eat it on its own with Ezekiel bread for lunch. Delicious!

INGREDIENTS:

4 large ripe tomatoes, chopped, preferably vine
    ripened, otherwise cluster tomatoes will do
2 medium cucumbers, seeded and cut into chunks,
    or 1 English cucumber
1 small purple onion or Vidalia onion, peeled and
    chopped
2 Tbsp / 30 ml fresh cilantro, chopped fine
4 oz / 112 g low-fat feta cheese, crumbled
2 cloves garlic, passed through a garlic press
2 Tbsp / 30 ml dried oregano
2 Tbsp / 30 ml fresh lemon juice
1 Tbsp / 15 ml extra virgin olive oil
²/₃ cup / 160 ml pitted black olives
Sea salt and fresh ground black pepper to taste

PREPARATION:

1   Find a brightly colored decorative bowl for serving this salad. Place first six ingredients in the bowl. Rub the oregano between your hands and sprinkle over the vegetables.

2   Drizzle lemon juice and olive oil over the salad. Add olives and toss gently.

MAKE IT A GREEK PASTA SALAD:

Measure 1 cup / 240 ml pasta, such as macaroni or fusilli. Use GF (gluten free) if required. Brown rice pasta is excellent, too. Bring 4 cups / 960 ml water to a boil and cook pasta until al dente. Rinse under cold water and drain well. Place in large serving bowl. Add above mixture and toss until vegetables are uniformly distributed. You may find you will have to increase the amount of lemon juice and olive oil in the pasta version of this recipe. Add sea salt and black pepper as necessary.

NUTRITIONAL VALUE PER SERVING:
Calories: 96 | Calories from Fat: 52 | Protein: 4g | Carbs: 7g
Dietary Fiber: 2g | Sugars: 3g | Fat: 5g | Sodium: 305mg

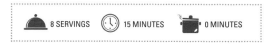 8 SERVINGS   15 MINUTES   0 MINUTES

PORTOBELLO MUSHROOM PASTA

Can I tell you how much I love Portobello mushrooms? These big brown fungi just do it for me. They are completely satisfying and taste as if I am really cheating – but I am not because Portobello mushrooms are so nourishing. The meaty texture and strong flavor satisfies even the biggest carnivore in your house. This recipe shares how I love them prepared best.

INGREDIENTS:

4 quarts / 3.8 L water

Sea salt and black pepper

1 cup / 240 ml shelled frozen edamame

4 Tbsp / 60 ml extra virgin olive oil, divided

2 cups / 480 ml brown rice penne or macaroni

2 Tbsp / 60 ml toasted sesame seeds

2 or 3 large Portobello mushrooms

4 cloves garlic, passed through a garlic press

2 Tbsp / 30 ml rice wine vinegar

1 cup / 240 ml Roma tomatoes, chopped and drained

½ cup / 120 ml fresh chopped basil

½ cup / 120 ml fresh chopped cilantro

PREPARATION:

1   Mushrooms are easy to clean. Simply remove the stalk and lift the outer skin from the cap using a small paring knife. It peels off readily. Slice the caps into quarter-inch pieces.

2   In a large saucepan bring about 4 quarts (about 3.8 L) of water to a full boil. Add a pinch of sea salt. Drop the frozen edamame into the boiling water and cook until the beans turn bright green. Immediately lift them out of the boiling water with a slotted spoon. Transfer to a small bowl and set aside.

3   In the still-boiling water add 2 Tbsp / 30 ml olive oil and the penne and cook al dente. Drain the penne, leaving behind about 1 cup / 240 ml of the cooking liquid. Put the penne back into the saucepan and cover.

4   Toast sesame seeds by placing in small skillet and cooking until fragrant.

5   In a large nonstick skillet heat remaining olive oil over medium-high heat. Add mushrooms and sauté until they become soft. Add the minced garlic and rice wine vinegar. Stir. Cover and let cook over low heat for about 5 minutes.

6   Place edamame in skillet along with tomatoes and herbs. Heat through. Pour mushroom mixture in pot with penne. Add sea salt and black pepper. Sprinkle with toasted sesame seeds. Place pasta in heated serving dish.

NUTRITIONAL VALUE PER SERVING:

Calories: 681 | Calories from Fat: 193 | Protein: 20g | Carbs: 100g | Dietary Fiber: 16g | Sugars: 7g | Fat: 7g | Sodium: 279mg

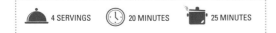

4 SERVINGS   20 MINUTES   25 MINUTES

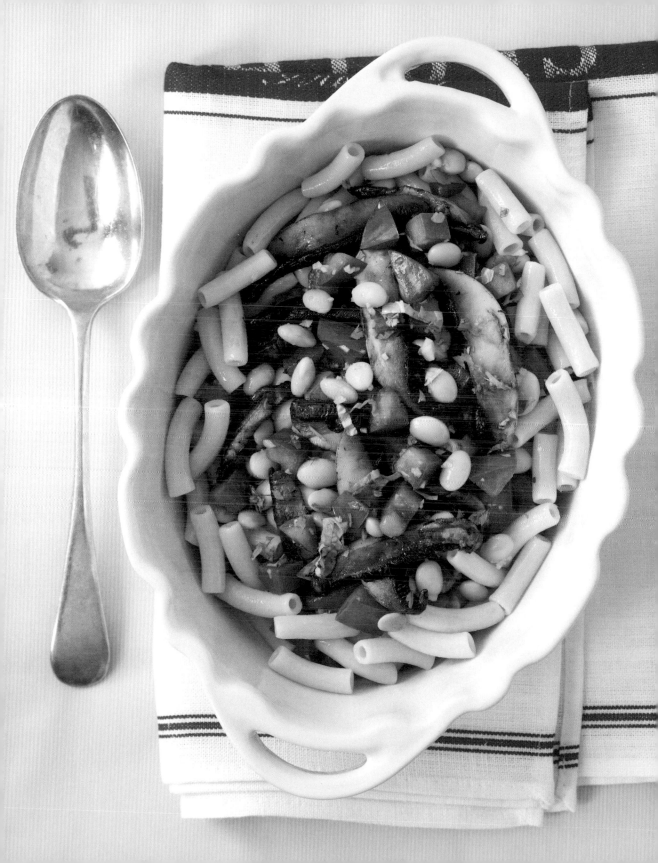

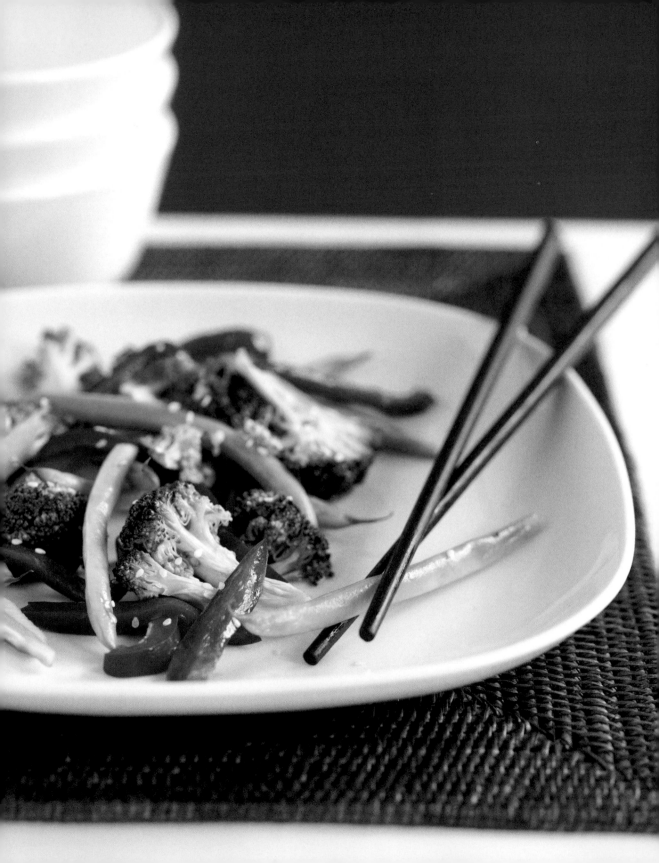

SESAME-ROASTED BROCCOLI AND GREEN BEANS

Want to serve something interesting for a festive occasion? Preparing broccoli and green beans this way makes the flavors pop and is less boring than the usual steamed version. The red pepper makes the dish look festive.

INGREDIENTS:

2 Tbsp / 30 ml olive oil

1 lb / 454 g green beans, trimmed

1 lb / 454 g broccoli, trimmed and cut into florets

2 sweet red bell peppers, sliced in strips

2 Tbsp / 30 ml oyster sauce or hoisin sauce

2 Tbsp / 30 ml maple syrup

1 Tbsp / 15 ml roasted sesame oil

2 Tbsp / 30 ml white sesame seeds

PREPARATION:

1 Preheat oven to 400°F / 204°C. Prepare a roasting pan by coating it lightly with oil. Place all vegetables in the roasting pan. Mix the oyster or hoisin sauce, maple syrup and sesame oil in a small bowl. Pour over the vegetables. Toss gently to coat the vegetables.

2 Place in the oven and bake for 10 minutes. Don't let the vegetables get burned. Remove the roasting pan from the oven and turn the vegetables over. Sprinkle with sesame seeds and return to the oven for another 5 minutes.

NUTRITIONAL VALUE PER SERVING:

Calories: 111 | Calories from Fat: 61 | Protein: 3g | Carbs: 10g
Dietary Fiber: 3g | Sugars: 4g | Fat: 6g | Sodium: 87mg

8 SERVINGS   10 MINUTES   15 MINUTES

EASY-TO-ASSEMBLE SNACKS FOR
KIDS & GROWN UPS ALIKE

You don't have to be a chef extraordinaire to Eat Clean. All you need is an assortment of fresh, wholesome ingredients on hand.

INGREDIENTS:

- Homemade hummus (the white peanut butter)
- Black bean spread
- Salsa
- An assortment of nut butters
- Sprouts – there are loads of varieties, so experiment a little
- Baby spinach or mesclun mix
- Fresh tomatoes – vine-ripened cluster tomatoes are best in the winter
- Ground flax seeds
- Bananas
- Apples
- Avocado
- Grilled or roasted turkey breast
- Grilled or roasted chicken breast
- Hardboiled eggs
- Leftover brown rice

WRAPS – brown rice, whole grain, pita, Ezekiel bread or wraps or any you prefer

ASSEMBLY:

1 **Choose your outer wrapping** – essentially the container you will be using.

2 **Choose the spread you want to use** – I love almond butter sprinkled with ground flax seeds, hummus, or herbed yogurt cheese.

3 **Choose the filling** – banana, sliced apple, grilled chicken, sprouts, salsa … the combinations are endless! That's why it's so nice to have leftovers on hand.

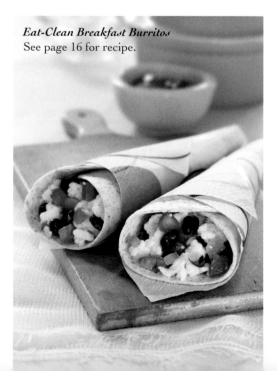

Eat-Clean Breakfast Burritos
See page 16 for recipe.

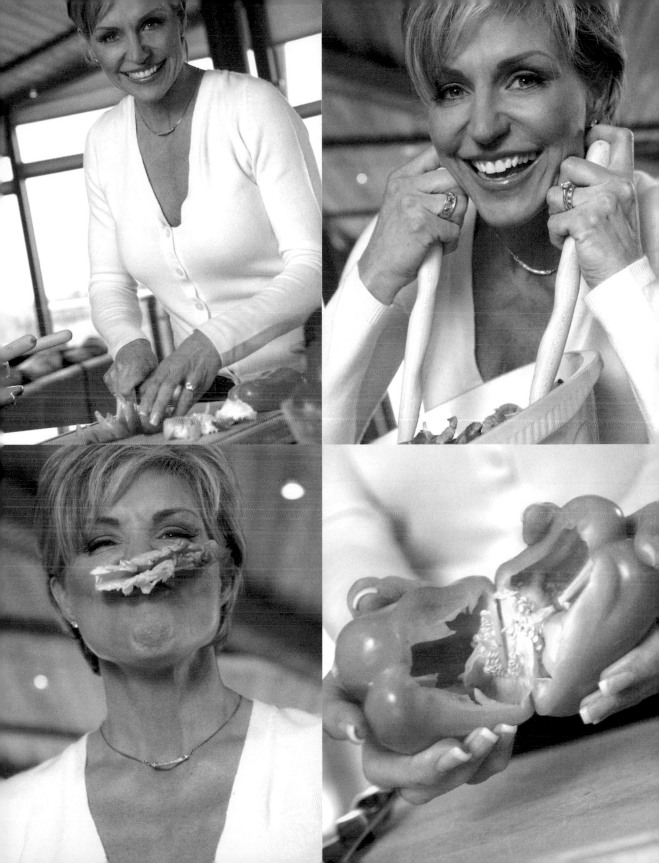

SWEET POTATO OVEN FRIES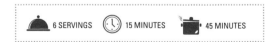

Nothing beats the aroma of these delicious wedges. They come out of the oven golden and crispy with just the right amount of seasoning. You'll feel like you're cheating when you take a bite, but this version of the sweet potato is chock full of healthy nutrients eager to make your body the best it can be!

INGREDIENTS:

Olive oil cooking spray

Enough sprigs of fresh rosemary to cover a baking sheet

1 tsp / 5 ml chili powder

1 tsp / 5 ml ground cumin

1 tsp / 5 ml paprika

1 tsp / 5 ml Kosher salt

1 tsp / 5 ml freshly ground black pepper

2 medium sweet potatoes (about 1 lb), scrubbed and blotted dry

PREPARATION:

1 Preheat oven to 400°F / 204°C.

2 Spray a baking sheet with olive oil spray. Spread rosemary sprigs on sheet in a single layer, making sure entire surface is covered. Mix together all other ingredients, except sweet potatoes, in small bowl.

3 Square off potatoes and slice into "steak fries." Lay strips of potato on rosemary in single layer. Sprinkle generously with seasoning mixture. Spray generously with olive oil spray. Bake 20 minutes.

4 Spray again. Return to oven for about 25 minutes more or until fries are golden and puffed.

NUTRITIONAL VALUE PER SERVING:

Calories: 44 | Calories from Fat: 1 | Protein: 1g | Carbs: 13g
Dietary Fiber: 1g | Sugars: 1g | Fat: 0g | Sodium: 288mg

6 SERVINGS   15 MINUTES   45 MINUTES

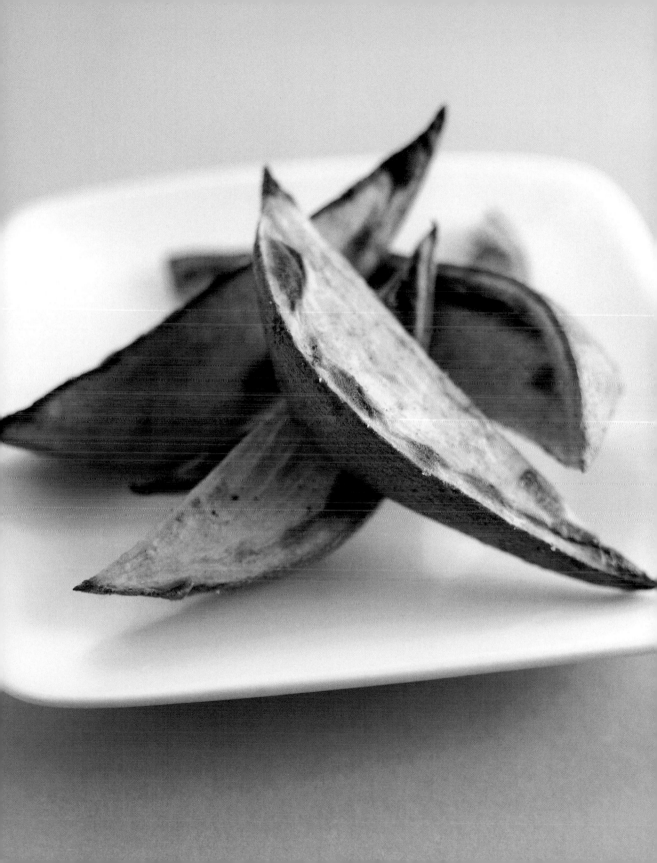

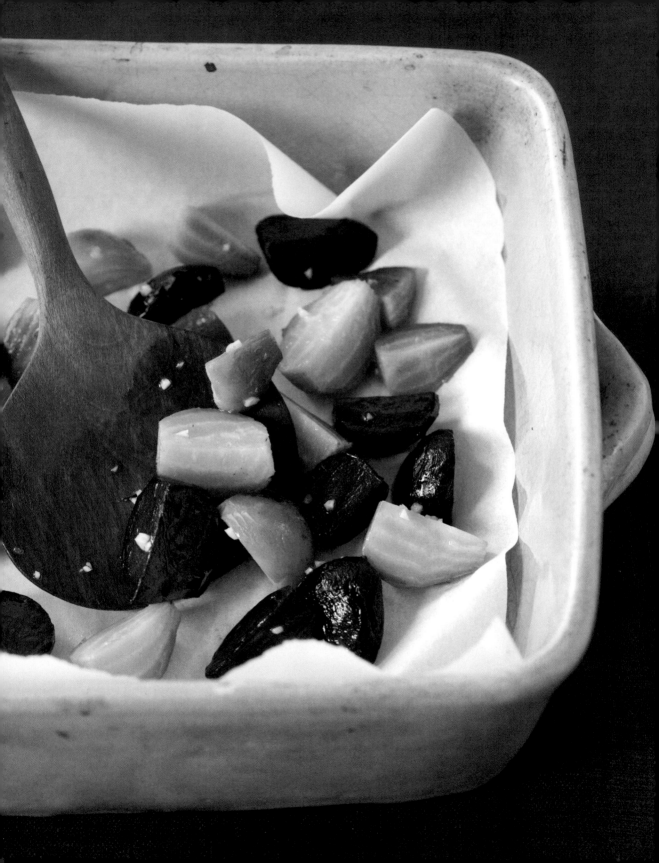

OVEN-ROASTED BEETS

Since we are on a roll and trying so many new wonderful flavors, add beets to your shopping list today. I want you to discover the nutty, warm taste of roasted beets. I enjoy pickled beets, but roasted beets should be on your dinner plate more often.

INGREDIENTS:

6 – 8 medium-sized beets

Extra virgin olive oil

4 cloves garlic, passed through garlic press

Parchment paper

OTHER OVEN-ROASTED BEET IDEAS

• Beets come in a sunshiny golden color, too. If you want to jazz things up, roast a mix of beet colors.

• Add walnuts to roasted beets for another flavor and nutritional punch.

• Once you have the beets roasted, skinned and chopped they can be added to salads or other vegetable mixtures, especially green beans, snow peas and other greens that contrast well with the vivid beet color.

PREPARATION:

1 Preheat oven to 350°F / 177°C.

2 Wash and scrub beets. Remove any strings. Line a cookie sheet with parchment paper. Place beets on the lined cookie sheet. Drizzle with olive oil and sprinkle minced garlic over beets. Cover tightly with tin foil and place in the oven.

3 Bake 1 hour.

4 Remove from heat. Let cool enough that you can handle the beets. The skins slip off easily at this point. Slice and place on a dinner plate next to your main course. Beets keep well in the fridge.

NUTRITIONAL VALUE PER SERVING:
Calories: 78 | Calories from Fat: 43 | Protein: 1g | Carbs: 8g
Dietary Fiber: 2g | Sugars: 5g | Fat: 4g | Sodium: 64mg

 6 SERVINGS   10 MINUTES   1 HOUR

LENTIL SALAD

On a day when you just don't feel like a hot meal but still want your Clean-Eating protein and complex carbohydrates, try this colorful and delicious salad.

INGREDIENTS:

3 cups / 725 ml water

1 cup / 240 ml Puy lentils, rinsed and picked over (watch for little stones)

2 cloves garlic, passed through garlic press

½ tsp / 2.5 ml dried thyme

3 bay leaves

¼ tsp / 1.25 ml sage

½ cup / 120 ml peeled, chopped carrots (sweet loose carrots are best)

Sea salt

1 cup / 240 ml green beans, cut into 1-inch pieces

1 cup / 240 ml frozen shelled edamame

½ cup / 120 ml scallions, chopped

DRESSING:

3 Tbsp / 45 ml rice wine vinegar

1 Roma tomato, chopped

1 clove garlic, passed through garlic press

2 Tbsp / 30 ml fresh basil, coarsely chopped

2 Tbsp / 30 ml fresh oregano, chopped

Sea salt and black pepper

PREPARATION:

1   In large saucepan place water, lentils, garlic, thyme, bay leaves and sage. Bring to a boil and reduce heat. Continue to cook for 30 minutes, covered. Lentils should be chewy, not soft. Add carrots and sea salt and cook 3 minutes. Then add green beans and edamame. Cook 5 minutes. Remove from heat. Drain cooking liquid into a bowl and set aside. Place lentil mixture in large pretty serving bowl. Add chopped scallions.

2   In a small bowl combine rice wine vinegar, tomato, garlic, basil, oregano and sea salt and pepper. Whisk briefly and pour over lentils. Add reserved cooking liquid if salad is dry. Toss all ingredients lightly until just combined.

NUTRITIONAL VALUE PER SERVING:
Calories: 188 | Calories from Fat: 29 | Protein: 14g | Carbs: 30g
Dietary Fiber: 12g | Sugars: 4g | Fat: 3g | Sodium: 284mg

6 SERVINGS   20 MINUTES   40 MINUTES

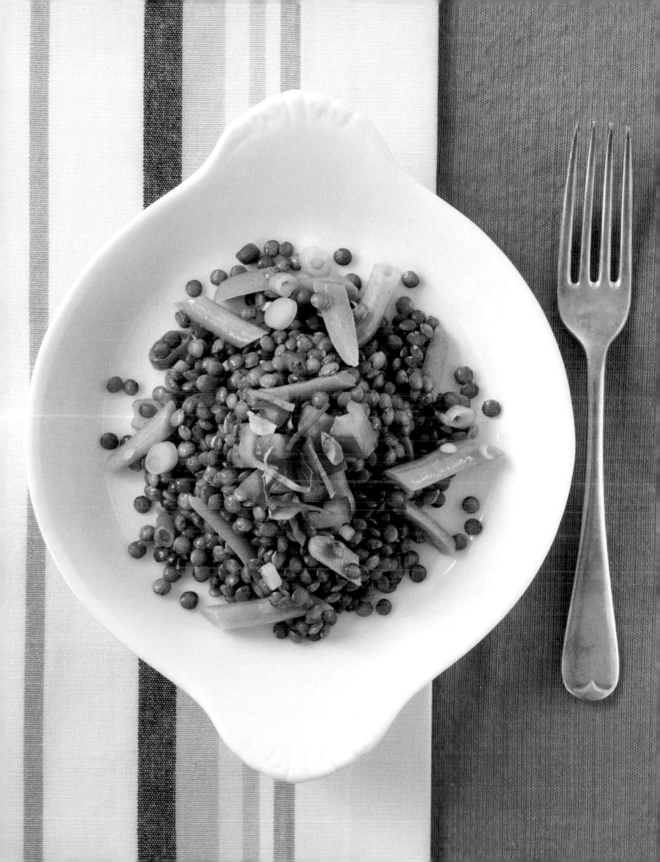

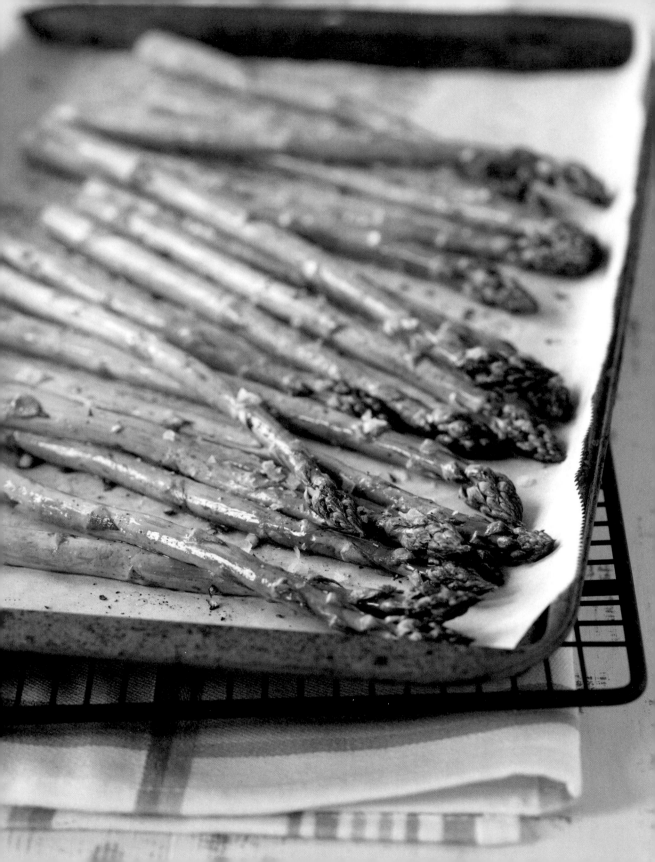

ROASTED ASPARAGUS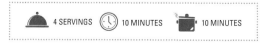

When spring rolls around there is nothing more delicious than tender asparagus. You can do a lot with this delightfully green vegetable, even eat it raw. Try it! It is a pleasant surprise. I also love this way of preparing asparagus. You don't need to cook the spears very long as they are tender in a flash. But roasting imparts an especially delicious flavor. Be careful not to overcook asparagus. It's better to undercook than overcook.

INGREDIENTS:

1 lb / 454 g asparagus, firm and bright green

2 Tbsp / 30 ml extra virgin olive oil

1 Tbsp / 15 ml balsamic vinegar

1 clove garlic

Sea salt and ground black pepper to taste

Cooking spray

PREPARATION:

1   Preheat oven to 425°F / 218°C. Break off woody stems of each asparagus spear. Rinse well under running water. Asparagus grows in sand and needs a good washing if you don't want your final dish to be gritty.

2   Toss spears in olive oil, vinegar and garlic. Season with salt and pepper. Lay in a single layer in a shallow baking dish coated with cooking spray. Bake 6 – 10 minutes until just done. Superb!

TIP

Just double the recipe if you have more to feed.

NUTRITIONAL VALUE PER SERVING:
Calories: 88 | Calories from Fat: 65 | Protein: 2g | Carbs: 5g
Dietary Fiber: 2g | Sugars: 1g | Fat: 7g | Sodium: 17mg

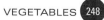

4 SERVINGS   10 MINUTES   10 MINUTES

SWEET POTATO SALAD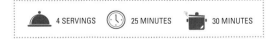

Sweet potatoes and I get along very well. My taste buds enjoy their pleasant sweet flavor, while my tongue loves the soft, dessert-like texture. They pack a serious nutritional resume. This salad makes good use of their firm flesh.

INGREDIENTS:

4 quarts / 3.8 L water

2 large sweet potatoes, scrubbed clean, fibers removed

2 Tbsp / 30 ml white vinegar

1 Tbsp / 15 ml fresh lemon juice – juice of half a lemon

5 green onions, trimmed and chopped

3 stalks celery, trimmed and chopped

½ firm English cucumber, chopped

½ cup / 120 ml fresh cilantro, chopped

½ cup / 120 ml nonfat plain yogurt or soy yogurt

Rind of one fresh lemon, grated

Sea salt and freshly ground black pepper

¼ cup / 60 ml toasted unsalted sunflower seeds

PREPARATION:

1   Peel and cut sweet potatoes into half-inch cubes. In medium saucepan place 4 quarts water (3.8 L) and chopped sweet potatoes. Bring water to a boil and reduce heat. Cook potatoes over low heat until they are tender – about 20 - 30 minutes. Do not let potatoes get too soft or mushy. Remove from heat and drain. Transfer to medium bowl. Set aside and let cool.

2   Meanwhile, place vinegar and lemon juice into a large decorative serving bowl. Mix and add all chopped vegetables – onion, celery, cucumber – and cilantro. Toss to coat veggies with vinegar and lemon juice. Now add cooled sweet potatoes and nonfat yogurt and gently toss. Season with salt and pepper.

3   Divide among four salad bowls and sprinkle with toasted sunflower seeds and lemon zest.

NUTRITIONAL VALUE PER SERVING:

Calories: 128 | Calories from Fat: 35 | Protein: 4g | Carbs: 18g
Dietary Fiber: 3g | Sugars: 5g | Fat: 3g | Sodium: 64mg

4 SERVINGS   25 MINUTES   30 MINUTES

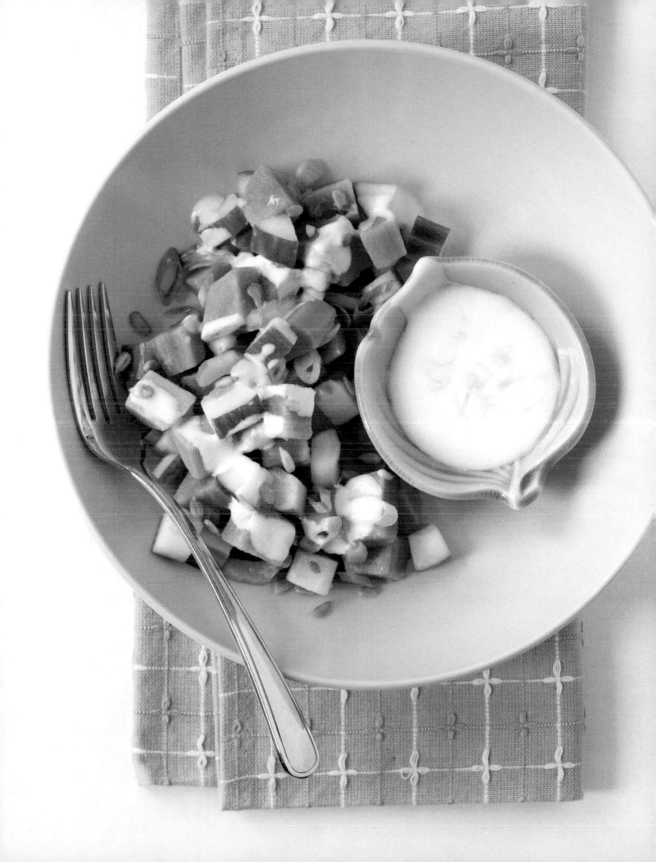

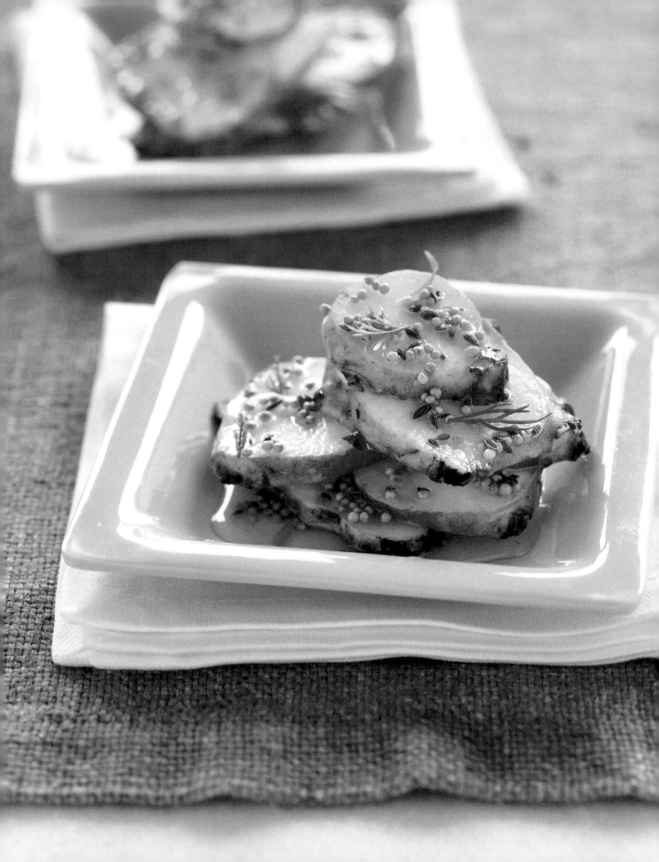

JERUSALEM ARTICHOKES

The Jerusalem artichoke is also known as the sunchoke. It is native to North America and is the tuber of the perennial sunflower. Valued by First Nations peoples for its nourishing flesh, the Jerusalem artichoke tastes much like the globe artichoke and is high in phosphorus and potassium. This version of the artichoke is available in the winter and spring.

INGREDIENTS:

1 lb / 454 g Jerusalem artichokes
½ cup / 120 ml cider vinegar
¼ cup / 60 ml organic honey
¼ tsp / 1.25 ml dill seeds
½ tsp / 2.5 ml mustard seeds
1 tsp / 5 ml tarragon
1 tsp / 5 ml chervil
1 tsp / 5 ml chopped fresh dill
Sea salt and black pepper to taste

PREPARATION:

1 Scrub the Jerusalem artichokes well. Do not peel. Slice into quarter-inch thick slices. Blanch the slices in boiling water for a minute or so. Drain and set aside in decorative serving bowl.

2 In a small saucepan, place vinegar, honey, and dill and mustard seeds. Bring to a boil. Remove from heat. Pour over blanched Jerusalem artichokes. Add remaining tarragon, chervil and fresh dill to the dish. Season with salt and pepper. Toss lightly. Refrigerate.

3 Serve as a chilled salad on a bed of baby spinach or serve as an accompaniment to grilled or roasted chicken and turkey.

NUTRITIONAL VALUE PER SERVING:

Calories: 95 | Calories from Fat: 9 | Protein: 4g | Carbs: 14g
Dietary Fiber: 1g | Sugars: 0.5g | Fat: 1g | Sodium: 66mg

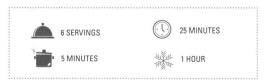

6 SERVINGS   25 MINUTES
5 MINUTES   1 HOUR

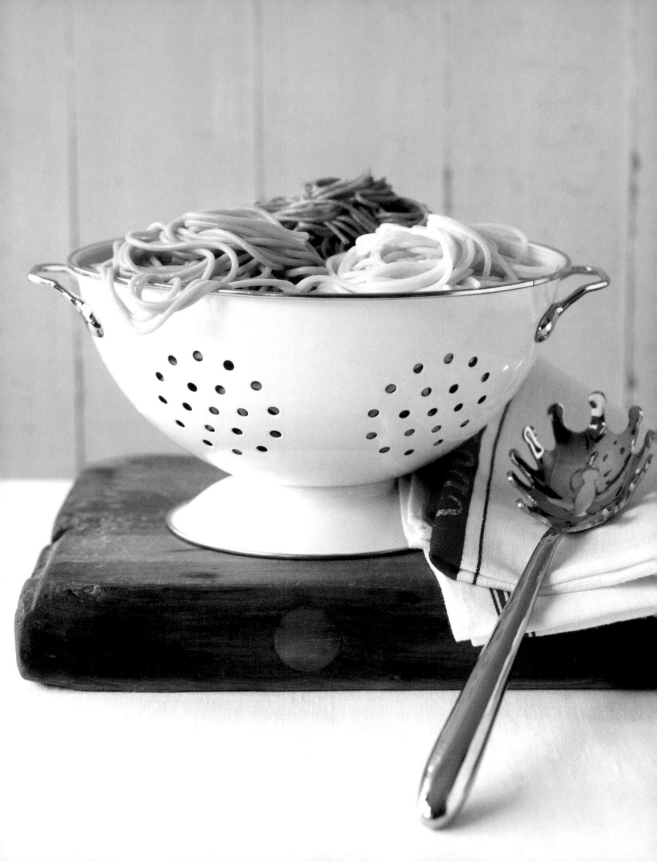

8

Pasta

This ubiquitous food finds itself on every menu with its pleasing and abundant shapes. Today there is a virtual explosion of this versatile fare. You can find glass noodles, rice noodles, spelt, kamut and many more to please your pasta-loving palate. You could enjoy a different shape, size and color every night of the week.

And if that wasn't enough, the variations of toppings, sauces and accompaniments are endless. Pasta is a forgiving dish that really allows you to flex your creative culinary muscle.

LINGUINE
with Jumbo Shrimp and Spinach

Jumbo shrimp are wonderful sources of protein and deserve a place on your dinner table. This combination of shrimp and spinach tastes fabulous, and these ingredients are loaded with superior nutrition – lycopene, calcium and folate, just to name a few.

INGREDIENTS:

1 lb / 454 g linguine – use brown rice, kamut, spelt
    or other type noodle
2 cups / 480 ml low-sodium chicken or vegetable
    stock (gluten free if necessary)
1 purple onion, minced
2 cloves garlic, passed through a garlic press
1 lb / 454 g large shrimp
2/3 cup / 160 ml yogurt cheese
    (see recipe page 141)
4 Tbsp / 60 ml fresh chopped basil
2 Tbsp / 30 ml fresh marjoram
2 tsp / 10 ml grated lemon rind (lemon zest)
Sea salt and fresh ground black pepper
1 cup / 240 ml cherry tomatoes, halved
4 cups / 960 ml shredded spinach

PREPARATION:

1 Bring 6 quarts / 5.7 L of salted water to a boil. Add pasta and cook al dente. Drain, rinse under cold water to prevent clumping, and return to the pot.

2 In a small saucepan heat chicken stock. Add onions, garlic and shrimp and let simmer, covered, for 3 to 5 minutes or until shrimp are heated through. Remove the shrimp from the cooking liquid and transfer to a glass bowl. Cover with a plate and wrap a clean kitchen towel around the bowl to keep warm.

3 In a small bowl, whisk together yogurt cheese, chopped basil, marjoram, lemon zest, sea salt and black pepper. Pour over pasta. Add cherry tomatoes, cooked shrimp and spinach. Toss gently to evenly distribute ingredients. Serve.

NUTRITIONAL VALUE PER SERVING:

Calories: 425 | Calories from Fat: 47 | Protein: 25g | Carbs: 68g
Dietary Fiber: 5g | Sugars: 8g | Fat: 5g | Sodium: 269mg

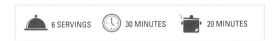 6 SERVINGS   30 MINUTES   20 MINUTES

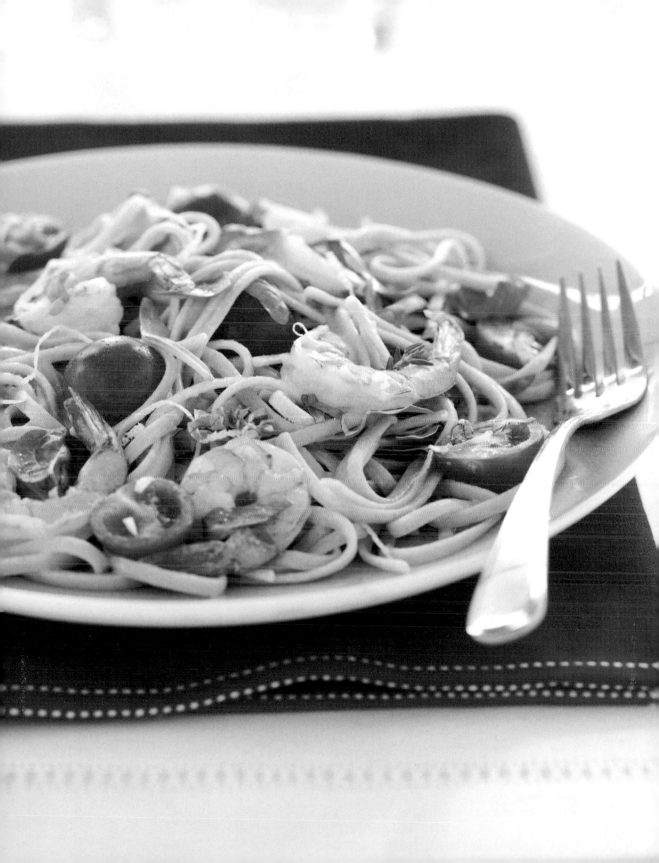

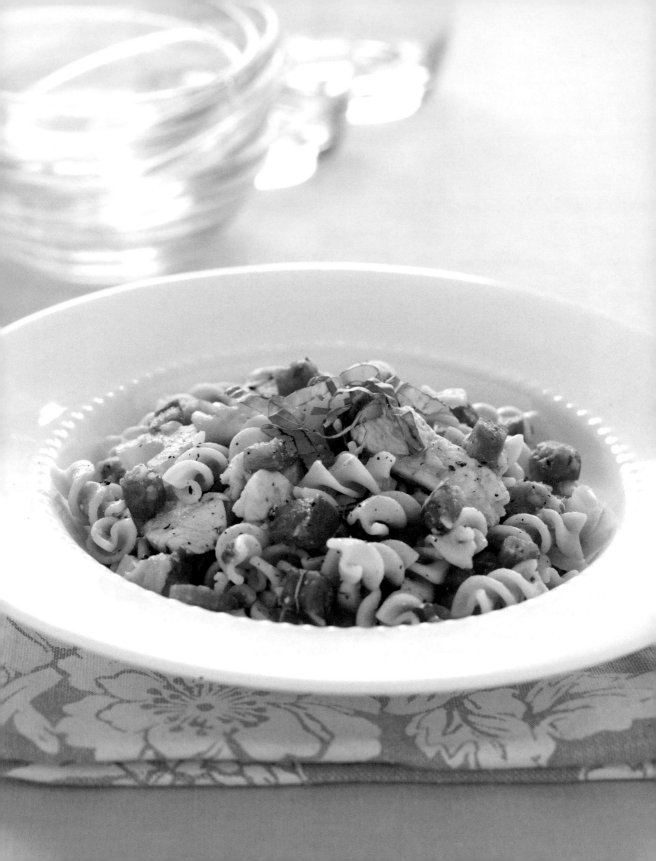

CHICKEN ROTINI
with Roma Tomato Sauce

For years I have prepared my own homemade tomato sauce. I would come home with bushels of tomatoes and make a disaster of the kitchen as I prepared a delicious, nutritious and preservative-free sauce. The Roma variety has always been my favorite. Their fruitful vines in addition to their peculiar egg shape and meaty texture make Roma tomatoes a perfect choice for home canning and tomato sauce. Give them a try tonight in your own homemade pasta delight!

INGREDIENTS:

6 lean chicken breasts, boneless and skinless or if
    vegetarian, use tofu, cut in 1" cubes

1 Tbsp / 15 ml extra virgin olive oil

1 large onion, peeled and chopped

1 large carrot, peeled and chopped

2 ribs celery, including leafy greens, chopped

½ cup / 120 ml fresh basil, chopped

2 tsp / 10 ml dried oregano leaves

4 cloves garlic, passed through a garlic press

8 Roma tomatoes, chopped

1 medium sweet potato, baked

¼ cup / 60 ml low-sodium chicken or vegetable
    broth (gluten free if necessary)

1 x 10 oz / 280 g package brown-rice rotini pasta

PREPARATION:

1   Cut chicken breasts into thin strips.

2   In a large skillet, heat olive oil over medium heat. Add onion, carrots and celery and cook until they become soft but not brown. Add herbs and garlic and continue cooking for 2 to 3 minutes. Add chopped Roma tomatoes and sweet potato pulp along with ¼ cup / 60 ml chicken broth. Add chicken strips and increase heat until mixture comes to full boil. Reduce heat and cover tightly. Let simmer for 20 minutes.

3   Meanwhile, in a large saucepan bring 6 quarts / 5.7 L water to a full boil. Add a pinch of salt and a splash of olive oil to the water to prevent pasta from sticking. Add pasta and cook al dente. Drain and return to the pot.

4   Add tomato mixture to pasta and mix until all ingredients are combined. Transfer to heated decorative serving bowl and serve.

NUTRITIONAL VALUE PER SERVING:
Calories: 355 | Calories from Fat: 53 | Protein: 28g | Carbs: 54g
Dietary Fiber: 4g | Sugars: 7g | Fat: 5g | Sodium: 294mg

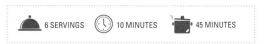
6 SERVINGS   10 MINUTES   45 MINUTES

PASTA WITH TUNA AND OLIVES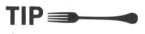

With a few standard ingredients it is simple to create a delicious Clean-Eating meal. Tuna and olives make a complete meal out of pasta and marinara sauce.

INGREDIENTS:

16 oz / 448 g spelt or Kamut pasta noodles
    (or gluten-free noodles of your choice)
1 Tbsp / 15 ml extra virgin olive oil
3 cloves garlic, passed through a garlic press
1 medium onion, peeled and chopped
2 stalks celery, trimmed and chopped
1 small carrot, peeled and chopped
¼ tsp / 1.25 ml red pepper flakes
1 x 28 oz / 784 g can tomato purée
Sea salt and fresh ground black pepper
2 Tbsp / 30 ml fresh chopped basil
2 Tbsp / 30 ml fresh chopped oregano
8 oz / 224 g albacore tuna, water packed
½ cup / 120 ml black, pitted Kalamata olives

PREPARATION:

1 Bring 8 cups / 1.9 L water to a boil in a large sauce pan. Put a little olive oil and sea salt into the boiling water. Drop the pasta noodles in the water and cook al dente or according to package instructions.

2 Place the olive oil in a Dutch oven and heat over medium heat. Add garlic, onions, celery, carrots and red pepper flakes. Sauté for 10 minutes or until vegetables become soft. Add tomatoes, sea salt, fresh black pepper and herbs. Add drained tuna and black olives. Let mixture heat through on low for 10 minutes. Serve over pasta.

TIP

Add a crisp salad loaded with the freshest ingredients to round out your pasta meal and increase your veggie intake.

NUTRITIONAL VALUE PER SERVING:
Calories: 426 | Calories from Fat: 62 | Protein: 23g | Carbs: 73g
Dietary Fiber: 9g | Sugars: 7g | Fat: 6g | Sodium: 228mg

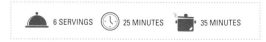

6 SERVINGS   25 MINUTES   35 MINUTES

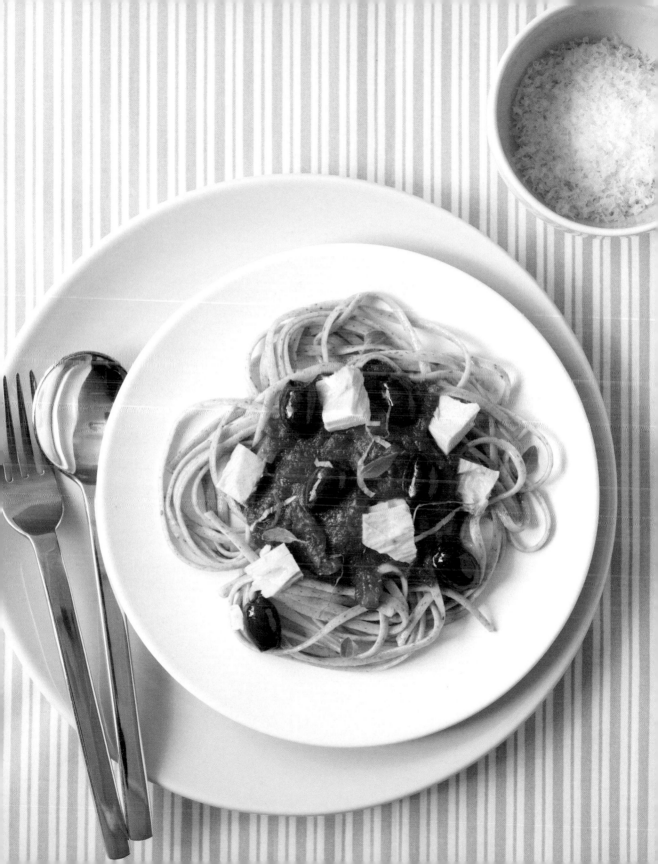

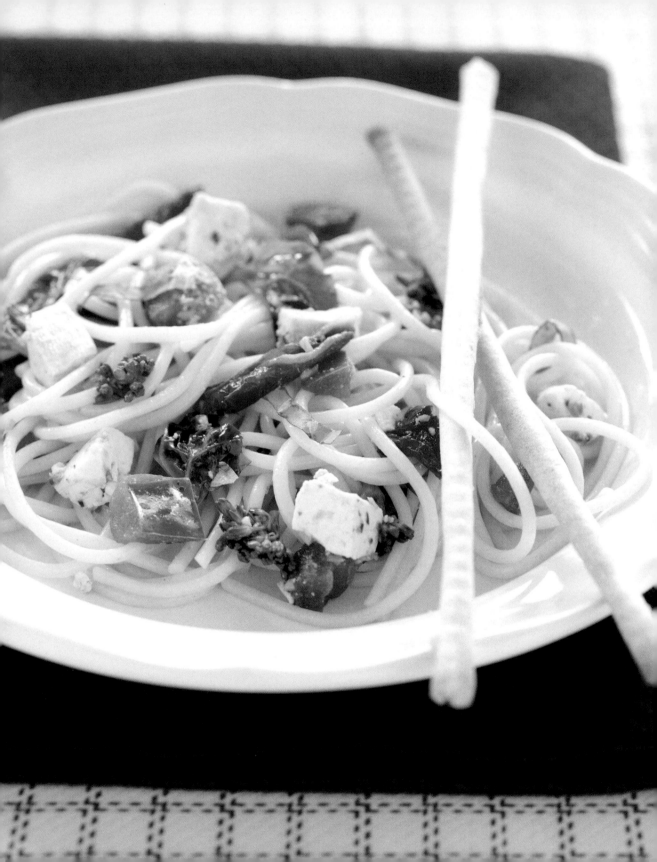

ITALIAN RICE-NOODLE PASTA
with Tofu and Sundried Tomatoes

For those who cannot tolerate gluten it is satisfying to know they can still enjoy pasta without the tummy ache. Rice noodles or brown rice noodles are a perfect gluten-free option to enjoy with any favorite pasta dish. This version incorporates the tangy flavor of sundried tomatoes and goes perfectly with tofu or strips of grilled chicken or turkey.

INGREDIENTS:

2 Tbsp / 30 ml (+ extra for pasta water) extra virgin olive oil

3 fresh garlic cloves, passed through a garlic press

3 Tbsp / 45 ml pesto, either homemade or commercial

2 lbs / 908 g firm tofu, rinsed, well drained and cut into cubes or strips

½ cup / 120 ml sundried tomatoes, chopped

1 cup / 240 ml fresh basil, coarsely chopped

5 or 6 large fresh Roma tomatoes, chopped

3 cups / 720 ml baby spinach leaves

1½ cups / 360 ml chopped broccolini

1 lb / 454 g brown rice pasta spaghetti noodles

Sea salt and freshly ground pepper

PREPARATION:

1 In a large nonstick sauté pan, heat olive oil and garlic over medium heat. Add pesto, tofu and sundried tomatoes and warm through. Add basil, fresh tomatoes, baby spinach and chopped broccolini. Simmer the tomato and vegetable mixture until you have a consistent sauce. Add more tomatoes if needed.

2 Meanwhile, in a large saucepan, boil about 6 quarts / 5.7 L water. Add a pinch of sea salt and a dash of olive oil to keep the pasta from sticking together. Add pasta and cook until al dente. Drain pasta and add sauce. Toss so that all ingredients are uniformly distributed. Transfer to a heated serving bowl and serve immediately.

TIP

You don't need to drown your noodles with oodles of sauce. Let the freshest ingredients speak for themselves.

NUTRITIONAL VALUE PER SERVING:
Calories: 444 | Calories from Fat: 145 | Protein: 24g | Carbs: 56g
Dietary Fiber: 8g | Sugars: 5g | Fat: 16g | Sodium: 118mg

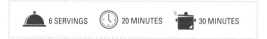 6 SERVINGS   20 MINUTES   30 MINUTES

BAKED ORZO AND SHRIMP

Don't limit your shrimp consumption to the typical shrimp cocktail hors d'oeuvre. It can be the perfect protein addition to many meals. This dish uses orzo to compliment the shrimp as a delicious complex carbohydrate. A variety of veggies and seasonings further enhance the flavor and texture of the meal, while yogurt cheese adds that perfect final touch!

INGREDIENTS:

2 lbs / 908 g large shrimp, peeled and deveined

1 Vidalia onion, peeled and chopped

1 red bell pepper, seeded and deveined, chopped

1 Tbsp / 15 ml extra virgin olive oil

Sea salt and fresh ground black pepper

4 cloves garlic, passed through a garlic press

1 lb / 454 g whole-wheat orzo

Pinch turmeric

4 cups / 906 ml low-sodium vegetable broth or
   water

1 cup / 240 ml water

3 cups / 720 ml chopped fresh Roma tomatoes, set
   in fine-mesh sieve and allowed to drain

1 cup / 240 ml frozen edamame

½ cup / 120 ml yogurt cheese
   (see recipe page 141)

¼ cup / 60 ml chopped fresh cilantro

1 tsp / 5 ml crumbled, dried oregano

4 green onions, trimmed and sliced thin

PREPARATION:

1   Preheat oven to 400°F / 205°C. Place all shrimp on a bed of paper towels. Season with sea salt and black pepper.

2   Place onion, pepper, olive oil and ½ teaspoon / 2.5 ml sea salt in a heavy skillet or Dutch oven. Cover and cook on low heat for 8 minutes. Add garlic and cook until you begin to smell it. Add orzo and turmeric. Stir well and cook 5 minutes. Add cooking liquids. Cook about 10 minutes. Add tomatoes, edamame and shrimp. Prepare a lasagna pan with a light coating of nonstick spray. Pour mixture into pan. Place a layer of yogurt cheese on top. Bake for 20 minutes. Divide among 6 plates and garnish with cilantro, oregano, and chopped green onions.

NUTRITIONAL VALUE PER SERVING:
Calories: 564 | Calories from Fat: 69 | Protein: 48g | Carbs: 74g
Dietary Fiber: 6g | Sugars: 11g | Fat: 7g | Sodium: 615mg

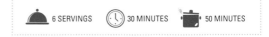 6 SERVINGS   30 MINUTES   50 MINUTES

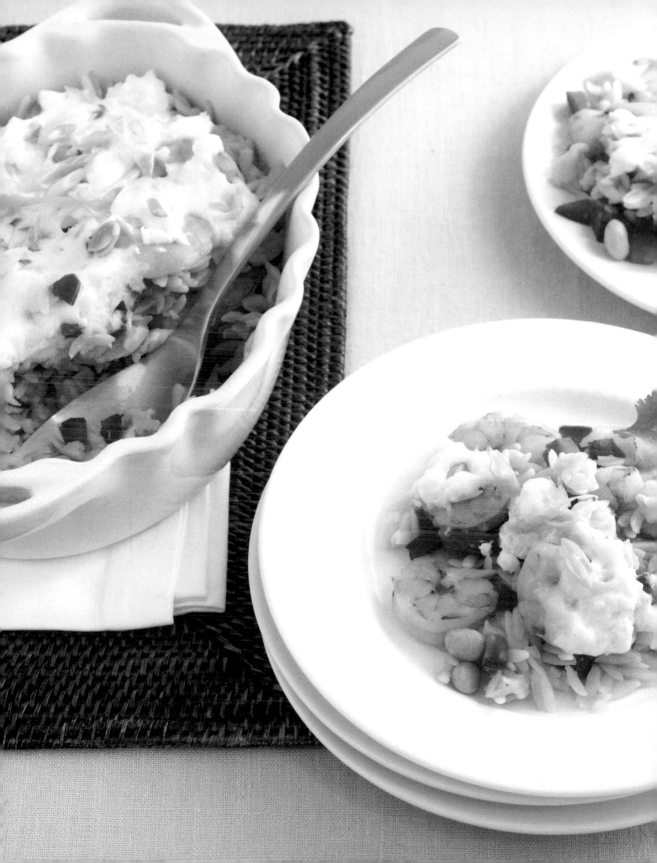

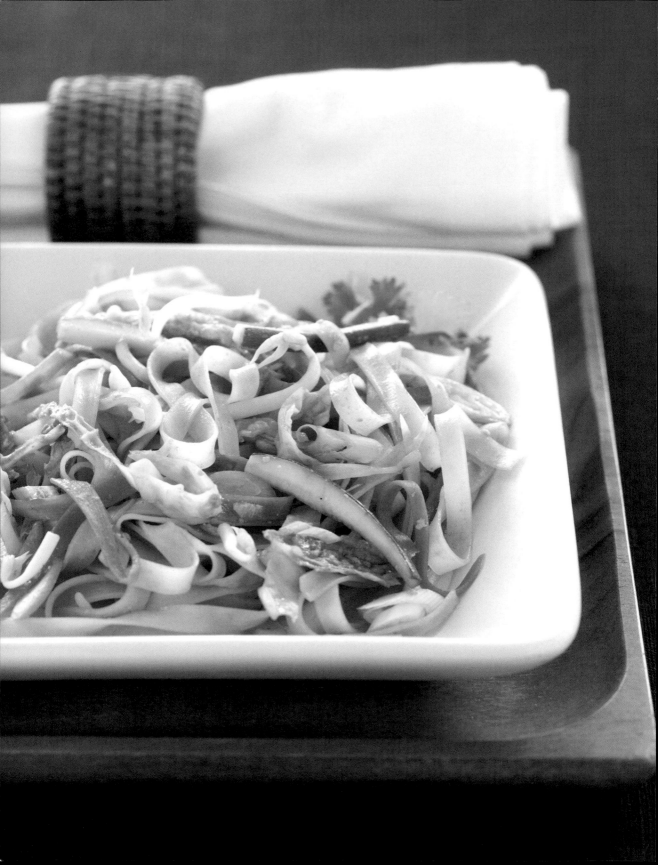

PAD THAI CLEAN-EATING STYLE

Pad Thai has innumerable versions, but the basic dish incorporates noodles, shrimp or some other meat and a host of vegetables. This is a vegetarian version. Use rice noodles to keep the dish at its healthiest and get creative with veggies, too.

INGREDIENTS:

8 oz / 224 g rice noodles, flat
   (Enough hot boiled water to cover noodles*)
1 Tbsp / 15 ml canola oil
2 cloves garlic, passed through a garlic press
2 cups / 480 ml shredded Savoy cabbage
2 thick carrots, peeled and cut into thin slices
5 egg whites, lightly beaten
3 cups / 720 ml bean sprouts
1 cup / 240 ml julienned green zucchini
1 cup / 240 ml green onions, chopped
¼ cup / 60 ml fresh cilantro, chopped for garnish
* Reserve 2 Tbsp / 30 ml of noodle water

FOR THE SAUCE:

3 Tbsp / 45 ml rice wine vinegar or rice vinegar
¼ cup / 60 ml tomato paste
2 Tbsp / 30 ml reserved noodle water
2 Tbsp / 30 ml unsulfured molasses
2 Tbsp / 30 ml low-sodium soy sauce or gluten-free
   tamari

PREPARATION:

1 Cover rice noodles with boiling water in a ceramic bowl. Cover and let stand for 20 minutes to soften noodles. Drain, reserving 2 tablespoons / 30 ml noodle water.

2 In a small bowl, whisk together all sauce ingredients. Set aside.

3 In a large skillet, heat oil over medium heat. Stir in garlic, cabbage and carrot. Stir-fry for 5 minutes. Make a well in the middle of the pan and scramble the egg whites. Add noodles and sauce and cook for 5 minutes. Add bean sprouts, zucchini and green onions and cook a little longer to heat through. Remove from heat and serve. Garnish each dish with chopped cilantro.

TIP

Pad Thai is über kid-friendly eating. Gather your kids and someone else's around the table for a spot-on meal.

NUTRITIONAL VALUE PER SERVING:

Calories: 158 | Calories from Fat: 19 | Protein: 5g | Carbs: 30g
Dietary Fiber: 2g | Sugars: 3g | Fat: 2g | Sodium: 102mg

8 SERVINGS   50 MINUTES   25 MINUTES

SPAGHETTI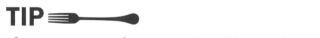
with Pesto Sauce

S paghetti is a family favorite any day of the week. Here's how to make it a Clean-Eating meal right from the start. Round out the meal with a verdant green salad.

INGREDIENTS:

1 lb / 454 g noodles (buckwheat or rice noodles)

3 quarts / 3 L water

1 tsp / 5 ml sea salt

PESTO INGREDIENTS:

3 cups / 720 ml fresh basil leaves

½ cup / 120 ml almonds, coarsely chopped

¾ cup / 180 ml parsley

2 cloves garlic, passed through a garlic press

¼ cup / 60 ml extra virgin olive oil

Sea salt

PREPARATION:

1   Bring water to a rolling boil. Add sea salt. Cook noodles al dente. Rinse under cold water to prevent clumping when cooking is complete. Place cooked noodles in large sauté pan or saucepan. Set aside.

2   Prepare pesto sauce by placing all ingredients in a food processor. Pulse until ingredients resemble a smooth paste. Scrape pesto out of food processor bowl and pour over cooked noodles. Over medium heat, toss noodles and pesto sauce until heated through. Serve hot.

TIP ⟶

Every summer I grow tubs of beautifully fragrant basil outside my kitchen door. I add it to everything!

NUTRITIONAL VALUE PER SERVING:
Calories: 421 | Calories from Fat: 127 | Protein: 8g | Carbs: 59g
Dietary Fiber: 3g | Sugars: 2g | Fat: 14g | Sodium: 282mg

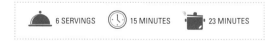
6 SERVINGS   15 MINUTES   23 MINUTES

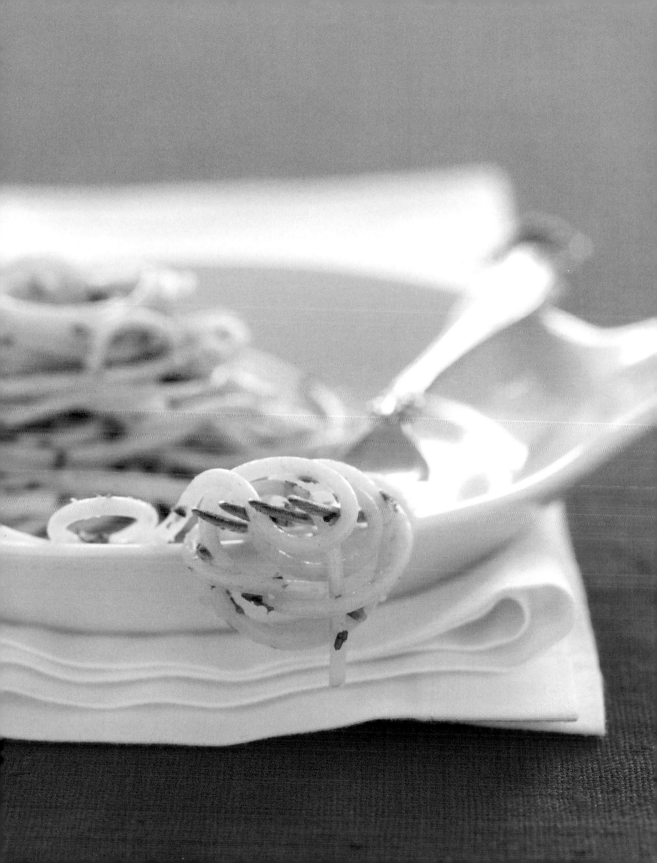

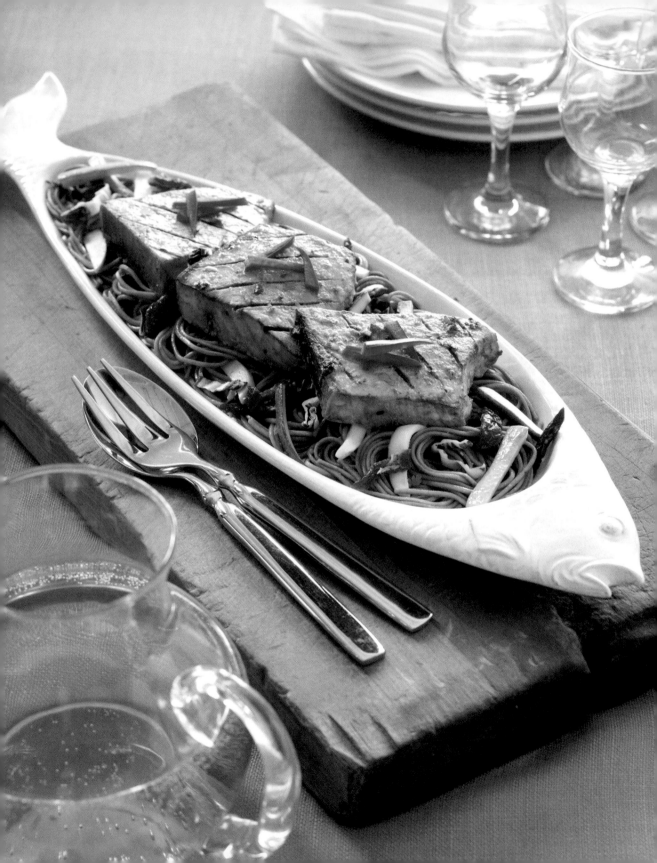

NEVIS-STYLE SWORDFISH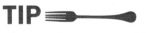
and Ginger Tahini Sauce on Soba Noodles

Nevis is a tiny island in the Caribbean. Lush with palm trees and idyllic scenery, the island is a must for those who love the quiet tropical life. This dish evokes the flavors of the island and is a perfect Clean-Eating entrée for yourself or when entertaining guests. Soba noodles are a healthier pasta alternative since they are made from buckwheat.

INGREDIENTS:

6 fresh swordfish fillets

3½ cups / 840 ml Ginger Garlic Tahini Sauce
  (recipe follows on next page)

3 Tbsp / 45 ml extra virgin olive oil

½ cup / 125 ml sundried tomatoes, slivered

2 small yellow zucchini, slivered

2 small green zucchini, slivered

1 small head radicchio, slivered

1 Tbsp / 15 ml capers *(optional)*

8 oz / 200 g buckwheat soba noodles

1 Tbsp / 15 ml toasted sesame oil

2 Tbsp / 30 ml low-sodium soy sauce or gluten-free
  tamari

½ cup / 120 ml fresh cilantro, chopped, for garnish

12 slivers of red bell pepper, for garnish

PREPARATION:

1 Place swordfish in large glass bowl with tight-fitting lid. Add 2½ cups / 600 ml of the Ginger Garlic Tahini Sauce for marinating. Allow to marinate in the fridge for several hours.

2 Remove fish from marinade and discard sauce. Prepare grill at medium-high heat. Grill fish for 5 minutes on one side and then flip over and cook the other side for another 4 minutes. Transfer swordfish to a platter and cover to keep warm.

3 Bring a large pot of water to a boil.

4 In large skillet over medium-high heat, add capers, and vegetables in batches, and stir-fry quickly.

5 Add soba noodles to boiling water and cook according to package directions or about 8 minutes. Return noodles to pot. Toss with toasted sesame oil and soy sauce. Add stir-fried vegetables and toss lightly. Transfer contents to large (preferably heated) serving platter or individual heated plates. Arrange grilled swordfish on top of noodles. Garnish with cilantro and red pepper. *Recipe continued...*

TIP 🍴

Go to the extra effort of buying the freshest tuna possible.

NUTRITIONAL VALUE PER SERVING:

Calories: 396 | Calories from Fat: 137 | Protein: 33g | Carbs: 32g
Dietary Fiber: 3g | Sugars: 3g | Fat: 0.15g | Sodium: 756mg

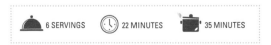

6 SERVINGS   22 MINUTES   35 MINUTES

GINGER GARLIC TAHINI SAUCE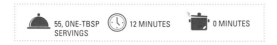

This delicious marinade can be used on chicken and turkey, too. Add it to stir-fries and use it on all seafood. It is enormously versatile.

INGREDIENTS:

1 cup / 240 ml low-sodium soy sauce or gluten-free
   tamari
½ cup / 125 ml rice vinegar
2 Tbsp / 30 ml tahini
2 Tbsp / 30 ml minced ginger
1 Tbsp / 15 ml minced garlic
1½ tsp / 8 ml dried red pepper flakes
¾ cup / 180 ml toasted sesame oil
¾ cup / 180 ml best-quality olive oil
Juice of 1 lemon

PREPARATION:

1 In a medium glass bowl, whisk all ingredients. Cover and refrigerate for a few weeks or until you need to make the next batch.

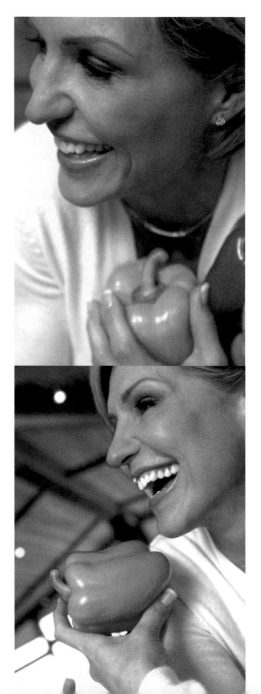

NUTRITIONAL VALUE PER ONE-TBSP SERVING:

Calories: 59 | Calories from Fat: 56 | Protein: 0.3g | Carbs: 0.58g
Dietary Fiber: 0.07g | Sugars: 0g | Fat: 0.6g | Sodium: 155mg

55, ONE-TBSP SERVINGS   12 MINUTES   0 MINUTES

CAN WE TALK NOODLES?

There are many, many kinds of noodles, so mix things up and get styling. Noodles are fun to eat, super easy to digest and take very little time to prepare. Introduce your family to one of these interesting varieties today.

RICE NOODLES, RICE VERMICELLI AND RICE STICKS

Who knew rice could be transformed into so many different shapes?

Rice noodles are a translucent white color when dry and become almost transparent when cooked. The noodles are usually thin but do come in varying widths and lengths. Rice noodles are, as you might have guessed, made from rice.

BEAN THREAD AND CELLOPHANE NOODLES

It's hard to believe noodles can be made from beans, but these transparent noodles are made from mung beans. The mung bean is native to India and is the seed of a plant. The mung bean is commonly used in Asian cooking. To make cellophane noodles the starch is removed from the ground beans. These noodles become soft and slippery when soaked in water.

WHEAT NOODLES

The best wheat noodles are those made fresh. They cook in a flash and packaged varieties do not compare. But for convenience, packaged varieties are a snap. There are countless shapes and variations of wheat noodles, which accounts for the ever-growing pasta aisle, at least in my grocery store.

DESIGNER NOODLES

This is my term for a host of noodles made from a range of flours including kamut, spelt, brown rice, artichoke, soybeans, spinach, tomato, corn and more. Flour and consequently noodles can be made from virtually any foodstuff, including beans, grains and vegetables. Once you get started experimenting with them you won't want to stop.

JAPANESE BUCKWHEAT OR SOBA NOODLES

These noodles are made from buckwheat and have a lovely textured tan color. Several variations of soba noodles are available, including jinenjo soba made with wild yam flour, cha soba made with tea leaves, and buckwheat and yomagi soba, which are made with buckwheat and mugwort.

SESAME TOFU ON SOBA NOODLES

Combining a delicious marinade with the nutty flavor of Japanese soba noodles makes this meal an Asian-fusion delight. Add in some colorful peppers and onions and you've got a complete Clean-Eating meal, perfect for when you're craving something a little different.

INGREDIENTS FOR MARINADE:

2 tsp / 10 ml rice vinegar

1 Tbsp / 15 ml black bean sauce, low sodium (check ingredients if gluten is a problem)

1 Tbsp / 15 ml gluten-free tamari

1 Tbsp / 15 ml water

INGREDIENTS FOR TOFU:

1 lb / 454g firm tofu, rinsed and well drained, cut into 2 ½" x 4 ½" strips

6 quarts / 5.7 L water

8 oz / 224g dry soba (buckwheat) noodles

2 cups / 480 ml arugula, rinsed and well drained

1 cup / 240 ml green onions, trimmed

1 cup / 240 ml red bell pepper, sliced into thin strips

2 Tbsp / 30 ml black bean sauce, low sodium and gluten free if necessary

3 Tbsp / 45 ml mixed white and black sesame seeds

2 tsp / 10 ml roasted sesame oil

¼ cup / 60 ml rice wine

2 Tbsp / 30 ml gluten-free tamari

PREPARATION FOR MARINADE :

1 Mix all ingredients together in shallow glass baking dish. Place tofu strips in marinade, ensuring they are well covered. Refrigerate.

PREPARATION FOR TOFU :

1 In a large saucepan bring 6 quarts / 5.7 L water to a rolling boil. Cook soba noodles al dente. Rinse and drain.

2 Remove tofu from marinade and place on paper towels to remove most of the marinade. Reserve marinade and add to soba noodles. Add arugula, green onions, red pepper and black bean sauce to soba noodles.

3 Spread sesame seeds on a flat platter or cutting board. Roll tofu slices in the sesame seeds. In a nonstick pan, add 1 teaspoon / 5 ml roasted sesame oil and fry or grill tofu slices until sesame seeds turn golden brown. Remove from pan.

4 In a small bowl combine rice wine, 1 teaspoon / 5 ml roasted sesame oil and tamari. Whisk until well blended and turn into pan. Warm gently. When heated through add soba noodles. Toss well.

5 Divide noodles among four dinner plates. Divide tofu among the four plates, arranging neatly beside soba noodles.

NUTRITIONAL VALUE PER SERVING:

Calories: 513 | Calories from Fat: 157 | Protein: 29g | Carbs: 66g
Dietary Fiber: 9g | Sugars: 11g | Fat: 17g | Sodium: 233mg

4 SERVINGS   35 MINUTES   10 MINUTES

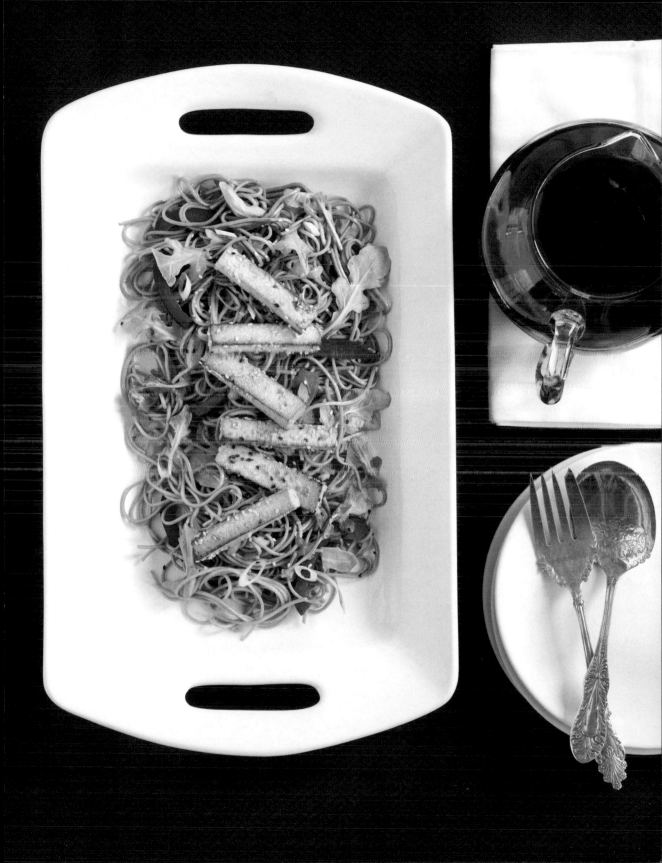

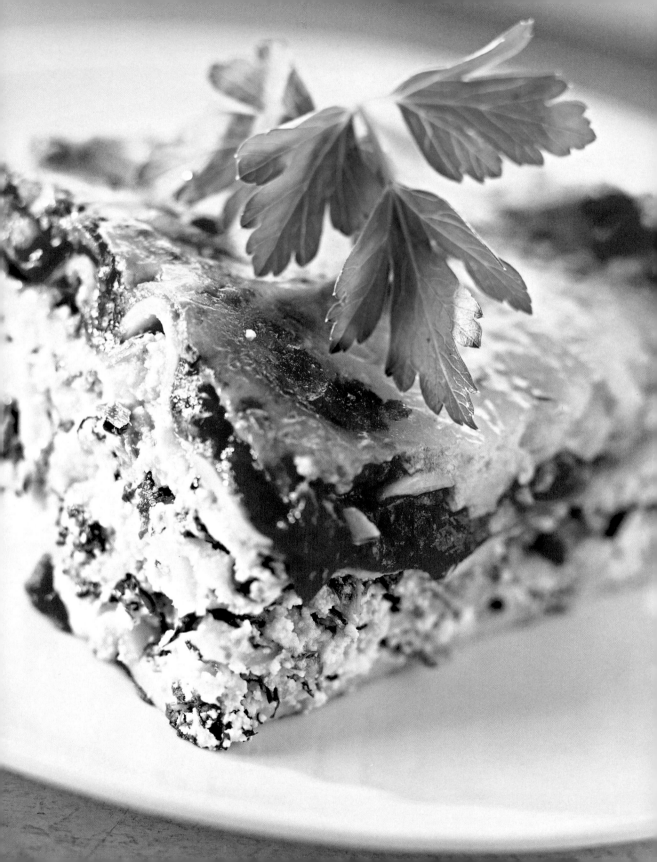

YOU-BUILD-IT LASAGNA

I love recipes that require building skills rather than fancy cooking skills. Although I do cook a lot I value the simplicity of putting things together that cook by themselves. These are the recipes I share with my university-aged daughters.

INGREDIENTS:

2½ quarts / 2.5 L water

4 Tbsp / 60 ml extra virgin olive oil

1 medium onion, peeled and chopped

3 cloves garlic, passed through a garlic press

3 ribs celery, trimmed and chopped

2 carrots, peeled and chopped

2 cups / 480 ml sliced mushrooms — *use a mixture of button, shiitake and Portobello or just your favorites*

1½ Tbsp / 25 ml low-sodium tamari (gluten free if necessary)

Freshly ground black pepper

4 cups / 960 ml fresh spinach

PASTA:

1 lb / 450 g dry lasagna noodles — *look for nutrient – dense pastas made from spinach, tomato, kamut, spelt, rice or gluten-free varieties ... there are many*

2 cups / 480 ml tomato sauce

(use Soup or Sauce recipe page 132)

2½ cups / 600 ml nonfat cottage cheese

6 cups / 1.4 L grated low- or nonfat mozzarella cheese

1½ cups / 360 ml goat cheese

NUTRITIONAL VALUE PER SERVING:

Calories: 408 | Calories from Fat: 70 | Protein: 39g | Carbs: 43g
Dietary Fiber: 4g | Sugars: 6g | Fat: 7g | Sodium: 823mg

🍽 10 SERVINGS   🕐 35 MINUTES   🍲 35 + 20 MINUTES

PREPARATION:

1 Preheat oven to 375°F / 190°C. In large skillet heat olive oil over medium heat. Add onion, garlic, celery and carrot. Cook 5 minutes until vegetables become soft. Add mushrooms and sauté for another few minutes. Stir in tamari, pepper and spinach. Let spinach wilt.

2 In a large saucepan bring 2½ quarts / 2.5 L water to a rolling boil. Pour a little olive oil into the water to prevent noodles from sticking. Add lasagna noodles and cook al dente. Drain noodles and run them under cold water.

3 Spread ½ cup / 125 ml or more tomato sauce on the bottom of a lasagna pan that's been coated with nonstick cooking spray. Place a layer of lasagna noodles on top. Spread ¾ cup / 180 ml cottage cheese on top of the lasagna noodles along with 1½ cups / 360 ml grated mozzarella cheese, ½ cup / 125 ml goat cheese and one third of the spinach and vegetable mixture. Repeat the layers until you run out of ingredients. End with tomato sauce on top.

4 Bake in hot oven for 35 minutes. Sprinkle more grated mozzarella cheese on top of lasagna and return to oven. Let cook for another 5 minutes. Remove from heat and let sit for 20 minutes before cutting and serving. Do not skip this step! It is much easier to cut set lasagna. Serve hot with a colorful green salad.

TRICOLORE LINGUINE
with Sundried Tomatoes

Tricolore noodles in plain, red (tomato) and green (spinach) mimic the Italian flag. They also add some variety to your typical pasta dish. Sundried tomatoes and green peas further compliment the multicolor theme while adding in delicious nutrients. So when you feel like going Italian for the night, whip up this dish and be in for a treat. Buon appetito!

INGREDIENTS:

2 cups / 480 ml fresh green peas *(or 1 cup green peas and 1 cup edamame)*

1 lb / 454 g tricolored rice or whole-wheat linguine

6 Tbsp / 90 ml extra virgin olive oil

6 cloves garlic, peeled and minced

2 shallots, peeled and minced

1 cup / 240 ml sundried tomatoes, not in oil, chopped

½ cup / 125 ml low-sodium, low-fat chicken or vegetable broth (gluten free if necessary)

Sea salt and freshly ground pepper to taste

½ cup / 125 ml fresh Italian parsley, chopped

PREPARATION:

1 Flash-cook peas and/or edamame until just tender but firm. Drain and set aside. Cook pasta al dente. Drain.

2 In a large skillet, sauté garlic and shallots in olive oil. Add sundried tomatoes, peas and chicken broth. Bring to a boil. Remove from heat and immediately add drained pasta to the skillet. Toss lightly until sauce and vegetables cover the linguine.

3 Add freshly ground black pepper and sea salt and garnish with chopped Italian parsley.

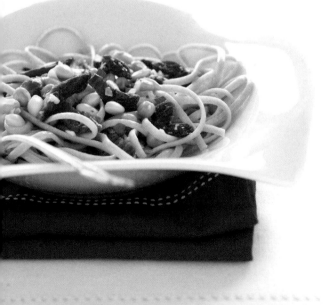

NUTRITIONAL VALUE PER SERVING:
Calories: 490 | Calories from Fat: 151 | Protein: 17g | Carbs: 75g
Dietary Fiber: 11g | Sugars: 7g | Fat: 17g | Sodium: 257mg

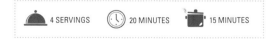

4 SERVINGS   20 MINUTES   15 MINUTES

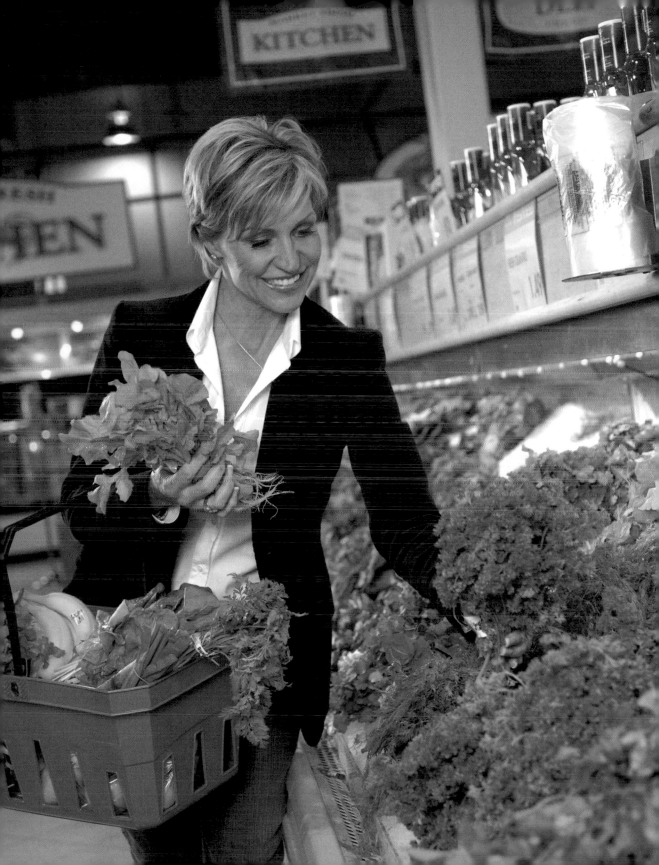

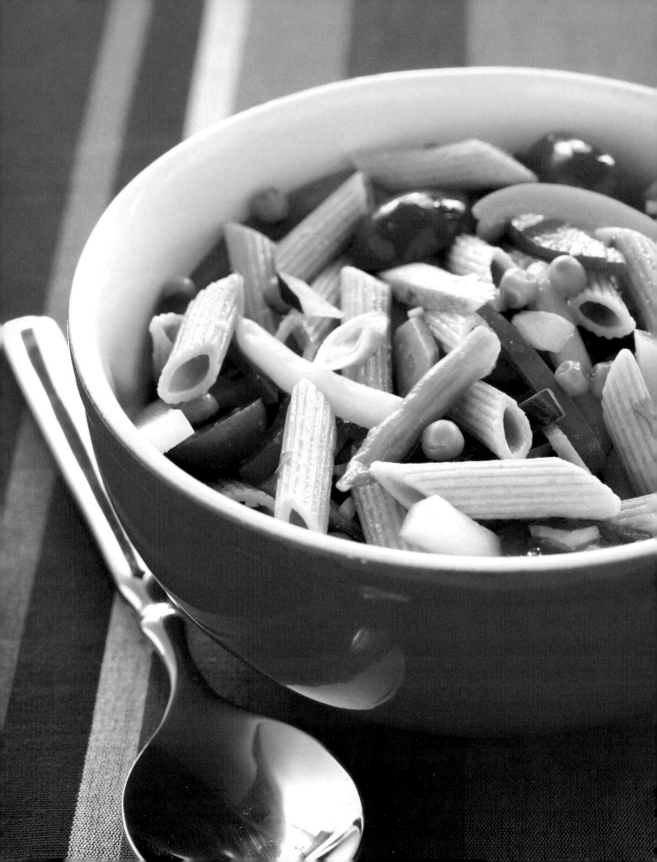

GARDEN PASTA SALAD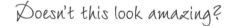

Pasta salads are the perfect dish to accompany or stand alone in hot summer weather. However, most pasta salads drown in greasy thick dressings that make them more like a goopy mess than the crisp delight they are supposed to be.

INGREDIENTS:

½ cup / 120 ml yellow beans, halved

½ cup / 120 ml green beans, halved

2 sweet carrots, peeled and penny sliced

3 cups / 720 ml cooked pasta* – bow tie,
    rotini, fusilli, penne, or gluten-free pasta

1 small yellow zucchini, thinly sliced

1 small green zucchini, thinly sliced

½ red pepper, seeded and deveined, cut into thin
    strips

½ orange pepper, seeded and deveined, cut into
    thin strips

1 vine-ripened tomato, chopped or ½ cup grape
    tomatoes, halved

¼ cup / 60 ml fresh cilantro, finely chopped

3 scallions, trimmed and chopped

¼ cup / 60 ml chives, finely chopped

¼ cup / 60 ml purple onion, finely diced

½ cup / 125 ml fresh peas

*reserve 3 Tbsp / 45 ml of the pasta cooking water
for dressing

DRESSING:

4 Tbsp / 60 ml rice wine vinegar

2 Tbsp / 30 ml avocado oil

3 Tbsp / 45 ml reserved pasta cooking liquid

¼ cup / 60 ml fresh basil, chopped

1 tsp / 5 ml Dijon mustard

1 garlic clove, passed through a garlic press

PREPARATION:

1 Blanch beans in a pot of boiling water for 3 minutes or until beans just begin to turn color. Place them in a bowl of ice water. Do the same for the carrots. Drain well and place in large decorative glass serving bowl. Using the same water, cook pasta al dente. Drain pasta, reserving 3 Tbsp / 45 ml of the cooking liquid for the dressing. Rinse pasta under cold water and drain well. Place pasta in bowl with carrots and beans. Add remaining zucchini, pepper, tomato, herbs, scallion, chives, onion and peas to the bowl.

2 In a small bowl, whisk together the dressing ingredients. Pour dressing over the salad. Toss until all ingredients are evenly distributed.

NUTRITIONAL VALUE PER SERVING:

Calories: 137 | Calories from Fat: 31 | Protein: 5g | Carbs: 21g
Dietary Fiber: 4g | Sugars: 2g | Fat: 3g | Sodium: 25mg

Doesn't this look amazing?

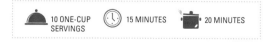

10 ONE-CUP SERVINGS   15 MINUTES   20 MINUTES

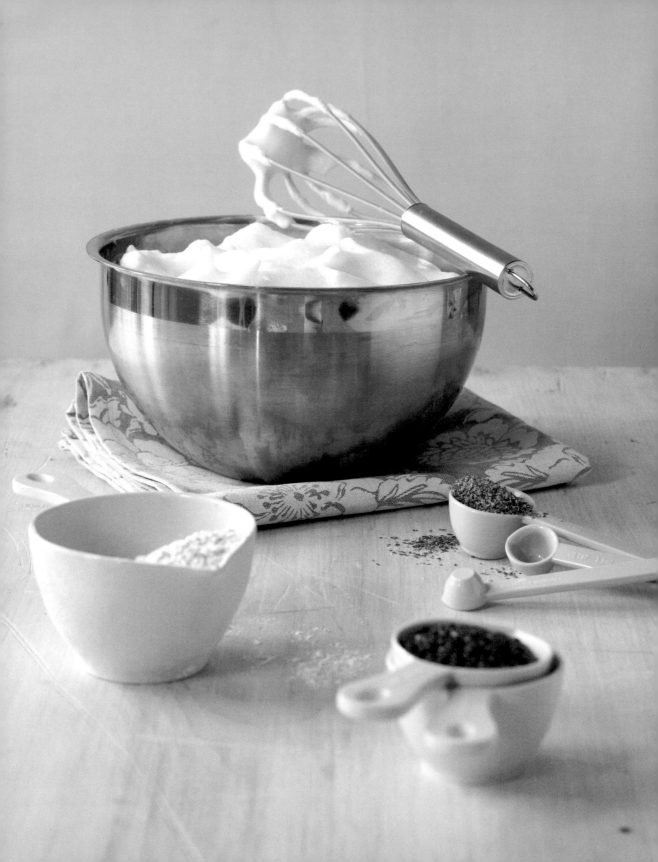

Sweets & Breads

When Eve was drawn to the apple in the Garden of Eden she was succumbing to many temptations, not the least of which was the delicious sweetness of the forbidden fruit. I understand this addiction, as I never travel far without apples! I love them so much. They are not only nutritious, but also easily portable and sweet. The perfect Clean-Eating food.

Make your sweets an occasional treat. Combine delicious and nutritious wholesome ingredients to make desserts that will fortify rather than debilitate your health.

SUPER PUDDING

If there were a super hero named after a seed, flax would be it! Flax The Super Seed is so versatile that it can even be incorporated into a delicious dessert. Dessert that satisfies your sweet tooth and provides incomparable nutrition – what more could you want? So when your sweet tooth is calling, it's Flax The Super Seed to the rescue!

INGREDIENTS:

6 Tbsp / 90 ml flax seeds
2 cups / 480 ml skim milk or soy milk
1 banana, peeled and mashed
1 Tbsp / 15 ml organic honey
Juice of one orange
1 apple, peeled and diced, core removed

TOPPING:

Sliced kiwi
Sliced fresh strawberries
Sliced banana

PREPARATION:

1 Grind flax seeds in a food mill or coffee grinder. Bring skim or soy milk to a boil in a medium saucepan. Add ground flax to boiling milk. Boil for about 30 seconds. Remove from heat and let cool in a medium-sized glass bowl.

2 The mixture will develop a consistency similar to pudding. Add remaining ingredients. Using a wire whisk or blender, whip mixture until it becomes fluffy.

NUTRITIONAL VALUE PER SERVING:

Calories: 206 | Calories from Fat: 44 | Protein: 7g | Carbs: 31g
Dietary Fiber: 5g | Sugars: 21g | Fat: 4g | Sodium: 65mg

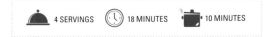

4 SERVINGS · 18 MINUTES · 10 MINUTES

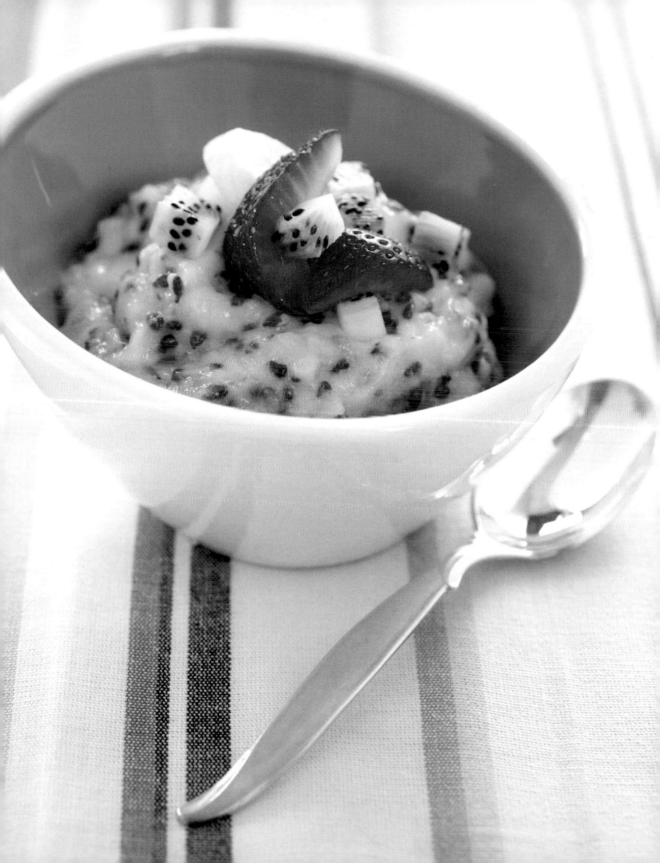

Makes about 6 dozen
smaller cookies or 3
dozen larger ones.
I like them bigger!

WHOLE-WHEAT FLAX COOKIES

Everyone likes a hearty cookie, especially a healthy one. And I admit to enjoying a cookie much more when I am certain it isn't crammed with ingredients that will only find their way to my waist. I also know that one cookie is enough. Just one!

INGREDIENTS:

½ cup / 120 ml whole flax seeds

1½ cups / 360 ml buttermilk (or skim milk soured with 1 Tbsp lemon juice)

2 cups / 480 ml whole-wheat flour **OR** 2 cups / 480 ml gluten-free flour combination of your liking

½ cup / 120 ml ground flax seeds (flax meal)

1 cup / 240 ml rolled oats (uncontaminated if necessary)

1 tsp / 5 ml baking powder

1 tsp / 5 ml baking soda

½ tsp / 2.5 ml sea salt

½ tsp / 2.5 ml cinnamon

¼ tsp / 1.25 ml ground nutmeg

¼ tsp / 1.25 ml ground mace

1 cup / 240 ml Olivina or Do-It-Yourself Olive Butter Spread (see pg. 117)

   OR 1 cup canola oil

1 cup / 240 ml Sucanat

2 eggs

2 Tbsp / 30 ml pure vanilla extract or bourbon vanilla extract

2 cups / 480 ml coarsely chopped, raw, unsalted almonds

½ cup / 120 ml dark, Sultana raisins

PREPARATION:

1 Preheat oven to 375°F / 190°C. In small bowl or glass measuring cup, soak whole flax seeds in buttermilk or soured skim milk. These are best soaked for about 2 hours at room temperature.

2 Meanwhile, in a large bowl, measure all dry ingredients including flour, flax meal, oats, baking powder, baking soda, sea salt and spices and combine with whisk until well blended. Don't add raisins or chopped almonds yet!

3 In another medium-sized bowl beat Olivina or olive oil-based margarine and Sucanat until fluffy. Add one egg at a time and beat well. Add vanilla and mix well again.

4 Combine liquid and dry ingredients and fold until all ingredients are evenly blended. Add raisins and chopped almonds and mix lightly until blended.

5 Prepare a cookie sheet with parchment paper or Silpat sheet or spray lightly with cooking spray. Using a large soup spoon, take dough and make balls. Place on cookie sheet and bake for 15 minutes.

NUTRITIONAL VALUE PER SERVING:

Calories: 182 | Calories from Fat: 98 | Protein: 4g | Carbs: 16g
Dietary Fiber: 3g | Sugars: 7g | Fat: 10g | Sodium: 35mg

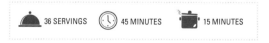 36 SERVINGS   45 MINUTES   15 MINUTES

TOFU CHOCOLATE MOUSSE

Y ou would not believe that this dessert is made with tofu. It is absolutely delicious and better still, is a cinch to make. My "picky eater" daughter, Kelsey-Lynn, loves to make this and it is done in no time. Guilt-free dessert! Who knew?

INGREDIENTS:

¾ cup / 180 ml dark chocolate chips or dark chocolate bars, broken into pieces

12 oz / 336 g silken tofu at room temperature, drained

½ cup / 120 ml warmed skim milk or soy, rice or almond milk

1 tsp / 5 ml best-quality vanilla

PREPARATION:

1 Melt chocolate chips in a double boiler or in the microwave. Make sure to let the chocolate melt slowly. Stir until chocolate is uniformly smooth.

2 In a food processor, combine tofu, melted chocolate, warmed milk and vanilla. Process until smooth. Place tofu mixture in fine-mesh strainer or sieve, pushing through with the back of a wooden spoon, into a medium decorative serving bowl. Serve from the bowl or ladle into individual serving bowls. Chill and serve.

NUTRITIONAL VALUE PER SERVING:

Calories: 281 | Calories from Fat: 144 | Protein: 9g | Carbs: 24g
Dietary Fiber: 4g | Sugars: 17g | Fat: 16g | Sodium: 77mg

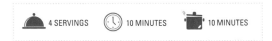 4 SERVINGS   10 MINUTES   10 MINUTES

TIP

Thanks Kelsey! You were the inspiration for this!

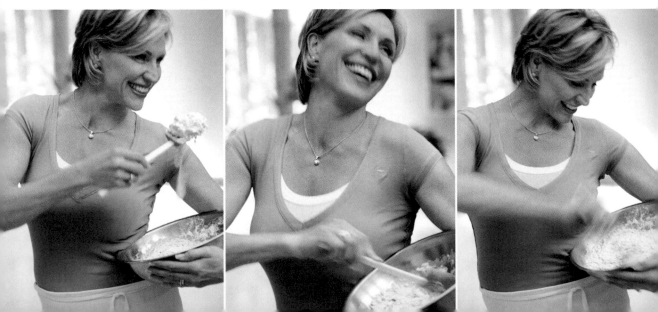

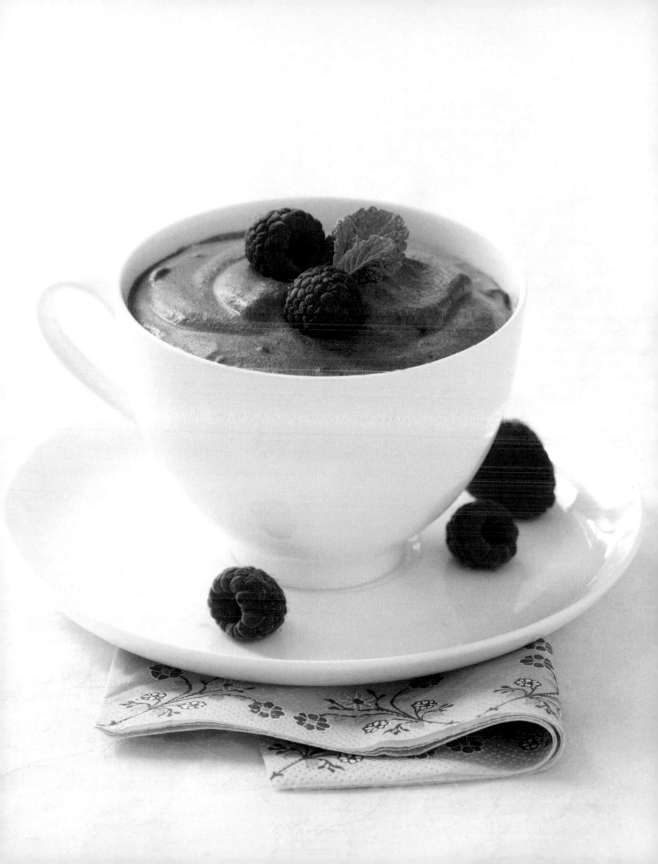

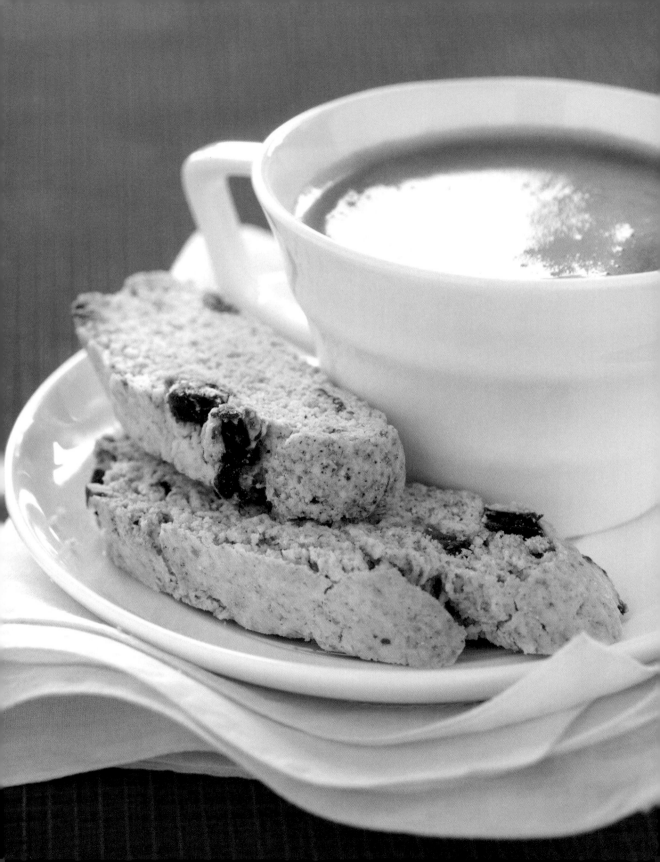

LOW-FAT ALMOND DATE BISCOTTI

Biscotti means twice baked. It is a wonderful Italian cookie made even better because it's low in fat and sugar. It is delicious with coffee or tea.

INGREDIENTS:

1 cup / 240 ml all-purpose flour

1 cup / 240 ml whole-wheat flour

⅓ cup / 80 ml sugar

2 tsp / 10 ml baking powder

4 Tbsp / 60 ml Olivina or reduced-fat margarine

3 egg whites

1 tsp / 5 ml best-quality vanilla extract

1 tsp / 5 ml best-quality almond extract

¼ cup / 60 ml finely chopped almonds

¼ cup / 60 ml finely chopped dates or other dried fruit (cranberry is nice)

Cooking spray

TIP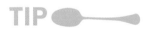

Using a serrated knife, slice the logs diagonally into half-inch slices.

PREPARATION:

1 Preheat oven to 350°F / 177°C. Combine dry ingredients. Stir to mix well. Use a pastry cutter to cut in the margarine until the mixture has the texture of coarse oatmeal. Stir in the egg whites and extracts. Fold in almonds and dates.

2 Turn the dough onto a lightly floured surface and shape into two 9" x 2" logs. Coat a baking sheet with nonstick cooking spray or line it with parchment paper. Place the logs on the sheet. Allow four inches of space between each log for spreading. Bake for about 25 minutes or until lightly browned.

3 Cool the logs at room temperature for 10 minutes. Using a serrated knife, slice the logs diagonally into half-inch-thick slices.

4 Place the slices on an ungreased baking sheet in a single layer, cut side down. Return to 350°F / 177°C oven for 18 – 20 minutes, or until dry and crisp. Turn the slices over after 10 minutes. Let cool completely. Serve or store.

NUTRITIONAL VALUE PER SERVING:

Calories: 47 | Calories from Fat: 18 | Protein: 1g | Carbs: 6g
Dietary Fiber: 0.3g | Sugars: 3g | Fat: 2g | Sodium: 6mg

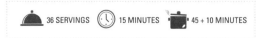

36 SERVINGS   15 MINUTES   45 + 10 MINUTES

PAPAYA FRUIT SALAD

You may think you are simply eating a delicious fruit salad – and you are! But did you know that savoring these incredible exotic fruits beautifies your skin, too? Enjoy a bowl early in the morning for breakfast or after dinner as a perfect ending to your day. You look better already!

INGREDIENTS:

Juice of one fresh lemon*

1 avocado

1 papaya

6 fresh figs

1 guava

2 nectarines (peaches will do if you can't find good nectarines)

1 Tbsp / 15 ml organic honey

½ Tbsp / 7.5 ml ground cinnamon

Pinch grated nutmeg

reserve 2 Tbsp of juice to use with honey

PREPARATION:

1 Have a large decorative glass bowl handy. Put the juice of the fresh lemon in the bowl first. I like to prepare the avocado first so it can sit in the lemon juice at the bottom of the bowl. That way it doesn't oxidize (turn brown) too quickly. Peel and chop the fruit into bite-sized pieces and put everything in the bowl.

2 In a small bowl soften the honey with 2 tablespoons / 30 ml of the lemon juice. This makes it easier to mix into the salad. Pour over salad and add spices. Toss gently. Serve!

TIP

I have made this beautiful salad countless times for TV cameras. The crew love it when I do because they get to eat it!

NUTRITIONAL VALUE PER SERVING:

Calories: 141 | Calories from Fat: 46 | Protein: 1g | Carbs: 23g
Dietary Fiber: 5g | Sugars: 11g | Fat: 5g | Sodium: 3mg

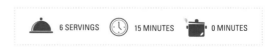

6 SERVINGS   15 MINUTES   0 MINUTES

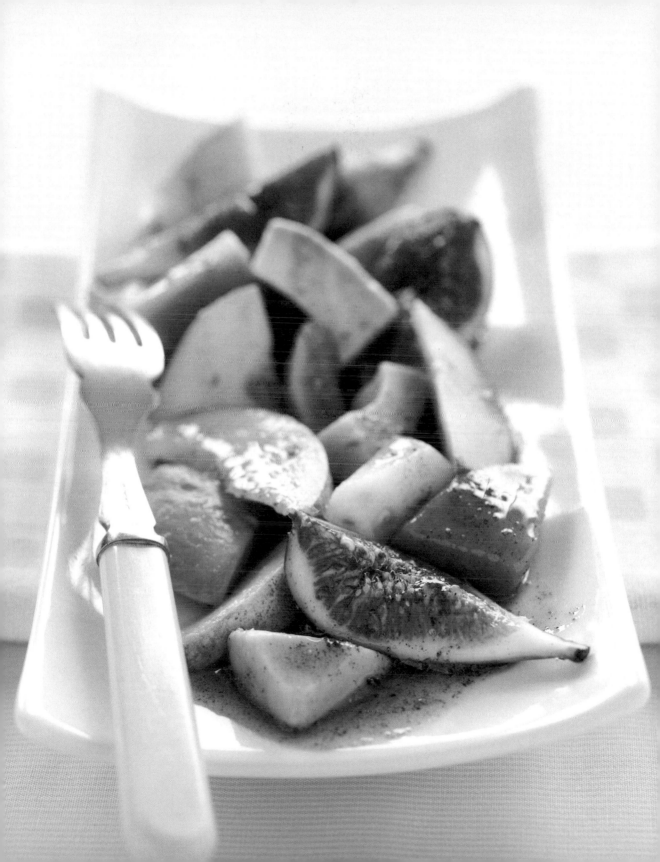

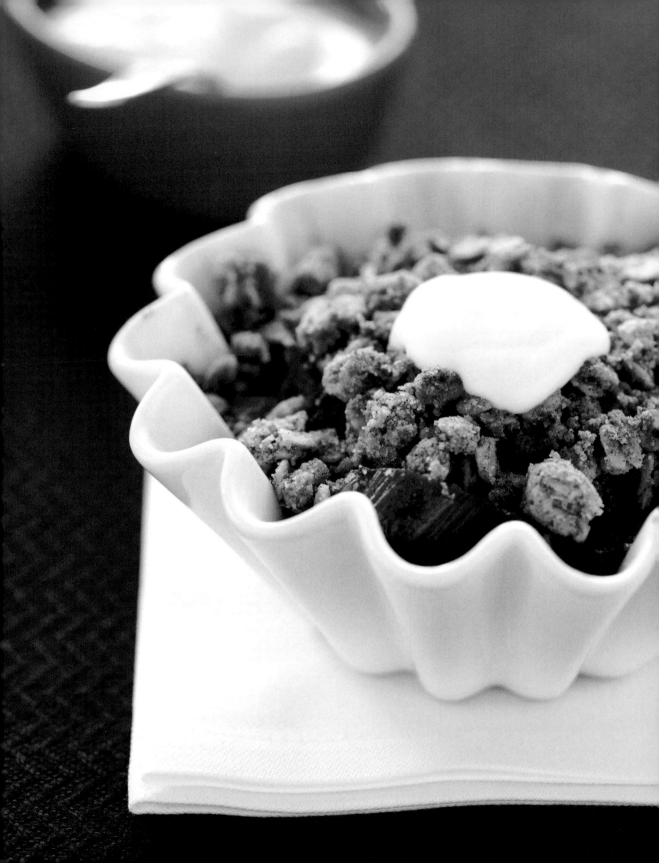

SPRINGTIME RHUBARB CRUMBLE

If you remember the name of this recipe you'll never forget when this vegetable is in season – springtime. Fresh rhubarb is absolutely divine in this crumble, and adds incredible nutritional punch. One cup / 240 ml of rhubarb alone contributes excellent amounts of vitamins C, A, and K and as much calcium as a glass of milk. Just be sure to sweeten with Sucanat since rhubarb is also known for its astringent effect on the mouth and nasal cavities. Pucker up!

INGREDIENTS:

1 lb / 454 g rhubarb, sliced

¼ cup / 60 ml Sucanat

1 tsp / 5 ml ground cinnamon

CRUMBLE:

½ cup / 120 ml canola oil

½ cup / 120 ml rolled oats (uncontaminted if necessary)

½ cup / 120 ml whole-wheat flour or gluten-free flour

1 tsp / 5 ml ground cinnamon

1 tsp / 5 ml Sucanat

Cooking spray

PREPARATION:

1 Preheat oven to 350°F / 177°C. Prepare a shallow baking dish with light coating of cooking spray.

2 Place rhubarb in baking dish. Dust with cinnamon and sugar.

3 In separate bowl, mix canola oil, oats, flour and cinnamon. Mix until concoction resembles bread crumbs. Stir in the sugar. Spoon over the rhubarb. Bake for 40 minutes. Remove from oven and serve hot!

TIP

I always get loads of fresh rhubarb in spring and freeze up big batches of it. It's easy to do and tastes like spring in the middle of winter.

NOTE: This recipe is easily doubled. You might want to make more since it tastes so good there are sure to be no leftovers.

NUTRITIONAL VALUE PER SERVING:
Calories: 326 | Calories from Fat: 172 | Protein: 3g | Carbs: 25g
Dietary Fiber: 3g | Sugars: 9g | Fat: 19g | Sodium: 9mg

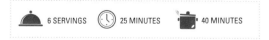
6 SERVINGS   25 MINUTES   40 MINUTES

SUMMER RICE PUDDING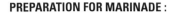

I love rice pudding. I don't eat it all the time, but when I am looking for the perfect sweet comfort food, rice pudding is it. This recipe is not as full of sins as many other versions, so I enjoy every bite, and now you can too.

INGREDIENTS:

1½ cups / 360 ml skim milk, soy milk, almond milk or milk of your preference

1 cup / 240 ml brown rice

2 Tbsp / 30 ml Sucanat sugar

Pinch ground nutmeg

¾ cup / 180 ml low-fat plain or vanilla yogurt or soy yogurt

1 cup / 240 ml fresh mixed berries or berries of your liking

Cooking spray

PREPARATION FOR MARINADE :

1 Preheat oven to 350°F / 177°C. Prepare a 6 cup / 1.4 L covered casserole dish with cooking spray. In a medium mixing bowl combine milk, rice and Sucanat. Pour into casserole dish, cover and bake for 35 minutes or until liquid is absorbed. Remove from oven. Transfer cooked rice into a bowl and let cool.

2 Once cool, fold yogurt into cooked rice.

3 Rinse and trim berries. If using strawberries, wash, hull and slice them into bite-sized pieces. Divide berries between four decorative dessert dishes or interesting glasses. Place equal amount of rice mixture on top of the berries in each dessert dish. Garnish with an attractive looking berry – or a sprig of fresh mint.

TIP

When winter limits your berry selection, choose zingy mandarin oranges, kiwi fruit and chopped apple.

NUTRITIONAL VALUE PER SERVING:
Calories: 274 | Calories from Fat: 16 | Protein: 9g | Carbs: 54g
Dietary Fiber: 3g | Sugars: 16g | Fat: 1g | Sodium: 87mg

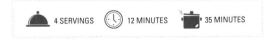
4 SERVINGS   12 MINUTES   35 MINUTES

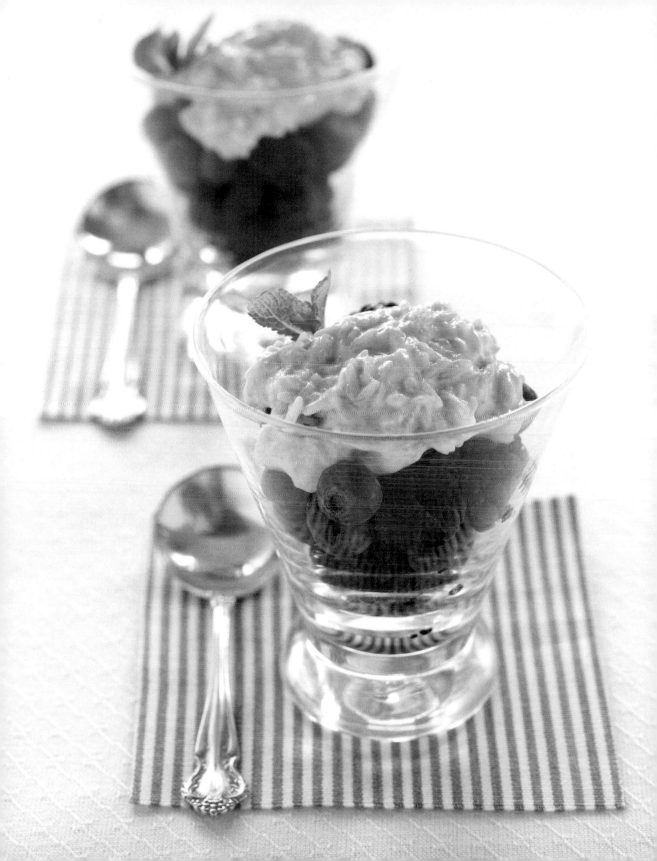

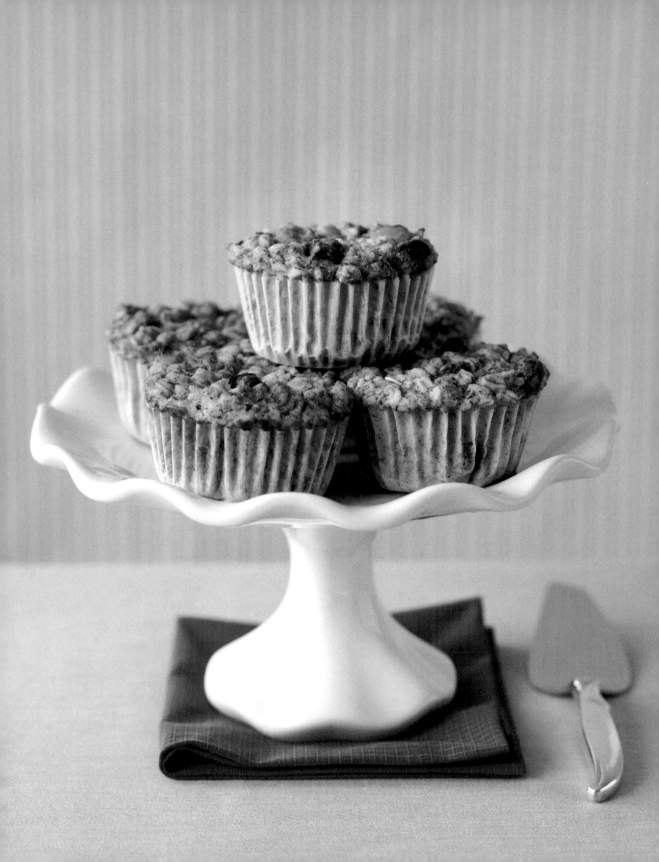

APPLESAUCE OATMEAL MUFFINS

Muffins are a wonderful quick snack but most commercial muffins are loaded with nasty surprises despite their healthy reputation. Extra saturated fats, sugars and sweeteners should not be part of a Clean-Eating plan. These muffins, loaded with Clean-Eating ingredients, are perfect for a quick snack or dessert.

INGREDIENTS:

1 cup / 240 ml dry old-fashioned oatmeal flakes

1 cup / 240 ml unsweetened applesauce

½ cup / 120 ml skim milk, soy milk, rice or almond
     milk *(your choice)*

2 egg whites, beaten

2 Tbsp / 30 ml ground flaxseed

2 Tbsp + 1 tsp / 35 ml canola oil

1 Tbsp / 15 ml baking powder

½ tsp / 2.5 ml baking soda

1 tsp / 5 ml cinnamon

½ tsp / 2.5 ml ground nutmeg

¾ cup / 180 ml whole-wheat flour

¼ cup / 60 ml dried cranberries

¼ cup / 60 ml dried cherries

¼ cup / 60 ml raisins

PREPARATION:

1 Preheat oven to 375°F / 190°C. Prepare muffin tin by lining with paper or silicon liners, or cooking spray.

2 Combine oatmeal, applesauce, milk, eggs, flax and oil in a medium bowl. In another medium bowl, combine dry ingredients, including dried fruit. Make a well in the center of the dry ingredients and pour wet ingredients into it. Stir until all ingredients are just combined.

3 Using a small ladle, fill muffin cups ⅔ full. Bake 15 to 20 minutes. Cool on wire rack. Serve with piping hot coffee and grab your Sunday paper.

TIP

Try a little unsweetened applesauce on your muffin rather than butter to add sweet moistness to it.

NUTRITIONAL VALUE PER MUFFIN:

Calories: 120 | Calories from Fat: 31 | Protein: 3g | Carbs: 20g
Dietary Fiber: 3g | Sugars: 3g | Fat: 3g | Sodium: 17mg

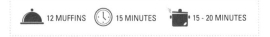

12 MUFFINS   15 MINUTES   15 - 20 MINUTES

BLUEBERRY CRUMBLE

On a recent trip to Nova Scotia I was amazed to discover wild blueberries growing virtually everywhere, hidden among dense green foliage near the Atlantic Ocean. They tasted like drops of sunshine. I used some of the wild blueberries in this delicious crumble recipe. This makes a humble but wholesome dessert. Make sure to check the label of your granola. Many packaged varieties look healthy but are loaded with unnecessary fat and sugar.

INGREDIENTS:

6 cups / 1.4 L blueberries, fresh or frozen

⅛ to ¼ cup (about 45 ml) natural organic sugar or organic honey

1 Tbsp / 15 ml arrowroot powder

4 Tbsp / 60 ml water

2 – 3 cups (about 600 ml) granola or muesli (made gluten free with uncontaminated oats if this is an issue)

PREPARATION:

1 Preheat oven to 375°F / 190°C.

2 Place berries in a deep oven-proof baking dish or in individual baking dishes. In a small bowl mix water and arrowroot powder thoroughly. Stir in the honey or sugar and pour over the blueberries. Top with granola. Bake uncovered for 30 to 40 minutes. Serve right from the oven or at room temperature.

TIP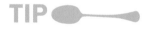

Place individual ramekins filled with crumble on a cookie sheet before baking. It will help keep your oven clean.

NUTRITIONAL VALUE PER SERVING:

Calories: 285 | Calories from Fat: 34 | Protein: 5g | Carbs: 63g
Dietary Fiber: 7g | Sugars: 26g | Fat: 3g | Sodium: 121mg

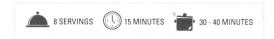
8 SERVINGS   15 MINUTES   30 - 40 MINUTES

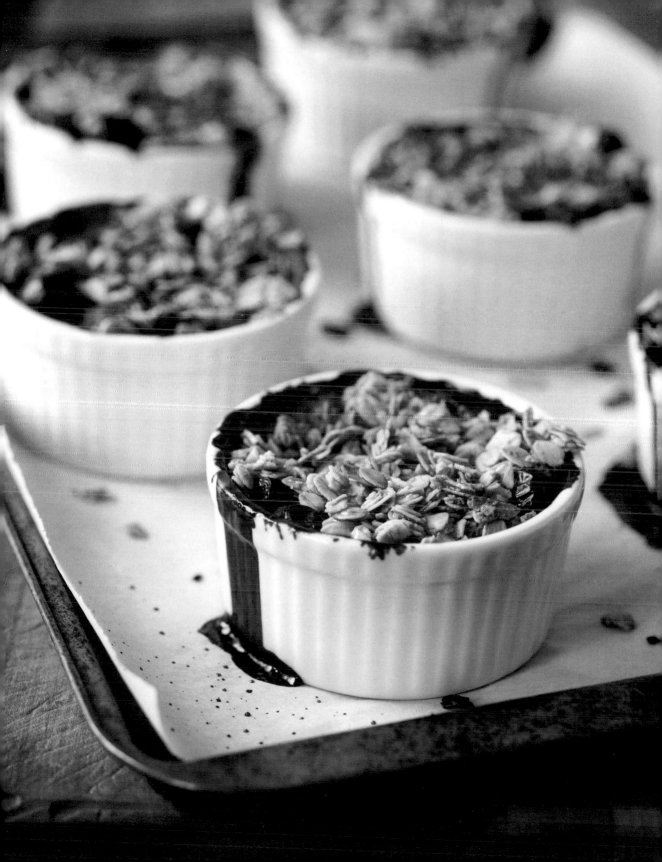

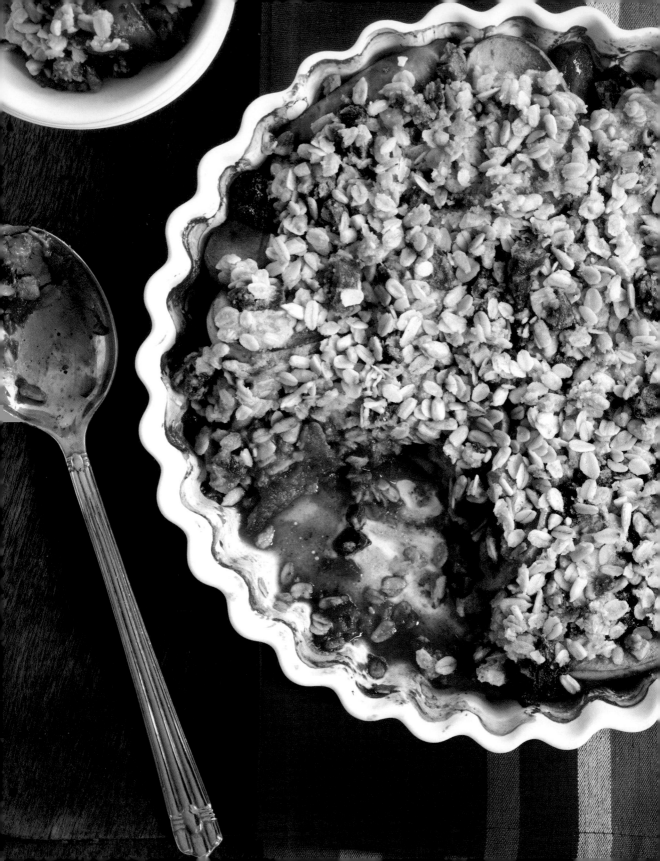

BLACKBERRY AND APPLE CRUMBLE

There is something about a crumble that just makes me say "Mmmmm!" Perhaps it's the sweet warmth of fruit juices or the lightness of the crumble topping or the thrill of eating something naturally sweet and nutritious. Whatever it is, crumbles of any sort satisfy my dessert craving. Prepare this dish in late summer when blackberries are ripe and early apples are just coming in. It is best with a cup of tea!

INGREDIENTS:

1 lb / 454 g cooking apples

Juice of 1 lemon

1 cup / 240 ml fresh blackberries

¼ cup / 60 ml whole-wheat flour or gluten-free flour

¼ cup / 60 ml rolled oats (uncontaminated if necessary)

3 Tbsp / 45 ml canola oil (extra may be needed)

¼ cup / 60 ml pitted dates, finely chopped

¼ cup / 60 ml unsalted sunflower seeds

Cooking spray

PREPARATION:

1 Preheat oven to 400°F / 204°C. Prepare an ovenproof dish by coating with cooking spray.

2 Core and slice the unpeeled apples and sprinkle with lemon juice. This helps prevent browning. Place in a medium saucepan with the blackberries. Cook over medium-low heat and bring to a simmer. Simmer for 5 minutes. Pour cooked fruit into baking dish.

3 In a separate bowl, mix the flour and oats. Rub in the oil and stir until mixture resembles crumbs. You may need to add more canola oil until desired texture is reached. Stir in dates and sunflower seeds. Sprinkle crumbly mixture over fruit.

4 Bake in the oven for 25 minutes.

TIP

Use leftover crumble in the morning as a base for breakfast. Simply add plain, nonfat yogurt and breakfast is served.

NUTRITIONAL VALUE PER SERVING:

Calories: 273 | Calories from Fat: 137 | Protein: 3g | Carbs: 35g
Dietary Fiber: 7g | Sugars: 21g | Fat: 15g | Sodium: 2mg

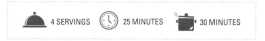

4 SERVINGS   25 MINUTES   30 MINUTES

CLEAN-EATING POWER PROTEIN BARS 🍃 🐄❋

I can't tell you the number of people who have asked me what kind of protein bar I eat. In fact I don't often eat commercial protein bars because they are hard on my stomach. I can clear a room, if you know what I mean. This recipe takes the pain out of protein.

INGREDIENTS:

1 cup / 240 ml whey or soy protein powder *(or use the kind you are already familiar with)*

½ cup / 120 ml quinoa flour or flour of your choice – amaranth, millet, spelt, kamut

2 cups / 480 ml rolled oats – *not instant*

½ cup / 120 ml oat bran

½ cup / 120 ml coarsely chopped flax seed

½ cup / 120 ml wheat germ

1 tsp / 5 ml sea salt *(don't skimp on this – sea salt provides valuable minerals and elements)*

1 tsp / 5 ml cinnamon

¼ tsp / 2.75 ml nutmeg

½ cup / 120 ml Sucanat or agave nectar or organic honey

1 cup / 240 ml dark chocolate, broken into pieces

1½ to 2 cups (about 420 ml) yogurt cheese or soy yogurt cheese (recipe see page 141)

¼ cup / 60 ml avocado oil, canola oil or healthy oil of your choice

2 tsp / 30 ml extra virgin olive oil

1 tsp / 15 ml best-quality vanilla

Cooking spray – *I prefer the olive oil based spray*

PREPARATION:

1 Preheat oven to 350°F / 177°C. Coat a 9 x 13-inch baking pan with cooking spray.

2 In large mixing bowl combine protein powder, flour, oats, oat bran, flax seed, wheat germ, sea salt, cinnamon, nutmeg, and Sucanat or other sweetener. Stir in broken chocolate pieces.

3 In another bowl mix the yogurt cheese, oils and vanilla. Mix well. Add the yogurt cheese mixture to the dry ingredients. Use your clean bare hands to combine these well. I like to coat my hands in olive oil to help prevent sticking.

4 Place mixture in prepared pan. Press it down and even out the top. Bake on middle rack in oven for 15 minutes. Remove from heat. Let cool and cut the dough into bars. Place these bars on a cookie sheet lined with Silpat and bake again for another 15 minutes. Remove from heat. Transfer to wire cooling rack and let cool. Place in airtight container and store in refrigerator. Makes anywhere from 20 to 24 bars, depending on how big you cut them.

NUTRITIONAL VALUE PER SERVING:
Calories: 290 | Calories from Fat: 73 | Protein: 15g | Carbs: 40g
Dietary Fiber: 5g | Sugars: 11g | Fat: 8g | Sodium: 80mg

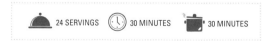
24 SERVINGS   30 MINUTES   30 MINUTES

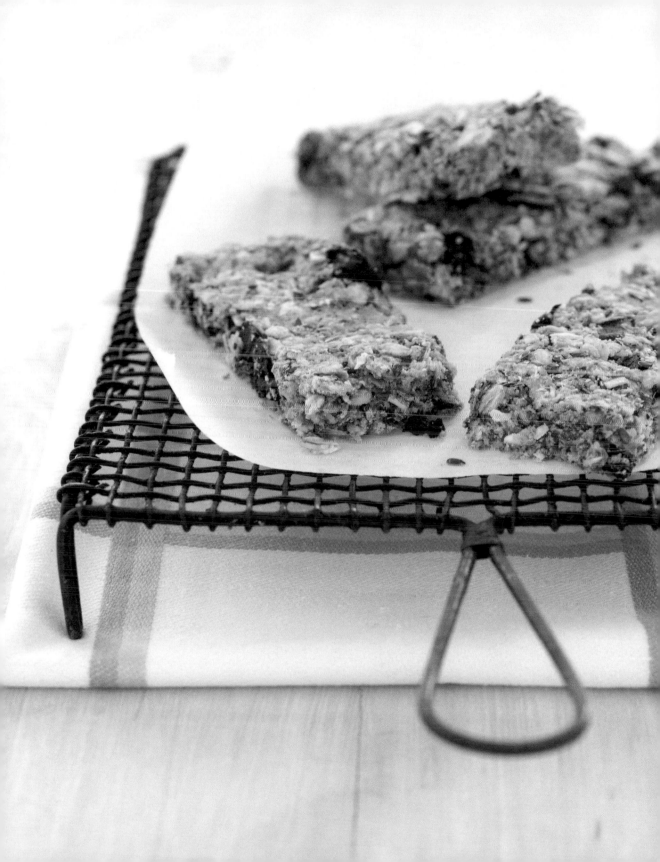

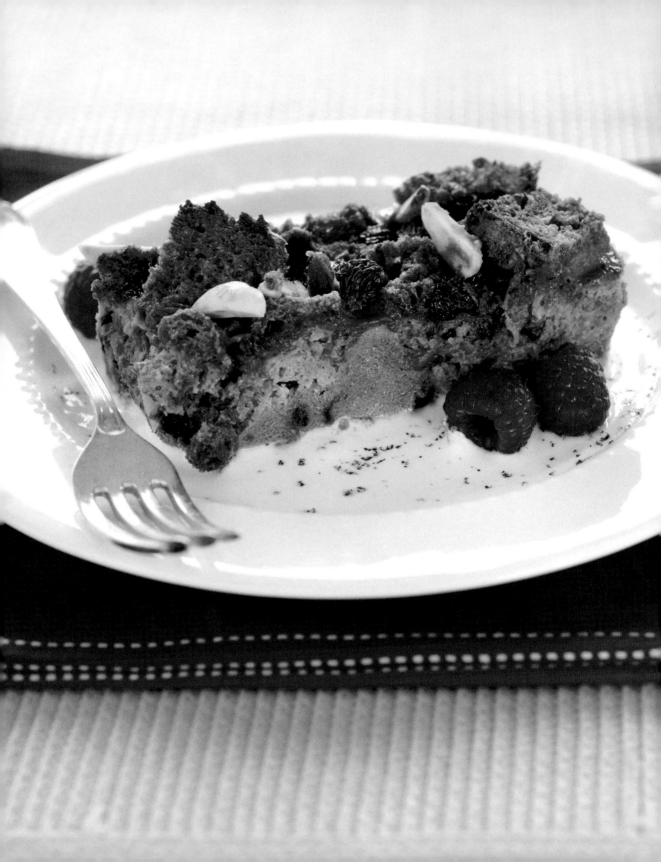

MOLASSES BREAD PUDDING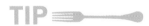

Molasses, the byproduct of cane sugar refining, is in my opinion an oft-overlooked nutritional powerhouse. The plant soaks up minerals from the ground, which then become available to you when it is harvested and processed in the form of molasses. Always look for unsulphured molasses!

INGREDIENTS:

4 cups / 960 ml Ezekiel bread, cubed *(I like raisin bread)*

¼ cup / 60 ml dried currants

¼ cup / 60 ml dark sultana raisins

¼ cup / 60 ml slivered raw almonds

2 eggs, beaten

⅓ cup / 80 ml molasses

Sea salt

2 cups / 480 ml low-fat soymilk *(or use any milk that suits your nutritional lifestyle)*

Cooking spray

PREPARATION:

1 Preheat oven to 350°F / 177°C. Prepare a loaf pan with cooking spray.

2 Place bread cubes in the bottom of the pan. Sprinkle dried fruits and almonds over bread cubes. In a medium mixing bowl, combine eggs, molasses and salt. Whisk well.

3 Transfer milk to medium saucepan. Bring to a boil. Remove from heat and whisk slowly into egg mixture. Pour over bread mixture in loaf pan.

4 Place loaf pan in shallow water bath and bake for one hour or until the bread mixture begins to look brown and the liquid has been absorbed. Remove from heat. Serve hot.

TIP

Serve with yogurt and fresh berries.
Sprinkle with nutmeg.

NUTRITIONAL VALUE PER SERVING:
Calories: 153 | Calories from Fat: 32 | Protein: 4g | Carbs: 26g
Dietary Fiber: 2g | Sugars: 15g | Fat: 3g | Sodium: 86mg

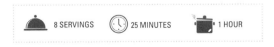

8 SERVINGS   25 MINUTES   1 HOUR

BANANA APPLESAUCE BREAD

Most of us often have a few brown spotted bananas lying around the kitchen. If I can't use them up right away I throw them in the freezer for use later. This recipe makes good use of overripe bananas. To thaw frozen bananas, place them in a sink of cold water. Cut the tough stem off the top after 5 minutes and squeeze thawed banana into a measuring cup. It's easy and rather fun to do!

INGREDIENTS:

1 cup / 240 ml all-purpose flour

½ cup / 120 ml whole-wheat flour

½ cup / 120 ml amaranth flour or flour of your choice

½ cup / 120 ml packed brown sugar

1 Tbsp / 15 ml baking powder

1 tsp / 5 ml cinnamon

¼ tsp / 1.25 ml baking soda

4 egg whites, beaten until fluffy

1 cup / 240 ml mashed bananas

½ cup / 120 ml buttermilk or skim milk soured with 1 Tbsp lemon juice

⅓ cup / 80 ml unsweetened applesauce

1 tsp / 5 ml vanilla

½ cup / 120 ml chopped walnuts

½ cup / 120 ml raisins

1 Tbsp / 15 ml grated orange zest

Cooking spray

PREPARATION:

1 Preheat oven to 350°F / 177°C. Lightly coat a 9 x 5-inch loaf pan with cooking spray and dust with flour.

2 In large bowl combine dry ingredients. In another medium bowl, beat egg whites until fluffy. Prepare soured milk at this time if using instead of buttermilk. Then pour bananas, buttermilk (or soured milk), applesauce and vanilla into a large bowl.

3 Add dry ingredients to wet and mix until just blended. Fold in egg whites, then add walnuts, raisins and grated orange zest. Pour into prepared loaf pan. Bake for 55 minutes.

TIP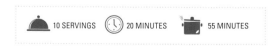

Give frozen bananas the slip — gently heat frozen banana in the microwave until skin just softens. Then peel and use the flesh.

NUTRITIONAL VALUE PER SERVING:
Calories: 211 | Calories from Fat: 32 | Protein: 5g | Carbs: 40g
Dietary Fiber: 1g | Sugars: 17g | Fat: 3g | Sodium: 34mg

10 SERVINGS   20 MINUTES   55 MINUTES

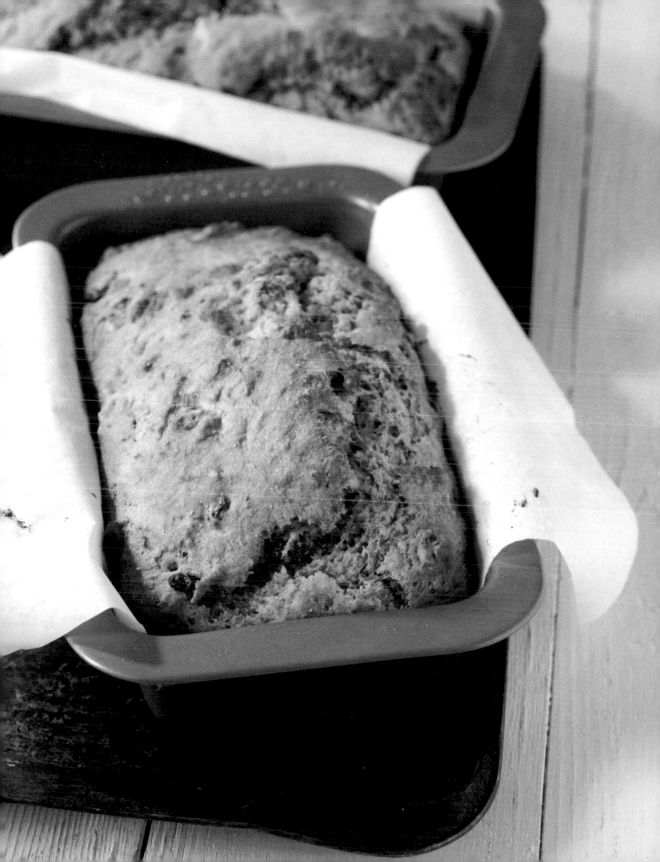

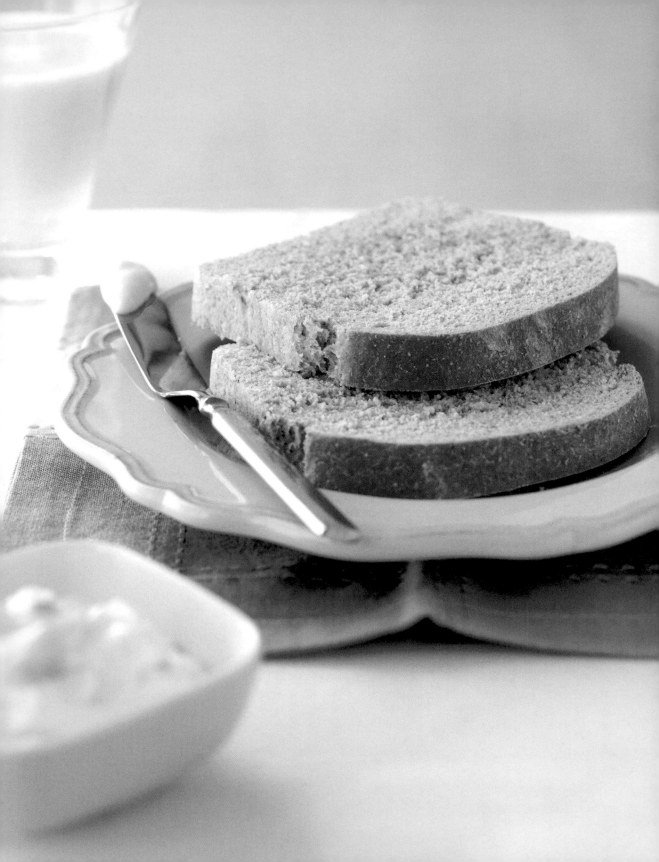

SCHOMMER'S WHOLE-GRAIN BREAD

This recipe comes from a reader who is passionate about making healthy bread. She wanted others to have access to this marvelous bread so here is her version just for you.

INGREDIENTS:

5½ cups / 1.3 L water
¼ cup / 60 ml organic honey
½ cup / 125 ml canola oil
1 Tbsp / 15 ml sea salt
¼ tsp / 1.25 ml ascorbic acid
3 Tbsp / 45 ml yeast

PREPARATION:

1 Combine above ingredients and let stand until the yeast is dissolved and starting to rise.

Add the following:

• 11 to 12 cups (about 2.7 L) whole-grain flour

2 Knead for 10 minutes.

3 Shape into loaves or buns and place into pans. Let rise until double in size.

4 Bake at 325°F / 163°C for 30-35 minutes until golden on top.

5 Remove from oven and turn out onto cooling racks immediately.

TIP

For an occasional treat, spread fresh-baked bread with some Do-It-Yourself Olive Butter Spread (page 117), a healthy alternative to regular butter.

NUTRITIONAL VALUE PER SERVING:

Calories: 83 | Calories from Fat: 18 | Protein: 2g | Carbs: 14g
Dietary Fiber: 2g | Sugars: 1g | Fat: 2g | Sodium: 142mg

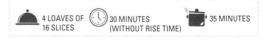

4 LOAVES OF 16 SLICES   30 MINUTES (WITHOUT RISE TIME)   35 MINUTES

EZEKIEL BREAD BY HAND

I f this is your first introduction to Ezekiel bread you will wonder at the unusual list of ingredients. Rest assured this is a wholesome complete food and tastes wonderful. In the end this does look like bread.

DRY FLOUR INGREDIENTS:

2 cups / 480 ml organic whole-wheat flour, unbleached

¾ cup / 180 ml amaranth flour

¼ cup / 60 ml millet flour

¼ cup / 60 ml lentil flour

1¾ cup / 420 ml rye flour

½ cup / 120 ml barley flour

2 Tbsp / 30 ml soybean flour*

2 Tbsp / 30 ml kidney-bean flour*

2 Tbsp / 30 ml lentil flour*

2 Tbsp / 30 ml sea salt

Combine all of these ingredients in a large mixing bowl. Set aside.

FOR YEAST MIXTURE:

4 Tbsp / 60 ml yeast

½ cup / 120 ml lukewarm water

4 Tbsp / 60 ml organic honey

In a small bowl combine all ingredients and set aside.

LIQUID FOR FLOUR MIXTURE:

¾ cup / 180 ml organic honey

½ cup / 120 ml safflower or olive oil

2 cups / 480 ml warm skim, soy, rice, goat or almond milk *(your preference)*

Combine these ingredients in a medium bowl.

NUTRITIONAL VALUE PER SERVING:

Calories: 99 | Calories from Fat: 19 | Protein: 3g | Carbs: 16g
Dietary Fiber: 2g | Sugars: 0.3g | Fat: 2g | Sodium: 12mg

* To make these flours: sprout dried beans (see page 55). Once they have sprouted, allow them to dry again by placing them in a colander in the fridge overnight (put a plate underneath to catch any drips). Grind to a flour-like consistency in a food mill or coffee grinder. If you don't want to bother with sprouting the beans, simply soak and cook dried beans. Allow them to cook until soft. Then rinse and drain them very well. Dry the beans as explained beforehand. Grind cooked beans in a food mill or coffee grinder.

PREPARATION:

1 Pour liquid for flour mixture over the flour mixture in the large bowl. Add the yeast mixture and mix until all ingredients are moistened. The dough needs to resemble a muffin batter at this point. Use more flour if the dough is too wet. If the dough is too dry use more warm milk. Do not overwork the dough.

2 Divide dough among four loaf pans sprayed lightly with cooking spray. Place loaf pans in a warm area with no cooling breeze nearby. Cover lightly with a damp tea towel. Let rise for one hour.

3 After an hour, place loaf pans in a preheated 375°F / 190°C oven. Bake for 30 to 45 minutes. A cake tester should come out clean and the top should bounce back when done.

P.S. This is a dense bread – don't expect it to rise high in the pan when baking.

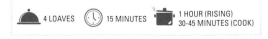

4 LOAVES   15 MINUTES   1 HOUR (RISING) 30-45 MINUTES (COOK)

EZEKIEL BREAD FOR
THE BREAD MACHINE

INGREDIENTS:

1 cup / 240 ml **water**

¼ cup / 60 ml **red kidney beans** (cooked and drained)

¼ cup / 60 ml **lentils** (cooked and drained)

1½ Tbsp / 22 ml **olive oil**

1½ Tbsp / 22 ml **organic honey**

¾ tsp / 4 ml **sea salt**

1 cup / 240 ml **amaranth flour**

1 cup / 240 ml **whole-wheat bread flour**

½ cup / 120 ml **barley flour**

½ cup / 120 ml **millet flour**

2 Tbsp / 30 ml **vital gluten**

1½ tsp / 22 ml **yeast**

PREPARATION:

1 Put all ingredients in the bread machine, choose a medium bake program, and press start.

NUTRITIONAL VALUE PER SERVING:

Calories: 99 | Calories from Fat: 19 | Protein: 3g | Carbs: 16g
Dietary Fiber: 2g | Sugar: 0.3g | Fat: 2g | Sodium: 12mg

| 1 LARGE LOAF | 10 MINUTES | 1 HOUR 15 MINUTES |

ADDITIONS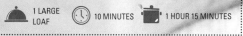

- Add 1 cup / 240 ml raisins to the recipe to increase the sweetness.
- Dust the top of the loaves with sesame seeds before baking.

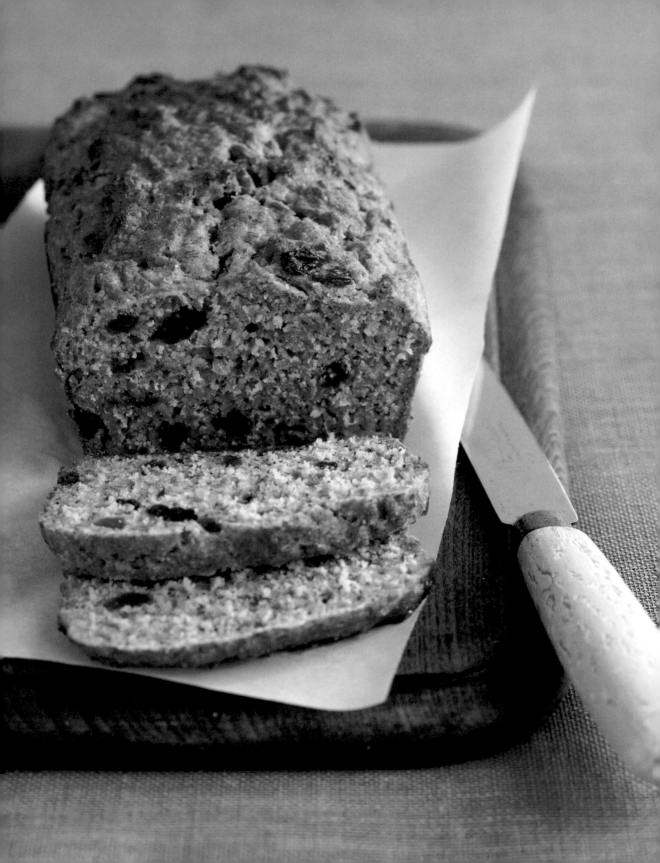

CARROT BREAD

Cornmeal is an often overlooked but deliciously versatile whole grain. It forms the basis of this moist bread which develops a pleasant orange color while baking. Enjoy it as a dessert or breakfast bread.

INGREDIENTS:

1 lb / 454 g loose sweet carrots, peeled and grated

1¼ cups / 300 ml whole-wheat flour

1¼ cups / 300 ml cornmeal

Pinch sea salt

¼ cup / 60 ml flax meal

1½ tsp / 8 ml baking powder

3 egg whites

1 yolk

2 Tbsp / 30 ml canola oil

½ cup / 125 ml organic honey

¾ cup / 180 ml skim milk or low-fat soy milk

¼ cup / 60 ml raisins

¼ cup / 60 ml dried cranberries

Cooking spray

PREPARATION:

1 Preheat oven to 375°F / 190°C.

2 In a small saucepan place carrots and enough water to just cover them. Bring to a boil and cook for 5 minutes. Remove from heat, drain, and let cool.

3 In a medium mixing bowl place dry ingredients: flour, cornmeal, salt, flax meal and baking powder.

4 In another bowl, whip egg whites until stiff.

5 In small bowl put egg yolk, oil, honey and milk. Mix well. Add to dry ingredients and mix until just combined. Add whipped egg whites and fold until just combined. Add dried fruits and cooked carrots and mix until just combined. Do not over-mix, or loaf will be tough.

6 Prepare a 5 x 9-inch loaf pan with cooking spray. Pour batter into loaf pan and bake for 60 minutes or until cake tester comes out clean. Makes 10 servings, more or less, depending how thick you slice the bread.

SWEET TIP

Top with unsweetened applesauce instead of butter. It's delicious!

NUTRITIONAL VALUE PER SERVING:

Calories: 288 | Calories from Fat: 53 | Protein: 6g | Carbs: 53g
Dietary Fiber: 6g | Sugars: 23g | Fat: 5g | Sodium: 67mg

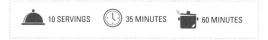

10 SERVINGS   35 MINUTES   60 MINUTES

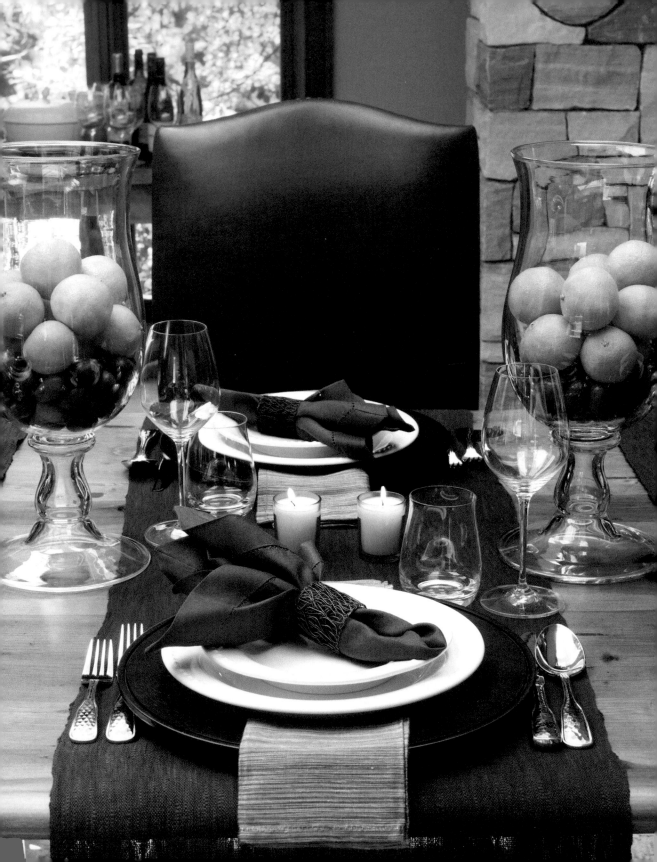

10

A Festive Occasion

I look forward to holidays and celebrations with glee. I enjoy them as much today as when I was a small child. The difference is that I now follow the Clean-Eating principles and guidelines to create my fabulous feast. A celebration may be a time to indulge just a little, but there is no need to go off the rails completely. So dig in and whoop it up, but be certain you will not have to loosen your belt at the end of the evening.

Wondering if your special occasions will be as "festive" if you Eat Clean? Don't worry. There are many ways to entertain and celebrate with flair, even when you choose to keep the menu fat free and clean. Why ruin all your hard work by noshing on foods that won't sit well? I have roasted enough family-sized turkeys and mouth-watering bison tenderloins to know you can pull it off.

CHRISTMAS DINNER – TURKEY AND ALL

Plan your menus ahead so you know what you are serving and can pull together the season's freshest ingredients. When my family comes for Christmas there are 21 or more at the dinner table. It is important to have a large bird, which I always order from my local butcher. The poultry he offers at his store is hormone free and never frozen.

I have experimented with various stuffings. My family still loves a bread-based stuffing but this brown-rice stuffing is delicious and cuts down on heavy carbs and starch. I love the color of sweet potatoes and always have them on hand to accompany a turkey dinner. This satisfies the little ones who demand mashed potatoes. Cranberry sauce and applesauce are a cinch to make so they are standbys that must appear when turkey is served. I prefer the taste of roasted Brussels sprouts to ordinary boiled ones so I serve them along with other vegetable side dishes

– with so many at the table I like to have plenty to choose from since everyone has different tastes.

A beautiful starting dish is shrimp cocktail served on a bed of butter lettuce and prepared to perfection with seafood sauce and lemon wedges. Some of my nieces and nephews don't like shrimp just yet, so I offer plenty of crudités along with hummus or another spread to keep them happy. The bread basket helps too. I fill it not only with bread, but with crisp crackers and interesting breadsticks, as well. I love the crackers from Duchy Originals – HRH Prince Charles produces these from organic ingredients. Delicious! Try the Oaten Biscuits with Cracked Black Pepper. You will love them.

Of course you are probably wondering what on earth a person could eat for dessert at a celebratory dinner that fits with Clean Eating. This is a special day, so do plan to enjoy something out of the ordinary. However, that treat does not have to be weighed down with cream and calories. Go for lighter fare that is rich on flavor. I always have a big bowl of mixed fresh berries on hand. They can be had on their own or served on the side with something a little more indulgent. Try roasted pears or even this lighter version of trifle – a family favorite. Desserts made with silken tofu are as sinful as those made with cream and butter. You don't even know those ingredients are missing, and the desserts don't sit heavily in your stomach.

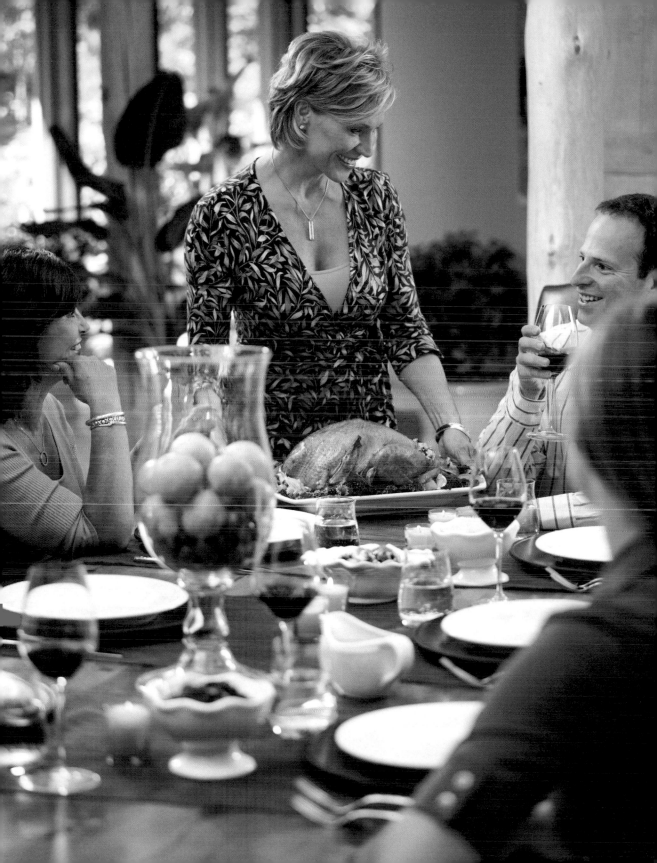

OTHER FESTIVE OCCASIONS

When considering alternatives to turkey, why not serve a beautifully roasted bison tenderloin? The meat is gorgeous and so nutritious you hardly know you are eating something good for you. You can, of course, roast beef tenderloin instead. It is also delicious and impressive.

Serve your favorite bottle of wine with your Clean-Eating meals. Enjoy a glass or two – again, this is a special occasion. When you decide to make a glass of wine your special treat this week, you don't have to feel guilty about having it. Just go easy.

In the beautiful little town near where I live there happens to be a lovely place to purchase wine. Not only do the merchants have a delightful assortment of wines but delicious vintage wines are also available. When I need advice about which wine to pair with a Clean Eating meal, I always seek the wisdom of the staff there. The following wine recommendations are sure to satisfy even the most discerning palates.

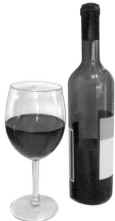

MENU

Hors D'oeuvres
Pumpkin Hummus

Shrimp Cocktail

Soup
Roasted Root Vegetable Soup

Main Course
Roasted Bison Tenderloin with Oven-Roasted Brussels Sprouts and Mashed Sweet Potatoes

Or

Oven-Roasted Turkey with Brown Rice and Apple Stuffing Low-fat Gravy, Homemade Applesauce and Cranberry Sauce

Dessert
Trifle

Fresh mixed berries and fresh fruit

WINE RECOMMENDATIONS

Compliments of Christine Barnes, product consultant specializing in vintages.

APPETIZERS

It is festive to start a meal on a sparkling note, so go for either a rosé champagne or a bottle of prosecco. *Prosecco* is a sparkling wine from *Italy*. *French Rosé* is more expensive but both are food friendly and delicious accompaniments for shrimp and hummus.

ROASTED ROOT VEGETABLE SOUP

You could carry a sparkling wine over to this dish, but a classic match is a dry *Spanish Sherry*. Another option would be *Innis and Gunn Beer*. It is oak aged and has a full-roasted feel, which would compliment the soup nicely. Serve non-alcoholic sparkling cider for children.

ROASTED BISON TENDERLOIN AND ROAST TURKEY

There is little fat in bison so it is best to stay away from wines with tannins. Ripe berry wines such as *New World Pinot Noir* from *Oregon* or *California* or a *Californian Zinfandel* are excellent choices. Both wines would also work well with roast turkey. Zinfandel can be high in alcohol, which may overwhelm the meal, so choose wisely. A good alternative is to serve a *Primitivo* from *Italy*, which is made with the same grape.

The sides of brown rice and apple stuffing and mashed sweet potatoes are wonderfully complimented by an *Ontario* or *Alsace Riesling* wine. This fruity wonder can work with the tart flavours of apples and cranberries and the sweetness of the sweet potatoes.

TRIFLE

Moscato d'Asti is a sweet Italian sparkler that is a perfect match for this classic Christmas treat.

An aged *Tawny Port* would go nicely, as would a *Framboise* – a sweet dessert wine made from raspberries. But my favourite would be a *Riesling Icewine* from *Ontario*.

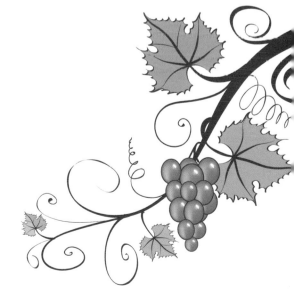

POMEGRANATE FIZZ

This colorful, fizzy cocktail is perfect for a get-together, as it offers variations for everyone. Pomegranate juice has been shown to improve cardiovascular health, reduce blood pressure and plaque build-up, act as an antioxidant, and even improve erectile function. Drink up!

INGREDIENTS:

2 oz pomegranate juice

½ to 1 oz triple sec or other orange liqueur

5 oz chilled champagne

Squeeze of fresh lemon juice

6 - 8 pomegranate seeds

Grated lemon rind (zest)

PREPARATION:

1 In a champagne flute pour the pomegranate juice. Add the liqueur, if using, then the champagne or sparkling water. Top with a few pomegranate seeds and grated lemon rind. Enjoy!

NUTRITIONAL VALUE PER SERVING:

Calories: 227 | Calories from Fat: 0 | Protein: 0g | Carbs: 21g
Dietary Fiber: 0g | Sugars: 19g | Fat: 0g | Sodium: 9mg

Other options:

CLEANER COCKTAIL

2 oz pomegranate juice

5 oz chilled champagne

Squeeze of fresh lemon juice

6 - 8 pomegranate seeds

Grated lemon rind (zest)

NUTRITIONAL VALUE PER SERVING:

Calories: 147 | Calories from Fat: 0 | Protein: 0g | Carbs: 13g
Dietary Fiber: 0g | Sugars: 11g | Fat: 0g | Sodium: 9mg

TRULY CLEAN COCKTAIL

2 oz pomegranate juice

5 oz chilled sparkling water

Squeeze of fresh lemon juice

6 - 8 pomegranate seeds

Grated lemon rind (zest)

NUTRITIONAL VALUE PER SERVING:

Calories: 41 | Calories from Fat: 0 | Protein: 0g | Carbs: 10.5g
Dietary Fiber: 0g | Sugars: 8.6g | Fat: 0g | Sodium: 41mg

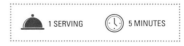 1 SERVING   5 MINUTES

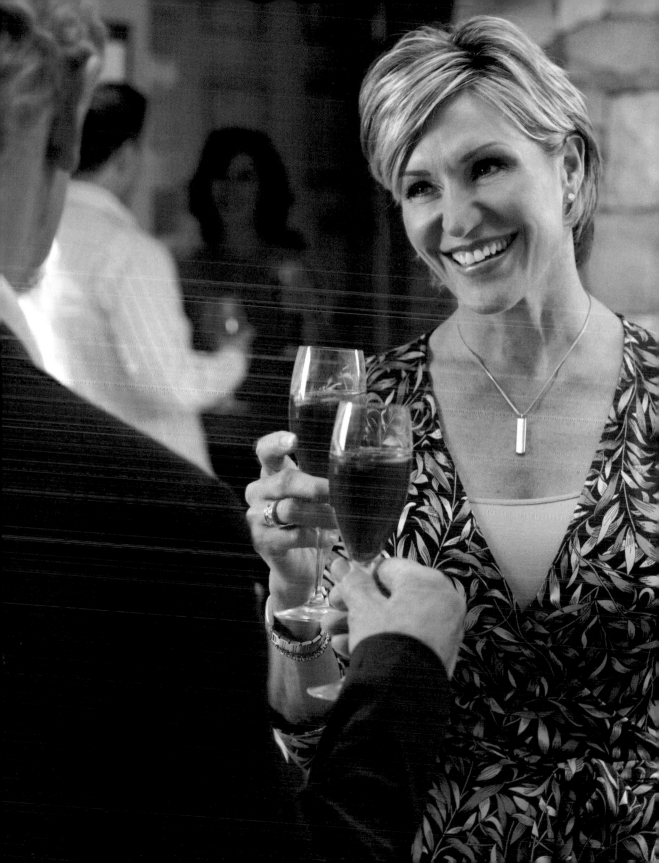

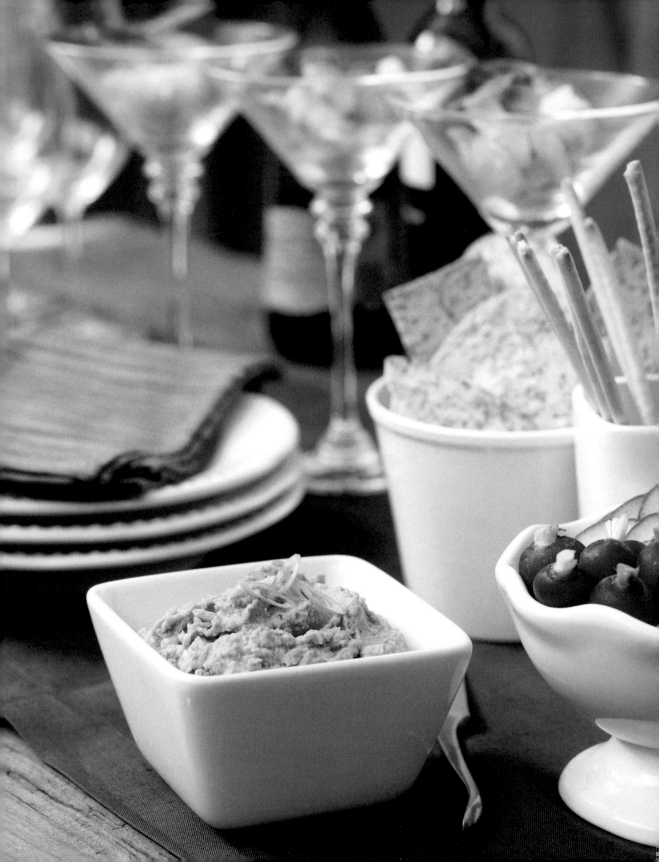

PUMPKIN HUMMUS

I s there any end to the delectable variations of pumpkin? This is a fabulous recipe for your festive table. Serve this with a basket of interesting breads, crackers and baked pita chips. This takes no more than 15 minutes to make if you have all ingredients handy. Make sure to buy the plain canned pumpkin, not the kind that already has pumpkin pie spices in it. Better yet, use fresh pumpkin. I like to bake a small pumpkin for this. If you don't have a pumpkin any small squash will do – butternut, acorn or even a large sweet potato. Makes 2½ cups.

INGREDIENTS:

2 Tbsp / 30 ml tahini

2 Tbsp / 30 ml fresh lemon juice

1 tsp / 5 ml ground cumin

1 tsp / 5 ml pumpkin oil

¾ tsp (about 4 ml) sea salt

⅛ tsp / 0.6 ml ground pepper

15 oz / 420 g pumpkin, baked or canned

4 cloves garlic, passed through a garlic press

2 Tbsp / 30 ml cilantro

PREPARATION:

1 Place all ingredients in a food processor. Process until smooth.

2 Spoon into a decorative stoneware serving bowl and serve chilled.

TIP

Make sure you buy the plain canned pumpkin, not the kind that has pumpkin pie spices in it.

NUTRITIONAL VALUE PER ONE TBSP SERVING:

Calories: 48 | Calories from Fat: 3 | Protein: 0.6g | Carbs: 9g
Dietary Fiber: 3g | Sugars: 1g | Fat: 1g | Sodium: 77mg

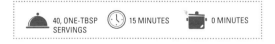

40, ONE-TBSP SERVINGS | 15 MINUTES | 0 MINUTES

SHRIMP COCKTAIL

If I am planning to serve this for a festive occasion I will head out of the house at an ungodly hour to get my hands on the best shrimp possible. There is a store one hour away from where I live that always has the best jumbo shrimp. The drive to Pusateri's is worth it. The lineup even at 7:00 am is proof of their unfailing high quality goods. They also have big, fat lemons close by so I don't forget to buy them.

Cocktail Sauce:

Buy a commercially made low-sodium variety or make your own. Cocktail sauce is virtually fat-free since it is made of ketchup, horseradish and lemon juice. Just watch the sugar and salt. Here's my recipe.

SHRIMP COCKTAIL INGREDIENTS:

5 cooked jumbo shrimp per person

Shredded iceberg lettuce – 1 cup / 240 ml per serving

Fresh whole lemons, cut into wedges, obvious
    seeds removed, ½ lemon per person

Cocktail sauce (see recipe) – 4 Tbsp per serving

COCKTAIL SAUCE INGREDIENTS:

1 small tin low-sodium tomato paste

¼ cup / 60 ml water

2 tsp / 10 ml organic honey

1 tsp / 5 ml sea salt

¼ tsp / 1.25 ml cumin

¼ tsp / 1.25 ml dry mustard

¼ tsp / 1.25 ml cinnamon

⅛ tsp / 0.6 ml cloves

2 tsp / 10 ml cider vinegar, organic is best

3 Tbsp / 45 ml prepared horseradish

2 Tbsp / 30 ml fresh lemon juice

¼ tsp / 1.25 ml hot sauce

SHRIMP COCKTAIL PREPARATION:

1 Count on 4 or 5 cooked jumbo shrimp for each person. Use a martini glass or another interesting glass dish for serving. Make a "nest" of shredded lettuce in each serving dish.

2 Arrange 5 cooked jumbo shrimp on each nest of lettuce. Arrange lemon wedges with the shrimp. Place a dollop of cocktail sauce in the center of each serving. Serve ice cold.

3 When I am having my whole family for dinner and am serving Shrimp Cocktail, I often prearrange the shrimp and lettuce in serving dishes. I cover them and refrigerate until I am ready to serve. Then I place the last minute touches of cocktail sauce and lemon wedges on each plate.

COCKTAIL SAUCE PREPARATION:

1 Mix all ingredients in a glass bowl. Cover and refrigerate until ready to use.

NUTRITIONAL VALUE PER SERVING:

Calories: 50 | Calories from Fat: 0 | Protein: 9g | Carbs: 11g
Dietary Fiber: 3g | Sugars: 5g | Fat: 0g | Sodium: 103mg

6 SERVINGS   10 MINUTES   0 MINUTES

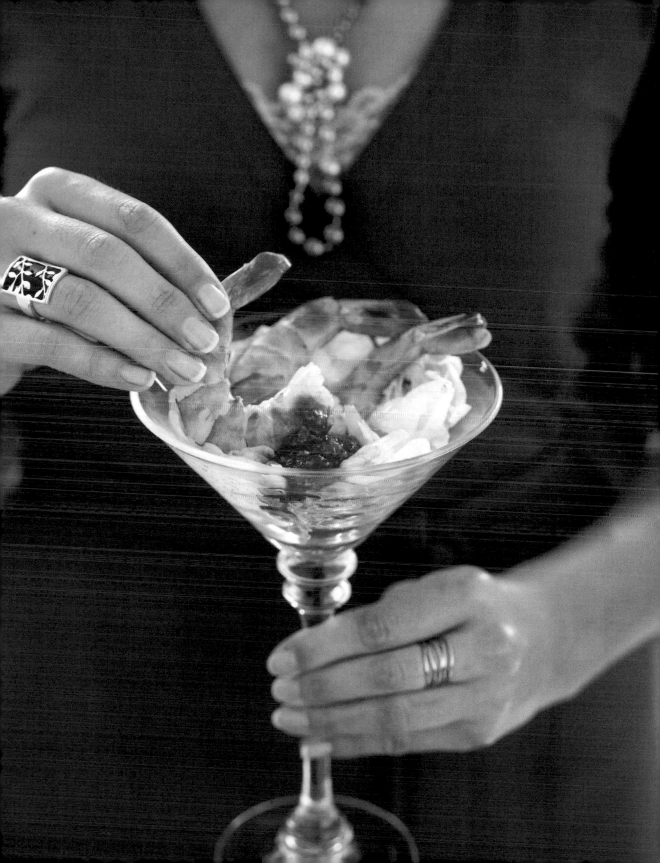

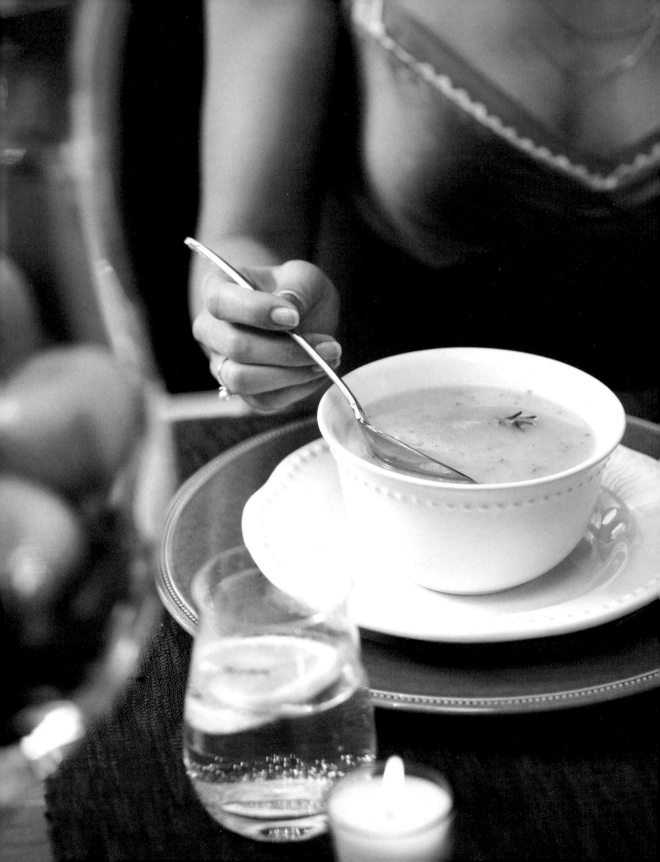

ROASTED ROOT VEGETABLE SOUP

Doesn't the title of this recipe just shout autumn? Take advantage of these delicious veggies when they are in peak season. Each one of them offers enough nutritional value to create a perfect Clean-Eating accompaniment to your holiday meal. Your soup bowl will be brimming with healthy goodies in palate-pleasing form. Canned soup just can't compare!

INGREDIENTS:

3 or 4 Tbsp (about 50 ml) extra virgin olive oil to coat vegetables while they roast

1 small butternut squash, peeled, seeded and cubed

2 large, sweet carrots, peeled and cut into chunks

1 large parsnip, peeled and cut into chunks

1 small turnip, peeled and cut into chunks

1 large cooking onion, peeled and cut into rings

1 head of garlic, loose skins removed and tops cut off

1 medium swede or rutabaga, peeled and cut into chunks

4 small red potatoes, scrubbed and cut into chunks

1 large sweet potato, peeled and cut into chunks

Sea salt and freshly ground black pepper

3 bay leaves

Parchment paper

8 cups / 2 L stock – low-sodium stock, either chicken or vegetable (gluten free if necessary)

Several fresh basil leaves

1 cup / 240 ml fresh chopped cilantro

1 tsp / 5 ml crumbled, dried thyme

1 tsp / 5 ml rosemary, fresh if possible

PREPARATION:

1 Preheat oven to 325°F / 163°C. Pour 2 tablespoons / 30 ml extra virgin olive oil in bottom of a roasting pan. Place all vegetables in the roasting pan and coat with a light misting of olive oil. Sprinkle with sea salt and freshly ground black pepper. Toss bay leaves on top. Cover vegetables with a layer of parchment. Just set it on top for the first 30 minutes of roasting. Then remove parchment paper and let roast for another 30 minutes. You will have to mix the veggies occasionally to roast them all properly. Your kitchen will smell divine while all of this is going on. Remove from oven. Remove any black bits and bay leaves, squeeze garlic out of its skin, and purée roasted vegetables in batches in a food processor or blender. Use the stock to help the process along; adding a cup of stock will make the blending easier. Place all puréed vegetables in large soup pan or Dutch oven and set over low heat on the stove. Add remaining stock (if any), basil, cilantro, thyme and rosemary.

2 Bring soup to gentle simmer and adjust seasonings. If you find the soup too thick simply add more stock and reheat. Serve in heated bowls with a sprig of rosemary or chives on each bowl for garnish.

NUTRITIONAL VALUE PER SERVING:

Calories: 201 | Calories from Fat: 60 | Protein: 7g | Carbs: 28g
Dietary Fiber: 3g | Sugars: 7g | Fat: 6g | Sodium: 305mg

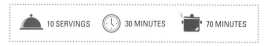

10 SERVINGS   30 MINUTES   70 MINUTES

ROASTED BISON TENDERLOIN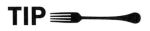
with Oven-Roasted Brussels Sprouts and Mashed Sweet Potatoes

....

There is no better way to enjoy your holiday occasion than with a perfectly prepared bison supper. The combination of juicy tenderloin, crisp Brussels sprouts and steaming mashed sweet potatoes (recipes follow) satisfies a big holiday appetite in a healthy way. Be amazed as the warm colors tempt you into seconds and even thirds. But watch those portion sizes! You don't want to fall completely off the wagon during the holidays.

INGREDIENTS:

1 good-sized bison tenderloin *(2 to 3 pounds or 1kg)*, use beef tenderloin if you can't find bison

1½ - 2 tsp / 7 ml sea salt

2 Tbsp / 30 ml cracked black peppercorns

¼ cup / 60 ml Dijon mustard

2 Tbsp / 30 ml finely chopped shallots

2 cloves garlic, passed through a garlic press

½ cup / 120 ml fresh rosemary

2 Tbsp / 30 ml extra virgin olive oil

¼ cup / 60 ml yogurt cheese (see recipe page 141)

PREPARATION:

1 Preheat oven to 275°F / 135°C.

2 Remove any silvery membranes from the meat. Shape the roast by binding it in several places with kitchen twine. This will also keep it from falling out of shape while it cooks. Mix the remaining ingredients together in a small bowl. With clean hands rub the seasoning mixture over the meat. Make sure it is well covered.

3 Set the bison in the oven and roast for 50 minutes. A meat thermometer should read about 130°F / 55°C for rare meat and 160°F / 71°C for medium rare. After cooking, allow the roast to sit covered tightly in foil for 20 minutes. Then it can be sliced and served.

TIP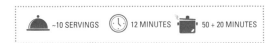

Be careful not to overcook bison. The meat is best served rare to medium.

recipes continued...

NUTRITIONAL VALUE PER SERVING:
Calories: 292 | Calories from Fat: 178 | Protein: 27g | Carbs: 1g
Dietary Fiber: 0g | Sugars: 0.48g | Fat: 20g | Sodium: 365mg

~10 SERVINGS   12 MINUTES   50 + 20 MINUTES

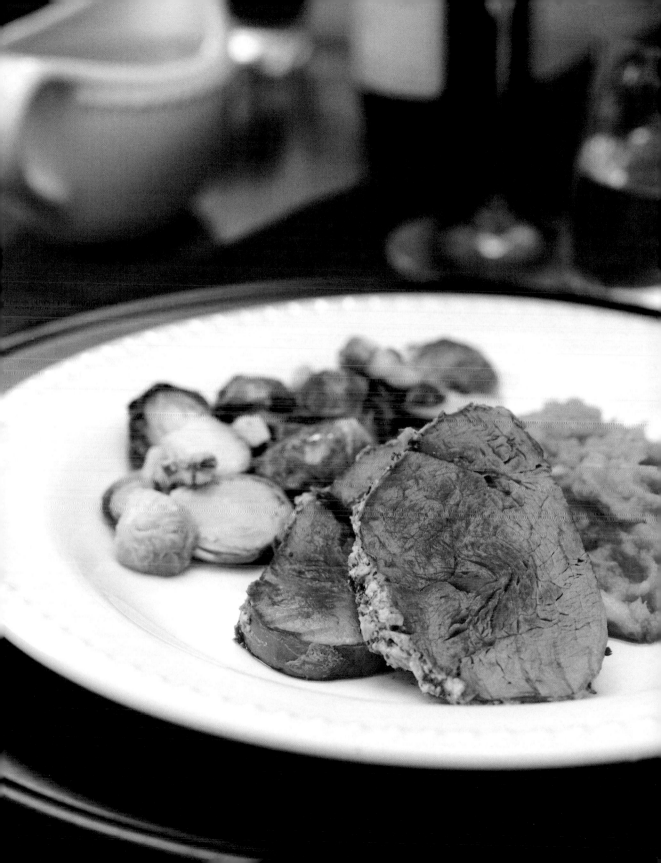

OVEN-ROASTED BRUSSELS SPROUTS

I may have to convince you that Brussels sprouts are a holiday treat. I certainly have to convince my daughters! But I don't think you'll be able to resist them when they are prepared like this. Walnuts and mushrooms make for an irresistible flavor combination that packs tons of nutritional value, while the olive oil leaves a brilliant, crisp green coat. You'll never turn Brussels sprouts down again!

INGREDIENTS:

1 lb / 454 g Brussels sprouts

3 Tbsp / 45 ml extra virgin olive oil

1 tsp / 5 ml sea salt, none other

1 tsp / 5 ml fresh ground black pepper

¼ cup / 60 ml walnuts, optional

¼ cup / 60 ml shiitake mushrooms, sliced *(optional)*

PREPARATION:

1   Place Brussels sprouts in a bowl of cold water with ice cubes. Sprinkle with salt. Let sit for 20 minutes. Meanwhile, preheat oven to 400°F / 205°C

2   Place a clean kitchen towel on the counter. One by one remove the Brussels sprouts and trim the hard end off the bottom. Trim off any loose or yellowed leaves. Make a small cross in the bottom of each sprout. Cut any large sprouts in half lengthwise. When all the sprouts have been cleaned and trimmed, place them in a medium bowl. Drizzle with olive oil, sea salt, black pepper, walnuts and shiitake mushrooms (if using). Toss lightly until all sprouts are well coated.

3   Line a baking sheet with parchment paper and gently transfer the sprouts to the baking sheet. Place any halved sprouts cut side down. Place in oven and bake until lightly browned for about 30 minutes. Serve hot.

TIP

Keep all sprout sizes uniform. If there are larger sprouts cut them in half so they cook thoroughly.

NUTRITIONAL VALUE PER SERVING WITH WALNUTS & MUSHROOMS:

Calories: 181 | Calories from Fat: 133 | Protein: 5g | Carbs: 12g
Dietary Fiber: 5g | Sugars: 2g | Fat: 14g | Sodium: 529mg

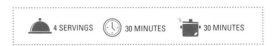

4 SERVINGS   30 MINUTES   30 MINUTES

MASHED SWEET POTATOES

Mashed potatoes are the ultimate comfort food. Their rich and creamy texture makes them an instant favorite that will warm you from the inside out. Unfortunately, the fat content of typical mashed potatoes is atrocious since they are packed with butter and cream. These sweet potatoes are much lighter and will still leave you feeling like you've eaten a decadent cream-filled cloud.

INGREDIENTS:

2 lbs / 908 g sweet potatoes, scrubbed, peeled and cut into chunks

2 medium parsnips, peeled and cut into chunks

½ tsp and 1 pinch (about 3 ml) sea salt

¼ cup / 60 ml low-sodium chicken or vegetable stock or water (gluten free if necessary)

1 Tbsp / 15 ml pumpkin oil

⅛ tsp / 0.6 ml ground nutmeg

⅛ tsp / 0.6 ml ground cinnamon

White pepper

TIP

This dish can be made up to two days ahead of time and refrigerated until you need it. Then pop in the oven to warm.

PREPARATION:

1   Place sweet potatoes and parsnips in a medium saucepan and cover with water. Add a pinch of salt and bring to a boil over high heat. Reduce heat and continue to cook for 15 to 20 minutes or until vegetables are tender. Remove from heat.

2   Drain, reserving cooking liquid. Add stock or water, pumpkin oil, sea salt, nutmeg, cinnamon and white pepper. Mash potatoes and parsnips with a potato masher until smooth. Add more reserved cooking liquid if the potato mixture is too stiff. Transfer mashed vegetables to a casserole dish that has been lightly coated with cooking spray. Cover and keep warm in low oven. Serve hot!

NUTRITIONAL VALUE PER SERVING:
Calories: 182 | Calories from Fat: 23 | Protein: 3g | Carbs: 37g
Dietary Fiber: 6g | Sugars: 8g | Fat: 2g | Sodium: 231mg

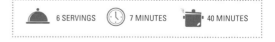

6 SERVINGS   7 MINUTES   40 MINUTES

HOW TO ROAST A TURKEY CLEAN-EATING STYLE!

Roasting a turkey can strike fear into the hearts of those who are inexperienced at cooking. When you discover how simple it really is you will wonder why you did not cook up a big bird sooner. It isn't hard to prepare turkey Clean-Eating style – poultry itself is very lean if you stick to the light meat. The extra calories and fat come from the many side dishes accompanying the feast. Serve a roasted turkey for Christmas, Thanksgiving or any special family gathering. Let's get started.

HOW TO BUY

I like to purchase a fresh bird from my local butcher. That way I can have the butcher trim the fat in advance. I also like to order a bird according to the number of guests sitting at the table – oh, and for leftovers! Leftovers are ideal for Clean Eating the next day. If you are buying a fresh bird make sure to place it in the refrigerator right away and keep it cold until you are going to cook it. I pick mine up two days before the big day. If you are using a frozen bird let it thaw for 24 to 48 hours in the fridge. Don't leave it on the counter.

Choose a bird that weighs about 15 pounds (about 7 kg) to feed 10 people. This size will still give you leftovers.

TO PREPARE

Give the bird a bath by rinsing it under cold running water and letting it drip in the sink. Use paper toweling to dry the inside cavity. Fill the cavities with stuffing. Seal the cavities with a skewer and rub olive oil all over the turkey. Place the bird in a roasting pan, breast side up. Season with your favorite poultry seasonings (see my tips below).

TO ROAST

Preheat oven to 325°F / 163°C. Make sure there is an oven rack on the lowest position in the oven. I like to use a meat thermometer so I get the cooking right every time. When it's done, the thermometer should read 185°F / 85°C when inserted into the center of the bird. On average the turkey will need 20 minutes of roasting time per pound. So if you have a 15 pound (7 kg) bird you will roast it for five hours.

Stuff the cavity with the Brown Rice and Apple Stuffing recipe on page 336. A 15-pound turkey will hold 5 cups (1.2 L) of stuffing in the main body cavity and you can put about 2 more cups into the neck cavity. Extra stuffing can be baked in a casserole dish. It will only take 30 to 40 minutes to bake.

Pour a little olive oil into clean hands and rub all over the gorgeous bird. I like to sprinkle a generous dusting of poultry seasonings – thyme, parsley and sage – over the bird. Add your favorite seasonings, too.

My mom had a trick of placing a layer of thick butcher bacon over the top of the turkey before popping it in the oven. This keeps the turkey moist while cooking. I don't ever eat the bacon or even the skin but somehow this helps retain any precious moisture.

Another trick is to put a whole apple at the opening of the body and neck cavity, again to keep moisture in. Give these little tricks a try for your optimum turkey-roasting experience!

Once your turkey has reached the correct temperature, remove it from the oven and cover it with foil. Arrange the foil so that it makes a tent over the meat. It is important to let the meat stand properly since this allows it to set, which makes for ideal carving.

TO CARVE

People in our house love the turkey legs. They are often the subject of heated debate when it is time to carve. Twist the legs off first. Place them on a heated platter or hand them out to winners of the "Turkey Leg Face Off." Using a sharp carving knife, begin to carve the breast meat. Start with the tip of the knife pointing towards the cavity. Slice thin slices of turkey, angling it as you work your way through the breast. Cover again with foil to keep warm. Remove the stuffing and place into warmed serving bowls. Scrape the cavities clean, as any stuffing left in the cavity can cause food poisoning. You don't want that!!

WHAT ABOUT THE GRAVY?

I don't often eat gravy – in fact I don't even eat it when I make a clean version of it. I just don't like gravy. But I do know how to make good gravy, so here goes!

GRAVY

What to do with the giblets? Never throw them out or give them to the dog! My mom would scold me if I ever did that. Instead use them to make a base stock for the gravy. In a saucepan place the giblets and cover them with water. Add one medium cooking onion and one carrot. Throw in a few bay leaves, peppercorns and celery greens. Simmer for about 3 hours and remove the foam as you go. Strain the liquid through a fine mesh sieve and reserve for the gravy. Cover and let sit until ready to use.

Once the turkey has been roasted, pour the pan drippings into a gravy separator and allow the strained, fat-free liquid to collect in a medium saucepan. Combine the strained giblet gravy with the turkey drippings. You should have about 3 to 4 cups (880 ml) of liquid. Another way to separate fat from healthy broth is to place all the pan drippings in a refrigerator and let the fat harden. Then remove it with a spoon and use the remaining liquid, which has probably turned into a jelly-like substance by now. Don't worry! That is a good sign because it means it is solid protein. Use this as gravy, or for an even lower-fat version use it as the broth for Low-Fat Gravy on page 337.

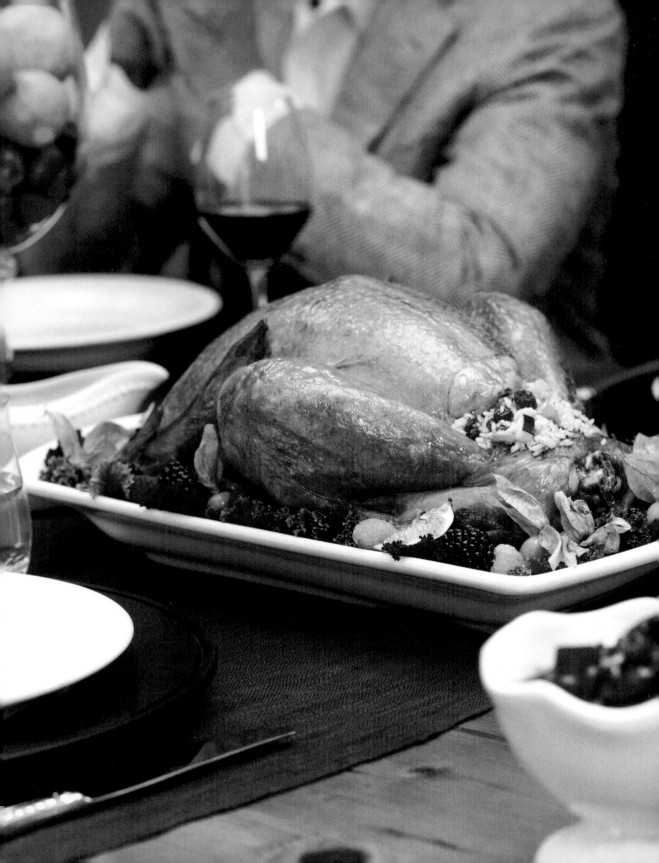

BROWN RICE AND APPLE STUFFING 🍃 🐟 Ⓢ

Stuffing always seems to be the favorite item around my holiday table. I just had to find a way to make it clean! Nutritionally-lacking white bread is cut from this recipe and replaced with brown rice. Switching to this grain not only ups the nutritional ante, it also provides a delicious nutty flavor. Now I know my family is getting the nutrition they need in their favorite holiday side-dish.

INGREDIENTS:

1½ cups / 360 ml brown rice, uncooked

2 cups / 480 ml natural apple juice plus 1½ cups
    water

2 tsp / 10 ml olive oil

1 crisp harvest apple, cored and diced

½ cup / 120 ml onion, diced

½ cup / 120 ml Brussels sprouts, chopped fine

4 cloves garlic, passed through a garlic press

1 carrot, peeled and chopped fine

1 cup / 240 ml celery, diced

⅓ cup / 80 ml uncontaminated oat bran or
    wheat bran

½ cup / 125 ml dried cranberries

⅓ cup / 80 ml slivered, raw almonds

½ tsp / 2.5 ml poultry seasoning

¼ tsp / 1.25 ml thyme

Freshly ground black pepper

PREPARATION:

1 Make rice according to package instructions. Use the combination of 2 cups / 480 ml natural apple juice and 1½ / 360 ml cups water for the cooking liquid.

2 Place olive oil in a large skillet and heat over medium heat. Cook all chopped fruits and vegetables until they are crisp, not soggy. Add cooked brown rice, bran, cranberries, almonds, poultry seasoning, pepper and thyme. Toss well.

3 Use as stuffing for poultry. Delicious!

recipes continued...

NUTRITIONAL VALUE PER SERVING:
Calories: 224 | Calories from Fat: 34 | Protein: 3g | Carbs: 45g
Dietary Fiber: 3g | Sugars: 16g | Fat: 5g | Sodium: 17mg

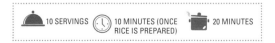
10 SERVINGS | 10 MINUTES (ONCE RICE IS PREPARED) | 20 MINUTES

LOW-FAT GRAVY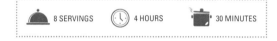

Gravy can be the downfall of an originally clean and healthy meal. Most gravy is drowning in fat, and most of us drown our turkey dinners in gravy! That's definitely not a Clean-Eating principle. I've worked out a recipe here that is absolutely delicious and still nutritious. So go ahead (if you must) and drown your turkey in a gravy you can feel good about.

INGREDIENTS:

1 Tbsp / 15 ml cornstarch or arrowroot powder

¼ cup / 60 ml cold broth (see Gravy on page 334) or water

PREPARATION:

1 Mix these ingredients well in a small bowl. Mix this solution into 1 to 1½ cups simmering broth (see Gravy on page 334). For every 1 to 1½ cups (about 500 ml) of broth make another solution of cornstarch or arrowroot. Season with sea salt. Serve hot!

NUTRITIONAL VALUE PER 2-TBSP SERVING:

Calories: 15 | Calories from Fat: 0 | Protein: 0g | Carbs: 3.5g
Dietary Fiber: 0g | Sugars: 1.5g | Fat: 0g | Sodium: 100mg

8 SERVINGS · 4 HOURS · 30 MINUTES

HOMEMADE APPLESAUCE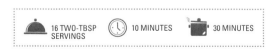

Is there anything better than homemade applesauce with freshly roasted turkey? Not really. Try this exquisite version for a gorgeous side dish. It is easy to do and can be prepared a few days ahead of time. I like it served room temperature. Apples are plentiful and at their peak in the autumn and early winter. Choose fruit that is as fresh as possible.

INGREDIENTS:

4 - 6 apples – firm cooking apples are best

1½ cups / 360 ml cooking water

1 Tbsp / 15 ml fresh lemon juice

Sea salt

2 Tbsp / 30 ml organic honey

PREPARATION:

1 Peel and core apples and place in medium saucepan. Add 1½ cups / 360 ml water, lemon juice and a pinch of sea salt. Bring to a boil and reduce heat. Let simmer for about 15 minutes or until soft. Remove from heat and put through a food mill. Stir in honey and you are done. If not using right away cover tightly with plastic wrap, otherwise serve hot.

NUTRITIONAL VALUE PER 2-TBSP SERVING:

Calories: 28 | Calories from Fat: 1 | Protein: 0g | Carbs: 8g
Dietary Fiber: 2g | Sugars: 6g | Fat: 0g | Sodium: 1mg

16 TWO-TBSP SERVINGS · 10 MINUTES · 30 MINUTES

CRANBERRY SAUCE

My husband loves this sauce so much he hopes for leftovers so he can spread it on toast the next morning for breakfast. It is a deeply colored sauce perfect for serving alongside turkey or chicken. Good luck on the leftovers! It tastes so good there usually isn't much left behind the next day.

INGREDIENTS:

4 cups / 960 ml fresh cranberries, picked over

1 hard, tart apple, peeled, cored and cut into chunks

1 cup / 240 ml orange juice

1 cup / 240 ml water

¼ cup / 60 ml organic honey

Rind of one orange, pith removed, minced

PREPARATION:

1 Rinse cranberries under running water. Place rinsed cranberries and apple in a medium saucepan with orange juice and water.

2 Cook berries over high heat until they burst. You will hear them popping. Reduce heat to low and add honey and orange peel. Continue cooking over low heat for another 15 minutes. The liquid should stick to the back of a spoon.

3 Remove from heat and let cool. Transfer to a bowl and cover with plastic wrap. Keep refrigerated until ready to use.

TIP

Stock up on fresh cranberries when they are in season and freeze them. Now you can make cranberry sauce to accompany any poultry dish throughout the year.

NUTRITIONAL VALUE PER 2-TBSP SERVING:
Calories: 18 | Calories from Fat: 0 | Protein: 0g | Carbs: 4.5g
Dietary Fiber: 1g | Sugars: 4g | Fat: 0g | Sodium: 0mg

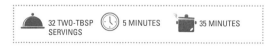

32 TWO-TBSP SERVINGS   5 MINUTES   35 MINUTES

TRIFLE— *The Truly Elegant Finishing Touch*

There are few desserts as delicious and festive as a stunning English trifle. There are, however, many decidedly non-Clean-Eating ingredients in most trifle recipes. Here is one I like that isn't too soggy or too loaded with alcohol. It looks magnificent on your dessert table.

INGREDIENTS:

2 packages Italian lady fingers or 1 angel food cake

½ cup / 125 ml raspberry juice

1 package each frozen unsweetened blueberries
    and raspberries, thawed and well drained

6 - 8 kiwi, peeled and cut into ¼-inch slices

INGREDIENTS FOR CUSTARD:

3 Tbsp / 45 ml Bird's Eye Custard powder

1 Tbsp / 15 ml Sucanat or organic honey

2½ cups / 600 ml skim milk

Pinch nutmeg

1 tsp / 5 ml vanilla

1 cup / 240 ml fresh raspberries for garnish

1 cup / 240 ml fresh kiwi slices for garnish

NOTE: I always have a huge bowl of fresh mixed berries on hand in addition to any other desserts I may be serving. You would be surprised at how popular they are. Everyone seems to love them.

NUTRITIONAL VALUE PER SERVING:

Calories: 207 | Calories from Fat: 21 | Protein: 5g | Carbs: 44g
Dietary Fiber: 5g | Sugars: 19g | Fat: 2g | Sodium: 76mg

12 SERVINGS   15 MINUTES   0 MINUTES

PREPARATION FOR CUSTARD:

1 Place custard powder and honey or Sucanat in large saucepan. Using a wire whisk gradually add milk and stir well. Place saucepan over medium heat. Bring custard to a gentle boil, stirring constantly. If you don't stir the custard it will stick to the bottom of the pan. Let cook until mixture thickens. Makes 2½ cups / 600 ml of custard. You may need to make more depending on the size of your trifle dish.

PREPARATION FOR TRIFLE:

1 Line the bottom of your trifle dish with lady fingers, or angel food cake cut into fingers. Sprinkle with raspberry juice and blueberries. Place a layer of kiwi slices over the blueberries. Spoon half of the custard over this layer.

2 Repeat the layering process, using raspberries this time.

3 Finish with a custard layer. Then arrange the fresh raspberries and kiwi to your liking on top. Cover with plastic wrap and refrigerate until ready to use. Keeps for three days – if it lasts that long.

4 Some people end the dish with a layer of whipped cream, but I like to top it with custard for obvious reasons. You can always offer whipped cream on the side but know that it doesn't exactly fit the Clean-Eating standard.

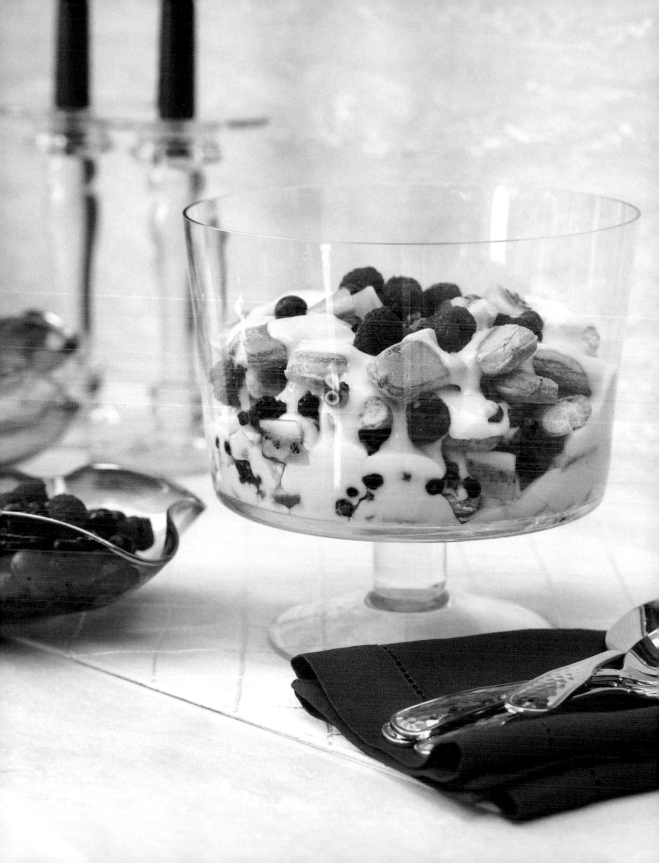

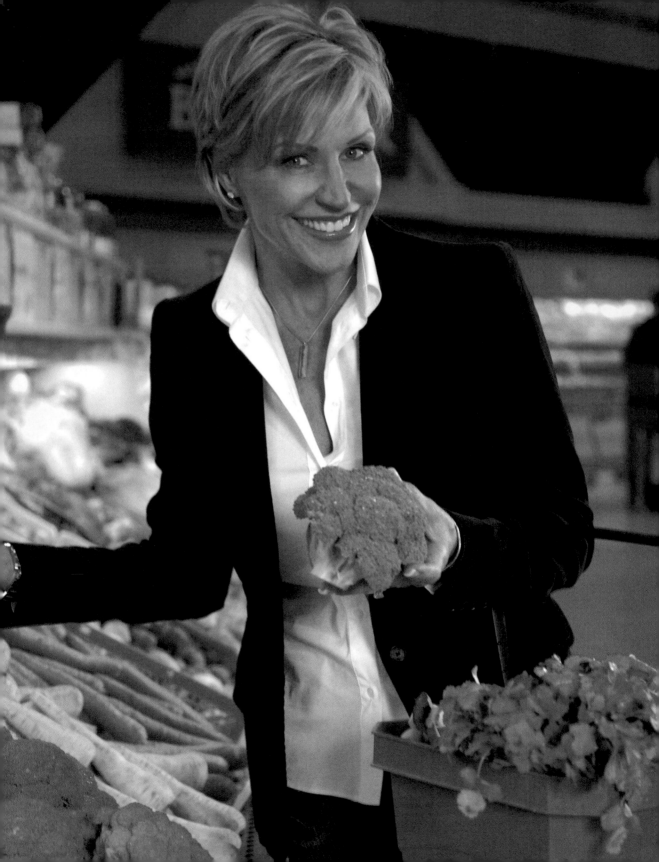

Q&A

It's funny I have written hundreds of thousands of words telling my story and that of Clean Eating, yet the demand for more information and specific details about nutrition is enormous. In this chapter you will find the answers to questions that were asked over and over again. I celebrate this natural curiosity – no question is a dumb question.

Q. Which yogurt is best?

A. There are so many types of yogurt available it is nearly impossible to make a quick decision about which is best. You need information. I always recommend checking the label first, because some yogurt contains so much sugar, sweeteners and other chemical calories that it is no longer a Clean-Eating food.

The rule of thumb is to look for a nonfat yogurt. In order for a yogurt to be fat free or nonfat it must contain less than 0.5% butterfat. Then you have to ask yourself if you really need the extra fruit-bottom, sugary syrup, chemically flavored stuff. The answer should be no. Choose plain, nonfat yogurt. You can always add your own fruit.

Here are some of my favorites:
• Liberté
• Stonyfield Farms
• Cascade Fresh

Q. Can I use egg substitutes?

A. Several kinds of egg substitutes are out in the marketplace. Vegans like to use egg replacements such as Ener-G Egg Replacer, especially for baking. It does what eggs do in recipes but is animal and dairy free, if that is your concern. If you are planning to make an egg-white omelet and just can't face cracking and separating a dozen eggs to get so many egg whites, you can buy the liquid egg whites. They are convenient and taste excellent. Sometimes

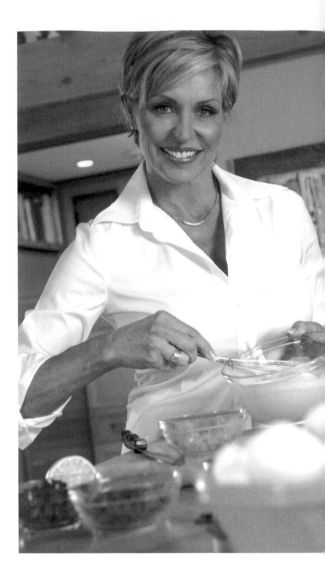

TIP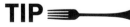

Make more egg whites on purpose so you can stuff them into a wrap at lunch.

I make more egg whites on purpose so I can stuff them into a wrap at lunch. I think you'll agree the convenience is worth it. Once again, I will caution you: quickly scan the label for unnecessary added sodium and any ingredients other than egg whites.

Q. Why does Eating Clean make me gassy?

A. Thank you for getting right down to the delicate details! Yes, we can make intense smells! Clean Eating takes a bit of getting used to with all that protein and fiber. If you haven't been eating these foods you will notice your body making a big stink about it. The good news is that it settles down after a few weeks. Here are some things you can do to ease the transition:

1. **Water will be your best friend.** Drink water with every meal. Not only will water provide the necessary liquid environment to deliver nutrients to all parts of the body, it will help move waste and its by-products (gas) out as well.

2. **Chew your food very well!** When Mom said not to gobble your food, she knew what she was talking about. By grinding food down, especially protein and fibrous foods, there is a better chance you will not offend your friends.

3. I often take **digestive enzymes** to assist my body in assimilating Clean Foods. There are many varieties available but the key ingredients are protease, amylase, lipase, glucoamylase, peptidase, bromelain, papain and cellulase.

Q. Is hemp a Clean Eating protein?

A. Hemp protein powder is a healthy, natural, complete protein, and best of all it usually comes with absolutely no additives, few carbs and a small amount of essential fats. This protein powder is created when hemp seeds, otherwise known as hemp hearts, are pressed to take the oil out. Hemp hearts are becoming ever more popular. Many people enjoy the benefits of hemp because it improves energy, stabilizes appetite, and improves digestion. Hemp hearts are half oil and one-third protein. A four-tablespoon serving contains 15 grams of lean protein, 1.5 grams of fiber, 4.5 grams carbohydrates and loads of natural minerals and vitamins. Hemp hearts are more readily digestible than most meat and dairy products. This is good news for those who cannot eat gluten, lactose, sugars, meats, nuts, shellfish and beans.

Hemp hearts or hemp protein powder can be added to cold or hot cereals, salads, sandwiches, pitas, wraps, desserts, stir-fries and baked goods.

Q. Can kids eat flax, wheat germ and bee pollen?

A. It's true some kids can be allergic to bees and hence possibly bee pollen. As I mentioned in

The Eat-Clean Diet book, use caution if you suspect your child is allergic. Try a few granules and watch your child closely. If all is well, begin by introducing a teaspoon into your child's breakfast cereal or yogurt.

Flax can have a powerful laxative effect, which is good news for those who need this kind of power. Again, introduce a teaspoon of ground or coarsely chopped seeds into breakfast cereal, yogurt or on salad. Flax is my number-one health/super food. I even take it with me when I travel.

Wheat germ is safe and easy to incorporate into everyday nutrition, unless the child is celiac or has a wheat sensitivity. I always add it to cold or hot cereal and baking.

Q. When should the last meal of the day be?

A. In *The Eat-Clean Diet* book I advocate eating the last meal of the day by 5:00 or 6:00 in the evening or a few hours before your bedtime, whenever that may be. I also suggest that if you are still hungry you can have a small snack before bedtime. Apparently some of you are confused.

What I am saying is that the last substantial meal of the day, where you are having lean protein and complex carbs from vegetables and whole grains or a sweet potato, should be a good four to five hours before bedtime. Then if you need something you can have a small snack – say a few almonds and an apple – before you jump under the covers. Some

of you will need the snack and some of you won't. Let your stomach be your guide. Don't eat the snack because I said so, eat it because you need it – you're hungry. But make sure the snack is small.

Q. Portion sizes: Can men and women eat the same amount of food and lose or maintain weight?

A. I love that readers are asking such intelligent questions! This is an excellent one. Eating Clean is the process of reeducating yourself about nutrition. Interesting things happen along the way. You learn to listen to your tummy, and once again feel what it means to be hungry or full. The sample menus in *The Eat-Clean Diet* book are for suggestion only. You may be a petite woman who cannot even begin to eat the suggested amount of food. On the other hand, you may be a 6' 2" man who requires more food. This is where you become responsible for your food intake. Eat when you are hungry and stop eating when you are full. It's simple stuff really! The portion sizes on page 16 in *The Eat-Clean Diet* are helpful – the bigger you are the bigger your hands are, so portions are automatically adjusted to your size. And remember, extra food, even if it is Clean Food, will be stored as fat. End of story.

Q. Is peanut butter okay?

A. Nuts and nut butters provide a valuable source of protein and other essential nutrients. By all means include them in your Clean-Eating nutrition plan. The problem with most commercial peanut butters is that they don't contain peanuts alone. Instead, they are full of sugars, stabilizers, preservatives, hydrogenated oils and other chemical calories and ingredients that are not good for you.

Nuts and nut butters are calorie-dense foods, but they are invaluable for their protein and essential fatty acid content. Be certain you are using all-natural nut butter, whether it is peanut or some other kind of nut or seed.

I encourage you to measure the amount of nut butter you are planning to eat. Don't just scoop it from the jar, or you will eat more than you should. Two tablespoons of natural peanut butter eaten with grains is the right Clean-Eating protein portion.

Try these other natural nut and seed butters:

• Almond
• Peanut
• Hazelnut
• Pumpkin seed
• Sesame seed
• Soy nut
• Macadamia
• Sunflower
• Cashew
• Pistachio
• ... and the many combinations of these

TIP: Don't be disgusted by the layer of oil sitting on top of the actual butter. This oil is the healthy oil from the nut or seed and has simply separated after production because the product is non-hydrogenated. Use a stiff knife or spoon to thoroughly mix the ground nuts or seeds into the oil. It should stay mixed until the jar is empty.

Q. Can I eat ostrich, emu and veal?

A. There are so many interesting lean protein sources that I did not mention in my first book, *The Eat-Clean Diet*. I simply wanted to introduce the idea of Clean Eating to you. In this cookbook I attempt to offer a wider range of lean protein sources. You already know how nutritious bison is and many of you have tried it on my suggestion. The raves are still pouring in. Others want to know why I did not mention veal or ostrich and even alligator. If these foods are readily available in your neck of the woods and you know how to prepare them Clean-Eating style – that is, baked, broiled, grilled or steamed, then by all means do so. Have frog legs if you like. I suppose I let my own bias against veal slip into the pages of my book since I cannot stand to drive by the farms near where I live and see the veal "huts" housing the wretched creatures.

Some folks find ostrich and emu meat a bit gamey, and they are higher in cholesterol than lean chicken, turkey or fish. It is worth checking the nutrition profile of the particular specialty meat you are interested in. I do my search online at www.nutritiondata.com, but there are loads of informative sites.

Q. Are pre-packaged foods such as Lean Cuisine and Weight Watchers considered Clean Eating?

A. We live in a quick fix world where the idea of reaching into the freezer and pulling out a ready-made meal is all too appealing. It's appealing all right, but maybe this compulsion to quick fix our way through life is adding up to a very big problem ... oh, you're right, it already has.

Although I applaud the efforts of both of these companies in assisting women and men to lose weight – that really is a good thing – I worry about the chemical calories lurking in any pre-packaged meals. Honestly! How long can a package of pre-made lasagna live in the freezer and what is making it look so good long after the expiry date? I encourage you to check the nutrition labels for everything from excess sodium, sugar, artificial sweeteners, trans and saturated fats to preservatives and other ingredients I don't even know how to spell.

Q. Why carbs and proteins at every meal?

A. Part of the magic of Eating Clean is consuming lean protein and complex carbohydrates at each of the several small meals eaten over the course of the day. Why is this magic? Together they offset unstable insulin levels and slow the release of glucose into the bloodstream. This magical combination further slows the carb-to-fat conversion, since it takes more work to digest these foods. Make the team of Lean Protein and Complex Carbohydrates work for you!

Q. Can you recommend a brand of protein powder as a supplement?

A. There are many types of protein powder available. Always make sure you purchase from a reputable company – one that has done the research and is not selling you a container of garbage. Next, I suggest you read the nutrition label. Too many fake sweeteners, sugars, carbs and chemical calories will not work well with Clean Eating. Be extremely careful if you are pre-diabetic or diabetic, since added sugars, whether fake or real, are a no-no! Also be aware of your own needs. Some of you have medical conditions not conducive to consuming large amounts of protein, especially those with compromised kidneys.

Although I am not endorsed by any supplement company I use MuscleTech's protein powder. My favorite flavor is vanilla. I also use a vegan protein powder called Raw Power.

Q. Pre- and post-workout nutrition – energy before, protein after!

A. I can't even begin to tell you the number of questions I have fielded about what to eat or not to eat before or after a workout. People seem to think this is dangerous territory. Now, I will shock you – I don't make a big fuss about it at all. I stick to eating every two to three hours and if that happens to fall on or around my workout I just factor in the "energy-before, protein-after" rule.

The simple rule of thumb is: energy foods are best consumed before the workout and protein foods are better after the workout. Complex carbohydrates break down into glucose, the energy used to fuel your machine. Protein is the repair molecule and is needed to rebuild the trillions of cells you have broken down during your workout.

If you have a big meal before a workout you need to wait at least an hour and a half before the workout. On the other hand you can eat a small meal up to half an hour before your training session.

REMEMBER:
Pre-workout nutrition should be high in complex carbohydrates. Post-workout meals should be high in lean protein.

Q. Is this statement true or false: *Rice cakes are the number-one diet food?*

A. Answer: FALSE.

Rice cakes are certainly consumed as if they were the number-one diet food, but the bad news is that they don't really work in your favor. It sure seems like they ought to be since they are made of virtually nothing but air and rice. Again that assumption is incorrect. In the true North American way, someone has figured out how to bestow rice cakes with every flavor from apple cinnamon to teriyaki. Some brands of rice cakes contain as many as 143 calories each while others carry a heavy dose of sodium. Those loaded with cheese pack extra unwanted fat and the sweet varieties often contain sweeteners. So how does the lowly rice cake qualify as a Clean-Eating food? It only works if you don't eat the loaded varieties, so you have to read the nutrition label (you knew I would say that). Oh! And of course you might want to pay attention to what you are piling on top of that rice cake, too.

If you are planning on eating rice cakes try some of the Lundberg or Quaker brands, but only the plain ones. This will serve as a whole-grain, complex-carbohydrate food.

Q. Why use sea salt?

A. Have you noticed the many varieties of salt available lately? There is ordinary table salt, kosher salt, sea salt, grey salt, pink salt and more. I recommend sea salt for Clean-Eating nutrition because it contains so many minerals necessary for optimum health. Ordinary table salt has been stripped of these elements, and even worse, contains added elements such as aluminum silicate to help keep the salt free running. The content of minerals and trace elements in sea salt closely resembles that of human blood. Sea salt contains approximately 80 of these – an excellent argument for using it.

From a cook's point of view sea salt and Kosher salt are preferred because of their irregular texture and milder flavor.

Q. What are Sucanat and other sugar substitutes?

A. Sugar can possess you. Its seductive sweetness is almost addictive. Sugar is ubiquitous. It's in virtually every food you eat, and most of it is unnecessary. Those who succumb to sugar find their taste buds do not respond to the normal flavor of foods any longer. They crave more and more sugar. Once you begin to Eat Clean you will notice your tongue becomes more sensitive to flavors and you can enjoy normal flavors once again without reaching for the sugar bowl.

Any of the following sweeteners can be used for cooking, or to sweeten your cup of coffee. Remember though, extra sugar, no matter what the source, can still lead to additional pounds.

It is occasionally necessary to use some sugar in baking and for other purposes. The idea is to use it only when necessary, and not in huge amounts. *Here is your list of alternatives:*

SUCANAT: The name stands for **Su**gar **Ca**ne **Nat**ural and is a natural sweetener made from crushing the sugar cane, extracting the juice and drying it. The result is dry, porous, richly colored Sucanat. It has a natural molasses flavor and can be substituted for sugar in any recipe. Sucanat is an excellent natural source of calcium, iron, vitamin B6, potassium and chromium. This product comes from Costa Rica.

RAPADURA SUGAR: Farmed in Brazil, rapadura organic sugar is an unbleached, unrefined sweetener that comes from molasses. Rapadura retains most of its essential nutrients, including vitamins and minerals. It has a mild caramel-like flavor and is perfect for baking.

AGAVE AND AGAVE NECTAR: Agave syrup or nectar is a sweetener produced from the native agave plant of Mexico. The core of the agave plant, called the piña, is where the juice comes from. The juice is squeezed out of the core, filtered and heated. The resulting liquid is filtered again and has a syrup-like quality. It is the perfect alternative to horrible white, refined sugars in baking. One-third cup / 80 ml of agave can be substituted for 1 cup / 240 ml of white sugar.

Q. HELP! I don't understand supplements.

A. In *The Eat-Clean Diet* I discuss supplements. A supplement is simply anything you consume over and above regular food, that helps fortify the body. I have listed the top-ten supplements in the book, but that does not mean you must take all of them. I don't and you don't have to either. There are some I use every day because I believe in them so strongly. These include Coenzyme Q10, bee pollen, flax seed, wheat germ, Tulsi tea, whey protein (by the way, whey protein already exists in milk and other dairy products), gamma-oryzanol in the form of brown rice, and omega-3 fatty acids. I also love maca but I don't take it everyday. I recently bought it in tea bag form and include it in one of the many cups of tea that I drink each day.

Clean Eating is the ideal way to incorporate most of these nutrients in the diet, so don't stress about the supplements unless you want to kick things up a notch.

Q. Are vegetables really carbohydrates?

A. You would be surprised how many people do not realize that vegetables are a good source of complex carbohydrates. I have received hundreds of emails questioning me about this, wondering why I would tell people to eat so many carbs and the answer is quite simple. You can eat carbs because these contain the high-quality nutrition prescribed for Clean Eating.

As you know there are two kinds of carbs: simple and complex. If you are uncertain about the difference, trust your taste buds. Simple carbs are easily identified by their sweet taste; think candy, ice cream, pastries and certain fruits. Complex carbs are delicious but certainly not sweet; think potatoes, asparagus, broccoli, oatmeal, and so on.

These two types of carbs both eventually break down to the same thing after digestion; glucose, which cells depend on for energy. However, it takes more work to digest complex carbs. For one, the molecular structure is more complex. Also, they tend to be accompanied by fiber. The healthiest form of energy comes from the complex carbohydrates present in high-fiber vegetables. Fiber allows proper absorption of sugars.

And while we are on the subject of sugars, fruit can be eaten when Eating Clean, but don't rely on fruit juice to do the job of an orange or an apple. Remember, the presence of fiber helps the body absorb sugars properly. So, eat the whole orange for breakfast, not just the juice.

Q. Can I drink flavored waters?

A. Eating Clean advocates drinking a lot of water. No one questions the benefits of H_2O. There are, however, many questions about drinking what I like to call "designer waters." Have you tried to buy a bottle of water lately? The grocery aisle for water has blossomed from non-existent into an explosion of choices. So what can you drink? Rather than telling you which brands to have and to stay away from, I will encourage you to read the label. Really read it! Many new "waters" contain carbohydrates, sugars, artificial sweeteners, preservatives, electrolytes and sodium. Have I forgotten anything? This is where you the consumer must take responsibility for what you put in your mouth. If in doubt about a product, drink plain water!

FRONT COVER PHOTO CREDIT

Cathy Chatterton (Make-up & hair by Franca Tarullo)

BACK COVER PHOTO CREDIT

Donna Griffith
(Food styling - Marianne Wren)

INTERIOR PHOTO CREDITS

Cathy Chatterton: pages 140, 240, 271, 278 **(Make-up & hair by Franca Tarullo)**

Robert Kennedy: pages 3, 100, 153-154, 188 **(Make-up & hair by Franca Tarullo)**

Robert Reiff: pages 11, 18, 31, 134, 144, 242, 275
(Food styling - Janet Miller)

istockphoto.com: pages 91, 319, 320

Donna Griffith: All other photos by Donna Griffith
(Food styling - Marianne Wren) (Make-up & hair by Franca Tarullo)

PROP-STYLING CREDITS

Rachel Corradetti & Gabriella Caruso Marques - A Festive Occasion chapter

Gabriella Caruso Marques: All other styling by Gabriella Caruso Marques

* Images of Tosca shopping were photographed in Zehrs, Orangeville, ON.